In *Mission and Method* Ann La Berge traces the development of the French public health movement within the sociopolitical context of early nineteenth-century France. Examining the community of hygienists that gathered on the Paris health council, La Berge shows how their competing ideologies – liberalism, conservatism, socialism, statism – fathered a movement that inspired and informed similar movements elsewhere, especially in Britain. She shows how the dialectic between liberalism, whose leading exponent was Villermé, and statism, the approach of Parent-Duchâtelet, characterized the movement and reflected the tension between liberal and social medicine that permeated nineteenth-century French medical discourse.

Cambridge History of Medicine

EDITORS: CHARLES WEBSTER AND CHARLES ROSENBERG

Mission and method

Mission and method
The early nineteenth-century French public health movement

ANN F. LA BERGE , *1944-*
Virginia Polytechnic Institute and State University

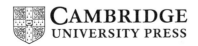
CAMBRIDGE
UNIVERSITY PRESS

Published by the Press Syndicate of the University of Cambridge
The Pitt Building, Trumpington Street, Cambridge CB2 1RP
40 West 20th Street, New York, NY 10011–4211, USA
10 Stamford Road, Oakleigh, Victoria 3166, Australia

© Cambridge University Press 1992

First published 1992

Printed in the United States of America

Library of Congress Cataloging-in-Publication Data
La Berge, Ann Elizabeth Fowler, 1944–
Mission and method: the early nineteenth-century French public
health movement/Ann F. La Berge.
p.   cm. – (Cambridge history of medicine)
Includes bibliographical references and index.
ISBN 0–521–40406–1 (hardback)
1. Public health – France – History – 19th century.   I. Title.
II. Series.
[DNLM: 1. Health Policy – history – France.   2. History of Medicine,
19th Cent. – France.   3. Public Health – history – France.   WA 11 GF7
L2m]
RA499.L23 1992
362.1′0944′09034 – dc20
DNLM/DLC
for Library of Congress   91–36335
                                                                  CIP

A catalog record for this book is available from the British Library.

ISBN 0–521–40406–1 hardback

For Bernard, Dora, and Moti
and to the memory of Bill Coleman

CONTENTS

TABLES AND ILLUSTRATIONS

PREFACE

The germ of this book was a doctoral dissertation entitled "Public Health in France and the French Public Health Movement, 1815–1848," written in the 1970s, when few secondary sources on nineteenth-century French public health were available. After reading Erwin Ackerknecht's pioneer article, "Hygiene in France, 1815–1848" (1948), his "Anticontagionism between 1821 and 1867" (1948), and George Rosen's *A History of Public Health* (1958), as well as some articles by Rosen, I set out to write a survey of public health in early nineteenth-century France. I wanted to write a descriptive account, providing the main outlines of the story by looking at public health theories, problems, institutions, and policies. I hoped to find out if the French hygienists actually accomplished anything, and to see how the French movement compared with the more familiar and already well-documented British movement. The dissertation succeeded, I believe, in providing the basic descriptive account I sought, and was, I am gratified to say, the starting point for a number of scholars who went on to write monographs about various aspects of nineteenth-century French public health.[1]

I was subsequently funded by the National Library of Medicine to do further research and write a book on the French public health movement. The present volume is the result of an additional year of research in France and the incorporation of many works that have appeared in the interim on nineteenth-century French medicine and public health. Indeed, in the 1980s, there was an outpouring of books and articles on French medicine, public health, and social welfare addressing such topics as public health and political economy, wet nursing, foundlings, vaccination, cholera, psychiatry, professional and popular medicine, housing, and water. Of all these works, clearly the most important in terms of the French public health movement was William Coleman's *Death Is a Social Disease: Public Health*

---

1 Erwin Ackerknecht, "Hygiene in France, 1815–1848," *Bull. Hist. Med.* 22 (1948): 117–155; Erwin Ackerknecht, "Anticontagionism between 1821 and 1867," *Bull. Hist. Med.* 22 (1948): 562–93; George Rosen, *A History of Public Health* (New York: MD Publications, 1958).

and Political Economy in Early Industrial France (1982), which focused on the contributions of Louis-René Villermé in statistics and political economy. Because Villermé was a liberal, Coleman analyzed public health primarily within the context of liberalism. He did not really deal with the public health movement as such, except for a brief section in his last chapter in which he referred to what I call the community of hygienists as the *parti d'hygiène*. Coleman's work made an important contribution by describing one of the main currents of early nineteenth-century French public health, but his account did not tell the whole story. One would get a distorted picture of the public health movement if it were viewed primarily within the context of liberalism. If any one approach dominated the public health movement, it was statism, the notion that it was the responsibility of the state to provide for public health through administrative, legislative, and institutional means. The main exponent of this viewpoint was Alexandre Parent-Duchâtelet, who was, along with Villermé, the other leading French hygienist specializing in urban and occupational hygiene. In his thinking, Parent-Duchâtelet was influenced by Félix Vicq d'Azyr, the architect of the eighteenth-century Royal Society of Medicine and the person who best articulated the statist approach to public health. The public health movement can best be characterized by a liberal–statist dialectic; the early nineteenth-century French public health movement flourished within the context of both liberalism and statism.[2]

This study focuses on the public health movement, the community of hygienists that gathered on the Paris health council and in the editorial society of the journal the *Annales d'hygiène publique et de médecine légale*, their mission, the theories they espoused, the problems they investigated, their efforts to institutionalize and professionalize public hygiene and transform it into a scientific discipline. I argue that the French public health movement, although incorporating liberal elements, was primarily statist in orientation. It was an Establishment movement operating within state-supported institutions and aiming at administrative and legislative reform, in addition to institutionalization of the public health idea and professionalization of public hygiene as a scientific discipline.

The tone of the study has been constrained by the sources available. Lack of personal papers and a paucity of archival sources would no doubt have discouraged other potential investigators. Indeed, personal papers are few, and archival sources, especially at the Archives Nationales, are not

---

2 For complete citations of these works published in the 1980s, see the Bibliographical Note; William Coleman, *Death Is a Social Disease: Public Health and Political Economy in Early Industrial France* (Madison: University of Wisconsin Press, 1982); on Vicq d'Azyr and statism, see Jan Goldstein, *Console and Classify: The French Psychiatric Profession in the Nineteenth Century* (New York: Cambridge University Press, 1987), pp. 20–8.

especially rich. There are, however, some good archival sources at the prefecture of police in Paris and in some of the departmental and municipal
archives. Archives aside, the number of printed sources is truly prodigious, and this study relies heavily on these sources: health council reports,
the *Annales d'hygiène publique*, other medical journals, newspaper accounts, and the numerous public health treatises. The present account is to
some extent official history, theoretical and institutional, policy oriented,
and descriptive, but lacking the familiarity and personal insights that
private papers might have provided. Rarely do we get behind the public
personae of the actors or behind their published works. Nevertheless, I
believe the present account conveys the essence of early nineteenth-century
French public health.

I hope this book will set the stage for further studies. It would be
interesting to see how the public health movement interfaced with clinical
medicine, at what levels, and in what individuals and institutions. George
Weisz's current work on the Royal Academy of Medicine, an institution in
which public hygienists and clinicians debated clinical and public health
questions, may move us closer to an integrated history of early nineteenth-
century French medicine. Historians have been interested in the growth of
professionalism in nineteenth-century French medicine. Martha Hildreth
has analyzed this development for the latter part of the century, and Jan
Goldstein and Matthew Ramsey have made important contributions to the
study of professionalization. What is now needed, it seems to me, is a
study discussing the rise of hygienism and the public health movement
within the context of the professionalization of medicine in nineteenth-
century France. A lacuna in the history of nineteenth-century French medicine and public health is the Second Empire. Most studies have focused on
the pre-1850 or post-1870 period, with the decades of the 1850s and 1860s
dropping out. Perhaps my brief epilogue will whet some investigator's
appetite to pursue the public health story into the 1850s and 1860s, a period
in need of further investigation in clinical medicine as well.[3]

In this book I argue that late eighteenth- and early nineteenth-century
France provided a model for public health theoretically, institutionally, and
practically. French hygienists articulated the public health idea and developed the scientific discipline of public hygiene. They possessed the administrative machinery and institutions through which their notions of public
health and public hygiene could be implemented.

---

3 George Weisz has published several articles on the Royal Academy of Medicine.
   For full citations, see the Bibliographical Note. Martha Hildreth, *Doctors,
   Bureaucrats, and Public Health in France, 1888–1902* (New York: Garland, 1987);
   Goldstein, *Console and Classify*; Matthew Ramsey, *Professional and Popular Medicine
   in France, 1770–1830: The Social World of Medical Practice* (New York: Cambridge
   University Press, 1988).

This then is the story of how a fairly small group of men, serving on the Paris health council and as editors of the *Annales d'hygiène publique et de médecine légale*, created and institutionalized the modern notion of public health and defined and delimited the concept of public hygiene. It is also the story of how they put these notions into practice in their day-to-day work on the health councils, as editors of the leading public health journal, and as individual investigators. The practice of public health in early nineteenth-century France meant primarily investigation, followed by recommendations for reform. By looking in detail at the major urban health problems of the era, the investigations carried out by the hygienists, and their recommendations for reform, we can arrive at a clear understanding of what the early nineteenth-century French public health movement actually was and what its practitioners did.

ACKNOWLEDGMENTS

This book has been through a number of permutations and reincarnations, and therefore there are many people to be thanked. First, I am grateful to the National Library of Medicine for funding the project (LM 02587). The administrators of the Extramural Grants Program have displayed much patience and understanding, qualities one doesn't always expect from a federal agency. I thank them for their financial support and their forbearance. I am indebted to so many friends and colleagues that one friend suggested that I should thank the whole history of medicine community. In fact, he was right. But I would especially like to acknowledge the support and encouragement of all my friends in the history of French medicine and public health: Evelyn Ackerman, Caroline Hannaway, Russ Maulitz, Toby Gelfand, Jackie Duffin, Martha Hildreth, George Weisz, Matt Ramsey, Dora Weiner, Joy Harvey, Othmar Keel, Jan Goldstein, and John Harley Warner, an honorary member of the subspecialty. I owe special thanks to Evelyn Ackerman, Martha Hildreth, Caroline Hannaway, and Joy Harvey for their unflagging support in recent months. I greatly appreciated the help of George Sussman in the early days of the project.

I would also like to mention other historians of medicine whose work has inspired me and had a great influence on my thinking: first of all, Erwin Ackerknecht, George Rosen, and Dora Weiner, the pioneers in French public health history; and second, as models of style, erudition, and collegiality in the history of medicine, Charles Rosenberg and John Harley Warner. Other historians of medicine whom I want to thank for their encouragement at various stages of the project are Toby Appel, Rima Apple, Antoinette Emch-Dériaz, and Mary Lindemann.

I owe special thanks to my colleagues at Virginia Tech, without whose support, encouragement, and sometimes even nagging this book would not have seen the light of day. First and foremost, I want to recognize the invaluable assistance of my close friends in the Women and Science Publication Support Group: Joy Harvey, Muriel Lederman, and Doris Zallen. Meeting with them on a regular basis, and having them enforce deadlines and read and critique my work, has been a great boon. In a real sense, this book is theirs as well as mine. Second, I would like to acknowledge the help and encouragement of my colleagues in the Science Studies Center: Peter Barker, Moti Feingold, Steve Fuller, Bob Paterson, Gary Downey, Skip Fuhrman, and Henry Bauer. Each of them in his own special way has helped me see this project through.

No doubt the book would not have been finished anywhere near the deadline without the help of Helen Graeff, Roger Ariew, and Marshall Fishwick in the Humanities Center and Richard Hirsh in the History Department. Roger and Richard have been my computer consultants, and I am deeply indebted to them for their willingness to share their technical expertise. The support of Helen and Marshall has been critical in bringing this project to closure. They have provided spiritual sustenance in the last phase of the book preparation, and their kind and loving support has made all the difference.

In the History Department, where I have many good friends, thanks go to Bert Moyer, David Lux, and Tom Dunlap, my colleagues in the history of science, and also to Tom Adriance and the former department head Harold Livesay. Through the years, all these friends have read my work, supported my research, and been helpful and encouraging.

Others who have cheered me on include Dick Burian, Joe Pitt, and Marjorie Grene of the Virginia Tech Philosophy Department. Marjorie offered to read the whole manuscript, and only lack of will to make any further revisions prevented me from accepting her generous offer.

A number of people have read earlier drafts of the manuscript and made many helpful suggestions, most of which I have taken. Susan Miller and Leslie Pomeroy read and made editorial suggestions. Erwin Ackerknecht read several chapters and gave them his blessing. Bill Coleman read an earlier version of the whole manuscript, and gave me many helpful comments and much encouragement. Caroline Hannaway read part of the manuscript and enabled me to make drastic cuts in the eighteenth-century background without feeling guilty. Moti Feingold read a couple of chapters and made very helpful stylistic and editorial suggestions, all of which I took. Charles Rosenberg has been unfailingly patient, having read a couple of drafts in their entirety. I have tried to incorporate all his suggestions. I have also taken the advice of the Cambridge referees, whom I thank for their insightful comments.

In France, the staffs at the libraries and archives where I worked have always been generous with their time and most helpful: the Bibliothèque nationale, the Archives nationales, the Archives de la préfecture de police, the Archives de la Seine, the Archives de l'assistance publique, the Bibliothèque centrale de médecine, and the Bibliothèque historique de la ville de Paris. For their hospitality, helpful conversations, and encouragement, thanks to Jean Théodoridès, Jean-Paul Sournia, Jean-Pierre Goubert,

the late Jacques Léonard, and especially Bernard Lécuyer, who was generous with his time and documents, and who welcomed me and made me
feel at home at the Maison des Sciences de l'Homme.

Many thanks to the people at Cambridge University Press who helped
me through various stages of book production: Helen Greenberg, who
copyedited the manuscript with skill and care; Louise Calabro Gruendel,
the production editor, whose advice and understanding were indispensable; and Helen Wheeler and her successor, John Kim, history of science
editors, who oversaw the whole project. Special thanks to John for his
patience in putting up with some unexpected delays.

I would also like to thank Dick Wolfe of the Countway Medical Library
at Harvard, who graciously assisted me in acquiring the illustrations for
this book. Several of my articles, published in *Clio Medica*, *Proceedings of
the Western Society for French History*, and *Bulletin of the History of Medicine*,
have been the sources for many of the ideas in this book. Portions of these
articles appear courtesy of the editors of these journals, to whom I say,
"Thank you."

Heartfelt appreciation to my family and close friends for their patience
and tolerance, as they politely asked, year in and year out, "How is the
book coming?" To my parents, Bill and Leigh Fowler, my sisters, Julia
Dunn and Jacque Clough, my nieces, Julie Dunn and Ellen Scott, my
daughters, Leigh Claire and Julia Louisa, and my good friends Harriet
Dorsey, Patty Foutz, and John Thomas, I simply say, "Thanks for your
patience and understanding."

In the last weeks of completing the book, when burnout could have set
in at any moment, the STS graduate students and some of my undergradu-
ate students at Virginia Tech were cheerful and supportive. Some of them
watched me working round the clock at Price House, and their friendliness
and good wishes made even the drudgery of renumbering footnotes en-
joyable. Thanks to all of you, but especially to Andrea Burrows, Lara
Blechschmidt, Sujatha Raman, Charlotte Webb, and Molly Patrick.

My greatest debt of gratitude is for my husband, Bernard La Berge; my
mentors in the history of medicine and public health, Dora Weiner and
the late Bill Coleman; and, most recently, my friend and colleague, Moti
Feingold. Bernard and Dora have provided unfailing support throughout
the whole project. They were always there when times were rough, were
never critical, and were always optimistic. Bernard has done more than his
share of child care and domestic service, and has in general put up with
me through every phase of the project. Without the time and effort he
contributed, I simply couldn't have finished the book. Dora has been with
me from the time I gave my first paper at an American Association for the
History of Medicine meeting. She has always been there when I needed
her, and her nonjudgmental and caring attitude has helped me through

some difficult times. Her scholarship and dedication have inspired me. Bill Coleman, like Dora, befriended me from the earliest days of the project. We shared similar interests in French public health, and his collegiality and willingness to share ideas contributed much to the success of this work. My ideas about French medicine and public health have been greatly influenced by Bill's many scholarly contributions. Finally, in the last reincarnation of the book, Moti Feingold forced my hand, pushed me to the limit, and set a standard of scholarly excellence and prodigious productivity that served as a model for me to emulate. To Bernard, Dora, and Moti, and to the memory of Bill, I dedicate this book.

INTRODUCTION

The first organized public health movement, composed of physicians, pharmacist-chemists, engineers, veterinarians, and administrators – all calling themselves *hygienists* – organized in Paris around the journal *Annales d'hygiène publique* and the Paris health council. Although the hygiene movement had no one leader comparable to Edwin Chadwick, the two most influential hygienists were Louis-René Villermé and Alexandre Parent-Duchâtelet.

The French public health movement was born and developed within the sociopolitical context of the Bourbon Restoration and the July Monarchy, with their national public health policies and programs, some of which were inherited from the Ancien Régime and the Revolutionary and Napoleonic eras. Several national health institutions and programs were already in place by the 1820s, when the movement began to coalesce. The Royal Academy of Medicine, for example, was founded in 1820 to replace the defunct Royal Society of Medicine, but it continued the traditions of its predecessor, whose interests focused on epidemics.

The public health movement also developed within the context of competing ideologies: liberalism, conservatism, socialism, and statism – all of them tracing their roots to the Ancien Régime and the Revolution. For the public health movement the two dominant ideologies were liberalism and statism. Liberalism was the political persuasion of the leaders of the July Monarchy, and many hygienists operated within the liberal framework, believing most reform was best handled at the individual level and that only limited state intervention to preserve the public health was justified. Villermé was the leading exponent of the liberal viewpoint within the community of hygienists.

Statism, an approach which appealed to persons of varying political persuasions, was characterized by the belief that the state, by administration and legislation, should assume the main role in public health reform and management. Public health could not be left up to individuals. Statists believed it was the state's responsibility to maintain the health of its citizenry, and public health experts should function as advisors to the state.

The dialectic between liberalism and statism, which characterized the public health movement, was reflected in the tension between liberal and social medicine that permeated nineteenth-century French medical discourse. Proponents of liberal medicine favored the private practice of medicine, whereas advocates of social medicine thought health care and preventive medicine could best be provided through a medical civil service. Medicine in the service of the state was their motto. The leading exponent of statism within the community of hygienists was Parent-Duchâtelet.[1]

The dialectic between liberalism and statism was played out within the broader context of scientism, an emerging creed that came to dominate French society by the late nineteenth century. With its roots in the combined empirical and rational tradition of the Enlightenment, scientism was the notion that science was the key to progress, and hence that all areas of investigation could and should be made "scientific." Proponents of scientism believed that a scientific approach was the best way to achieve positive knowledge that would provide an antidote to the power of authority and systems builders. Public hygiene was one of those areas that had to be transformed into a scientific discipline, and this was one of the most important aspects of the mission of the hygienists.

If the hygienists' method was scientific, their mission was hygienism, a kind of medical imperialism incorporating both the medicalization and moralization of society, whose goal was to preserve the fabric of society in the face of what many feared would be massive socioeconomic dislocation and fragmentation caused by industrialization and urbanization. Hygienism also included the notion that physicians and administrators should address traditional charitable-welfare concerns within the secular context of the state. In order to accomplish the hygienic mission, public hygienists had to increase their authority and legitimize their efforts. This was to be done by professionalization, institutionalization of the public health idea, and the development of a scientific discipline of public hygiene.

Two developments of the 1820s and 1830s created public health problems that demanded immediate attention: urbanization – the migration of rural inhabitants to the cities – and industrialization, or the application of steam power to industry and the concentration of large numbers of workers under one roof. The migration of many single, unskilled workers to Paris increased the pressure on reformers and administrators to address traditional urban health problems, such as an inadequate water supply and an outdated sewer system. At the same time, in the 1820s and 1830s, public health investigators brought to the attention of colleagues, administrators,

---

1 The statist approach is nicely developed by Jan Goldstein in *Console and Classify: The French Psychiatric Profession in the Nineteenth Century* (New York: Cambridge University Press, 1987), pp. 20–8.

and the informed public the urgency of public health reform in a city that was increasingly being referred to as "sick."

Before 1850, industrialization had less of an effect in Paris than in other regions of France. Indeed, most trades and crafts in Paris were preindustrial. The sociomedical investigations of Parent-Duchâtelet, the leading occupational hygienist of the era, analyzed the public health hazards of many local industries. Parent-Duchâtelet used these studies in order to reform occupational hygiene, arguing that if an investigator applied a scientific, sociological method to the study of occupations, he would find that many dangers traditionally associated with them did not exist, but that others that had been ignored needed to be addressed. Outside Paris, Villermé and the Lille physician Jean-Pierre Thouvenin directed their attention to the effects of industrialization on the health of the working classes. In his sociohygienic work *Tableau de l'état physique et moral des ouvriers employés dans les manufactures de coton, de laine et de soie*, Villermé concluded that the real problem of the French textile workers was not the work or long working hours, but that their income was too low to provide a basic standard of living.[2]

French public hygienists were influenced by and contributed to the early nineteenth-century statistics movement. Both Villermé and Parent-Duchâtelet sought to make every area of investigation scientific, or quantifiable. Especially important were the differential mortality studies of Villermé, Louis-François Benoiston de Châteauneuf, and others, whose statistical data indicated a strong correlation between standard of living and health and longevity. They concluded that affluent people lived longer and that the main causes of premature death were socioeconomic. This kind of thinking permeated the French public health movement and gave it a decidedly social tone.

In examining the social causes of disease, hygienists questioned the predominant theory of disease causation, which attributed disease mainly to climatic causes, environmental conditions, and especially miasma – loosely interpreted as bad smells. If filth was the primary cause of disease, then the solution was *assainissement*, or sanitary reform. Conversely, if social factors, mainly poverty, were the principal cause of disease and mortality, how should public health reform address the issue? Some hygienists, such as the Lyonnais venerealogist Ariste Potton, advocated far-reaching social reform. Most hygienists, however, stopped short of urging social reform, adopting instead a meliorist stance, according to which their responsibility was merely investigative. These hygienists believed that after they had investigated a public health problem and identified its causes, their work was over. They assumed that a problem,

2 Two vols. (Paris: J. Renouard, 1840).

once pointed out and understood, would either be addressed by the authorities or solved by long-term socioeconomic change. As William Coleman characterized the meliorist approach, hygienists were good on diagnosis but weak on therapy. Thus, although Villermé recognized the harmful effects of industrialization on the working classes, he still argued that in the long run industrialization would be beneficial, raising the standard of living and improving the health of the working classes.[3]

The scientific methodology of public hygiene was also central to the message of Parent-Duchâtelet and his colleague, pharmacist-chemist Alphonse Chevallier. Their program consisted of subjecting traditionally held views about occupational health and disease to critical examination in an attempt to verify or refute them. This led them to take radical and unpopular stands on several public health questions. For example, after the 1832 cholera epidemic, in which over 18,000 Parisians died, Parent-Duchâtelet became a member of the commission charged with investigating the correlation of the incidence of cholera with environmental and social conditions and with reaching conclusions about the course of the disease. Parent-Duchâtelet's investigations of the city dump and the workers who were exposed to it led him to conclude that the miasmatic theory was wrong. If bad smells caused disease, then the mortality rate of people living in and around the dump should have been higher than that of other residents. Yet, few of these people had even contracted cholera. This led Parent-Duchâtelet to challenge the predominant theory of disease causation and to suggest that other causes had to be considered.

The city of Paris was the public hygienists' principal "laboratory." Hygienists investigated and made policy recommendations on most urban health problems: the water supply; the system of sewers and cesspits; the city dump; the regulation of bathing establishments and of food and drink; horsebutchering and other offensive trades; and dissection amphitheaters. Other problems were addressed as well: prostitution, with its related problem of venereal disease; infant abandonment; and the wet-nursing industry. The published reports of the Paris health council, the published and manuscript reports of the provincial health councils, the *Annales d'hygiène publique*, and numerous hygienic treatises provide us with a detailed record of the practice of public health in early-nineteenth-century France, a clear understanding of the method of public health investigation, and the relationship between hygienic policy recommendations and implementation of policy. Using all of these sources, a clear picture of the activity and vitality of the French public health movement emerges.

---

3 William Coleman, *Death Is a Social Disease: Public Health and Political Economy in Early Industrial France* (Madison: University of Wisconsin Press, 1982), pp. 237–8.

The present study analyzes the theory, practice, institutional base, and national policy of public health in early-nineteenth-century France. Second, and in contrast to previous studies, it identifies clearly who the hygienists were. It analyzes the community of hygienists, their theories, investigations, methodology, and programs, including professionalization and disciplinary development. Third, this study allows us to view the 1832 cholera epidemic within the context of the public health movement. Such an analysis is greatly needed, since most treatments of that epidemic lack such contextual considerations.

Cholera has always posed methodological problems for historians of public health, epidemiology, and medicine. Numerous monographs have been written on the nineteenth-century cholera epidemic, and several have focused exclusively on the French experience. François Delaporte has argued that the cholera epidemic was a turning point, when the environmental theory of disease causation gave way to the social theory. Within the context of the public health movement, however, the social theory of epidemiology antedated the cholera epidemic, which served to strengthen support for an already widely accepted theory. Patrice Bourdelais and Jean-Yves Raulot also failed to place the 1832 epidemic within the preexisting public health movement, leading them to conclude that the epidemic provided the major stimulus initiating that movement. Viewed within the context of the public health movement, however, cholera appears as one of several catalysts for reform within an already ongoing movement. The epidemic served as a test case for theories already being widely debated and programs and policies that had long been recommended. Cholera was one of many factors, such as population pressure, which forced the issue of public health reform.[4]

Similarly, although many recent works have addressed various aspects of public health in early-nineteenth-century France – notably, William Coleman's work on Villermé, Jean-Pierre Goubert on water, Alain Corbin on the cultural shifts in the perception of odor and public health ramifications, Jill Harsin and Corbin on prostitution – none has analyzed the public health movement, the individual hygienists, their relationships, institutions, theories and programs. Scholars are aware of the hygiene movement but have not taken the trouble to analyze it in detail. Instead they have taken it for granted. This lack of a general study of public health in France and the French public health movement has led some historians to misinterpret the cholera experience, whereas others have provided

---

4 François Delaporte, *Disease and Civilization: The Cholera in Paris, 1832* (Cambridge, MA: MIT Press, 1986); Patrice Bourdelais and Jean-Yves Raulot, *Une peur bleue: Histoire du choléra en France, 1832–1854* (Paris: Payot, 1987).

particularistic accounts of various aspects of public health, but without placing them in the context either of the public health movement or of French national public health policies and programs.[5]

Furthermore, although we have Coleman's excellent study on Villermé, no equivalent treatment exists for Parent-Duchâtelet. Yet he was a more central figure than Villermé in the French public health movement. True, some attention has been given to Parent-Duchâtelet's landmark sociohygienic investigation of prostitution in Paris, but this research failed to integrate that work with his work in occupational and urban hygiene or to place his work on prostitution within the broader context of public health theory, methodology, and the public health movement. Although these historians have recognized the importance of Parent-Duchâtelet's methodology, they have not related it to his program of professionalization, institutionalization, and disciplinary development of *hygiène publique*. The present study places great emphasis on the role of Parent-Duchâtelet in the public health movement and offers a comprehensive account of the many facets of his public health work, analyzing his contributions in urban and occupational hygiene as well has his major theoretical and institutional contributions.[6]

By way of conclusion, the present study also considers some broader aspects of the history of public health by challenging the prevalent notion that the British were the leaders in the nineteenth-century public health movement and that the British example set the model for similar movements elsewhere. This study argues that an active and influential French public health movement not only antedated the British, but also that Chadwick and Smith were greatly influenced by French hygienic ideas and institutions.

5 Coleman, *Death Is a Social Disease*; Jean-Pierre Goubert, *The Conquest of Water: The Advent of Health in the Industrial Age* (Princeton, NJ: Princeton University Press, 1989); Alain Corbin, *Le miasme et la jonquille: l'odorat et l'imaginaire social, 18–19e siècles* (Paris: Aubier-Montaigne, 1982); Jill Harsin, *Prostitution in Nineteenth-Century Paris* (Princeton, NJ: Princeton University Press, 1985); Alain Corbin, "Présentation" to Alexandre Parent-Duchâtelet, *La Prostitution à Paris au XIXe siécle*, texte présenté et annoté par Alain Corbin (Paris: Seuil, 1981), pp. 9–42.
6 Harsin, *Prostitution in Paris*; Corbin, "Présentation."

I

Community, method, context

1

Public health and the community of hygienists

From the fall of the Roman Empire to the late eighteenth century, two kinds of public health measures dominated: emergency measures to deal with epidemic disease and specific measures relating to municipal nuisances such as offensive trades and waste disposal. The principal goal of public health was the prevention and management of epidemics, whose methods varied, but typically included emergency measures such as quarantines, sequestration, *cordons sanitaires*, and temporary institutions such as boards of health and sanitary intendancies. These measures were predicated upon two theories of disease causation: an environmentalist and climatic theory – the predominant theory – and a contagionist theory. Plague had traditionally been considered a contagious disease, and epidemic prevention and control were based upon that experience.[1] Epidemics posed severe problems for authorities and created a crisis mentality, demanding immediate attention. Once the crisis was over, however, the institutions established to manage the emergency were disbanded, and business as usual resumed. Endemic diseases received little attention from authorities, since they were a way of life and death known to all. There was little concern for permanent public health regulations and institutions in the rural areas and small towns where most people lived. In larger towns and cities, however, local authorities regulated "nuisances," such as refuse disposal and offensive trades. Enforcement varied widely from place to place, with many regulations not being enforced at all. If a particular situation became too troublesome, ad hoc action was taken.

Until the mid-eighteenth century in France public health was primarily

---

1 For background, see George Rosen, *A History of Public Health* (New York: MD Publications, 1958), pp. 81–130; George Rosen "Mercantilism and Health Policy in Eighteenth-Century French Thought," in *From Medical Police to Social Medicine: Essays on the History of Health Care* (New York: Science History Publications, 1974), pp. 201–19; Carlo Cipolla, *Public Health and the Medical Profession in the Renaissance* (Cambridge: Cambridge University Press, 1976). On the last great European plague epidemic, the 1720 Marseilles epidemic, see Charles Carrière, Marcel Cordurié, and Ferréol Rébuffat, *Marseille, ville morte. La peste de 1720* (Marseille: Garcon, 1968).

a local affair, and progress in establishing public health institutions was slow. The traditional public health concerns – epidemics and epizootics – were managed by royal decrees and local ordinances. Some cities had health offices (*bureaux de santé*) to handle local problems and advise administrative authorities, and coastal cities had sanitary institutions to enforce quarantine regulations. During the eighteenth century, intendants were in charge of public health in their districts and were expected to communicate with the central authority on public health matters – mainly epidemics. Some intendants appointed epidemic physicians (*médecins des épidémies*) to regular posts to assist during epidemics, but there was no uniform national public health administration or professional medical organization to investigate epidemic diseases and dispense information on their management. Although a few individuals articulated a modern concept of public health, they did not institutionalize it in any permanent way until the 1770s.

Standards of personal hygiene varied according to educational and economic levels, geographic location, availability of water, climate, and other physical factors. Although the tradition of private or individual hygiene dates from Hippocrates and Galen, before the mid-eighteenth century in France there was little interest in applying these rules to the public. Even in a forward-thinking collection like the *Encyclopédie*, only personal or individual hygiene was stressed. William Coleman has convincingly argued, for example, that the personal hygiene expounded in the *Encyclopédie*, based on the six Galenic nonnaturals, fitted neatly the prevailing individualistic, utilitarian outlook of the educated nobility and bourgeoisie of Ancien Régime France.[2]

Private or individual hygiene was the traditional area of hygienic interest in France until the last quarter of the eighteenth century, when a shift from a preoccupation with private hygiene to public health occurred. At that time, concepts of public health were being advanced concurrently in several areas of Europe. Johann Peter Frank began publishing his six-volume *System einer vollständigen medicinischen Polizey* in 1779, and Samuel-Auguste-André-David Tissot in Switzerland wrote (but did not publish) his "De la police médicale" sometime between 1787 and 1797.[3] In Scotland,

2 James Riley, *The Eighteenth-Century Campaign to Avoid Disease* (New York: St. Martin's, 1987); William Coleman, "Health and Hygiene in the *Encyclopédie*: A Medical Doctrine for the Bourgeoisie," *J. Hist. Med.* 29 (1974): 399–421; Caroline Hannaway, "From Private Hygiene to Public Health: A Transformation in Western Medicine in the Eighteenth and Nineteenth Centuries," in Teizo Ogawa, ed., *Public Health: Proceedings of the Fifth International Symposium on the Comparative History of Medicine – East and West* (Tokyo: Saikon Publishing for the Taniguchi Foundation, 1981), pp. 108–28.

3 Johann Peter Frank, *System einer vollständigen medicinischen Polizey*, 6 vols. (Mannheim: C. F. Schwann, 1779–1819). See the English translation by Erna Lesky, *A System of Complete Medical Police. Selections from Johann Peter Frank*, ed. and with an introduction by Erna Lesky (Baltimore: Johns Hopkins University

Andrew Duncan prepared a series of lectures on medical police, and in France, a modern concept of public health was articulated and institutionalized after 1776 by the founders and leaders of the Royal Society of Medicine.[4]

THE PUBLIC HEALTH IDEA

The public health idea espoused in late-eighteenth-century France was an Enlightenment approach to health, disease, and epidemics. It incorporated and was derived from many of the general currents of Enlightenment thought: the emphasis on progress, rational reform, education, natural law, orderliness, empiricism, and humanitarianism. The public health idea included, first, preventive medicine, for public health was not just to be invoked in response to medical emergencies, but was an ongoing administrative practice aimed at reducing mortality and morbidity and improving the quality of life. The environmental – or Hippocratic – approach to health and disease had for centuries been the prevailing notion of private hygiene. When raised to the public level by the founders of the Royal Society of Medicine in the 1770s, the result was an all-encompassing attitude toward public health. Reforming physicians of the Royal Society of Medicine broadened the scope of public health from epidemic prevention and control and nuisance regulation to include anything and everything related to health. After all, at a time when diseases could not be attributed to any one specific cause, anything could be potentially hazardous to health.

The notion of public health advanced by physicians was part of the rational reform of society and was dependent upon the Enlightenment idea of the progress of civilization. Condorcet articulated the Enlightenment belief in progress, arguing that humankind and civilization were always

Press, 1976); S. A. A. D. Tissot, "De la police médicale." On Tissot and this work, see Antoinette Emch-Dériaz, "Towards a Social Conception of Health in the Second Half of the Eighteenth Century: Tissot (1728–1797) and the New Preoccupation with Health and Well-Being" (Ph.D. dissertation, University of Rochester, 1983), pp. 308–66.

4 Andrew Duncan, *Heads of Lectures on Medical Police* (Edinburgh: Adam Neil and Co., 1801). There were, of course, some forerunners. See Rosen, *History of Public Health*, pp. 81–130. Interest in public health was evident much earlier in the century in some of the German states. See George Rosen, "Cameralism and the Concept of the Medical Police," *Bull. Hist. Med.* 27 (1953): 21–42. Interest in public health dated from the seventeenth century in England. See Riley, *Eighteenth Century Campaign*. See also Othmar Keel, "The Politics of Health and the Institutionalization of Clinical Practices in Europe in the Second Half of the Eighteenth Century," in William Bynum and Roy Porter, eds., *William Hunter and the Eighteenth-Century Medical World* (London: Cambridge University Press, 1985), pp. 214–24. For a good overview, see Hannaway, "From Hygiene to Public Health."

improving and would continue to do so, moving in the direction of per-fectibility. On the one hand, progress was inevitable. On the other hand, humans, confident of their power to change the environment and reform society, could speed up progress by social, political, economic, and edu-cational reforms. One of the most important aspects of the idea of the progress of civilization for public health reformers was the belief that as civilization advanced, public health improved. Public health was concomi-tant with progress and civilization. Condorcet expressed these ideas in his *Esquisse d'un tableau historique des progrès de l'esprit humain*, where he dis-cussed the physical perfectibility of the human species. He was confident that preventive medicine and better material conditions would increase the average length of life and ensure humans good health and strong con-stitutions. The spread of preventive medicine, advancing because of the progress of reason and social order, would eventually result in the disap-pearance of communicable epidemic diseases and common diseases caused by climate, food, and work. Although Condorcet did not predict immor-tality, he foresaw a continually increasing life span in which death would only result from accidents or the final slowing down of vital forces. Disease had no place in his prediction of human health improvement.[5]

Enlightenment attitudes toward nature were also important to the modern concept of public health. Rousseau emphasized humanity in the state of nature, suggesting that what was natural was good and in keeping with the harmony of the universe. Health was the natural state of humans, a desirable goal to be pursued by individuals, physicians, and the state for the benefit of the whole population. Beliefs about the underlying orderli-ness of nature and humanity's ability to control and manipulate nature also figured in the new notion of public health, for hygienists assumed there were natural laws governing disease and epidemics that would become apparent if enough empirical data were gathered. An example of an attempt to discover these laws was Vicq d'Azyr's program in the Royal Society of Medicine in which masses of meteorological and epidemio-logical data were collected in the hope that such patterns would emerge. The further assumption was that once the causes of disease and epidemics were known, the environment could be altered or controlled to prevent or decrease the incidence of disease.[6]

Influenced by humanitarianism, social and public health reformers

5 Condorcet, *Esquisse d'un tableau historique des progrès de l'esprit humain*. First published in 1795 after Condorcet's death. Preface and notes by Monique and François Hincker (Paris: Editions sociales, 1971). On Condorcet, see Keith Baker, *Condorcet: From Natural Philosophy to Social Mathematics* (Chicago: University of Chicago Press, 1975), and the older work by J. Salwyn Shapiro, *Condorcet and the Rise of Liberalism* (New York: Harcourt, Brace, & Co., 1934), pp. 234–70.

6 Riley, *Eighteenth-Century Campaign*; Jean-Paul Desaive, Jean-Pierre Goubert, et al., *Médecins, climat et épidémies à la fin du XVIIIe siècle* (Paris: Mouton, 1972).

dependent on any particular governmental form, although it did
n effective central administration.

ublic health idea was institutionalized in several organizations:
ational level, the Royal Society of Medicine and its nineteenth-
successor, the Royal Academy of Medicine, and at the local level,
th councils (*conseils de salubrité*). In France the institutionalization
c health followed from a general notion of the rational, scientific
g of society for which Keith Baker has argued and that was
fied in the work of both Anne-Robert-Jacques Turgot and Félix
Azyr, the architect of the Royal Society of Medicine. Furthermore,
yal Society of Medicine was conceived on the plan of the Royal
ny of Sciences, the continental model for scientific institutions.

to the institutionalization of public health was its day-to-day
stration. As a state agency, the Royal Society of Medicine was
e as a coordinating body at the apex of a national public health
stration. Indeed, many contemporaries conceived of it as a virtual
ry of Health. Certainly that was one of the goals of its founders.
gh historians do not agree on the effectiveness of the central
stration of Ancien Régime France, the royal intendants provided the
ramework for what became in the Revolutionary and Napoleonic
s a highly centralized, uniform national bureaucracy operating
the well-defined boundaries of a modern nation-state. One of the
al goals of public health reformers in the 1770s and 1780s was a
ized administration through which the public health could be
istered.[10]

nce and the scientific method as conceived by Enlightenment
istrators and the founders of the Royal Society of Medicine were
mental to the public health idea. Within the society, diseases and
mics were to be investigated by gathering quantitative data to
le an empirical basis for the development and implementation of
es and programs. The meteorological data collection program of the

o Baker, *Condorcet*, esp. ch. 1. On Turgot and Vicq d'Azyr, see Charles C. Gillispie,
    Science and Polity in France at the End of the Old Régime (Princeton, NJ: Princeton
    University Press, 1980), pp. 196–203, 12–33, 229. Douglas Dakin, *Turgot and the
    Ancien Régime in France* (New York: Octagon Books, 1965), esp. pp. 195–206.
    Caroline Hannaway, "The Société Royale de Médecine and Epidemics in the
    Ancien Régime," *Bull. Hist. Med.* 46 (1972): 257–73, and Caroline Hannaway,
    "Medicine, Public Welfare, and the State in Eighteenth-Century France: The
    Société Royale de Médecine of Paris (1776–1793)" (Ph.D. dissertation, Johns
    Hopkins, University, 1974). See also Keith Baker, "Scientism at the End of the
    Old Régime: Reflections on a Theory of Professor Charles Gillispie," *Minerva*
    25 (1987): 21–34. Coleman, "Health and Hygiene in the Encyclopédie"; Guy
    Thuillier, *Bureaucratie et bureaucrates en France au XIXe siècle* (Geneva: Droz, 1980),
    pp. ix–xi.

directed their attention to the treatment of pr
sanitary conditions in prisons and hospitals. T
prison reform was John Howard's *State of the*
(1777). In a 1780 appendix to that work, How
reporting on the state of prisons on the contin
read in France, and nineteenth-century refor
Villermé and Alexis de Tocqueville cited it as
topic.[7] The concern for humanitarian reform
Parisian hospital reform movement of the 1780
was the Hôtel-Dieu, the oldest, largest, and mos

Finally, the Enlightenment concept of medic
public health idea. The concept of medical
administration of an enlightened despot, had it
(cameralist) notion that public health was of cent
despots, since the health of the state was its
medical police was best described by Johann P
Complete Medical Police, in which he proclaime
people was the responsibility of the state and ou
of public and private hygiene from the cradle to
the theory of medical police, the state assumed th
responsibility of protecting citizens from epiden
all aspects of the nation's health by a medical civ
some of the German states by the institution of the

Yet it would be hard to argue that the concept
any direct influence on the founders of the Roya
on other French public health advocates. The pub
in late-eighteenth-century France was the French
continental phenomenon. Although the two had n
cal police was associated with enlightened despotis

was no
require
The
at the
century
the he:
of pub
planni
exemp
Vicq d
the R
Acade
Relate
admir
to ser
admir
Minis
Altho
admir
basic
perioc
withi
princ
centr
admir
Sci
admir
funda
epide
provi
polic

7 See Shelby T. McCloy, *The Humanitarian Movemen*
(Lexington: University of Kentucky Press, 1957); Lou
itarianism of Antoine-Laurent Lavoisier," *Studies o*
Century 88 (1972): 651–75; *Appendix to the State of*
further account of foreign prisons and hospitals (Warringtor

8 Louis S. Greenbaum, "Scientists and Politicians: Hosp
Eve of the French Revolution," *Proceedings of the Cons(*
(1973), ed. Claude Sturgill (Gainesville: University F
168–91; Louis Greenbaum, "Measure of Civilizatior
Jacques Tenon on the Eve of the French Revolution,"
43–66; and the original work, Jacques Tenon, *Mém*
(Paris: Pierres, 1788).

9 Rosen, *Public Health,* pp. 81–130; Rosen, "Mercan
Rosen, "Cameralism and the Concept of the Medical
Jordanova, "Policing Public Health in France, 1780–1
Public Health: Proceedings of the 5th International Syn
History of Medicine-East and West, pp. 12–32.

Royal Society of Medicine exemplifies this scientific approach to disease. In an attempt to find underlying patterns and laws of epidemic disease, the Royal Society of Medicine had its army of provincial correspondents send in quarterly reports providing meteorological data, gathered daily throughout the nation. The Revolution intervened and the society was abolished before this twenty-year data collection program was complete. Science and the scientific method were also central in a broader context, since public health constituted an important part of a general program of reforming society upon the basis of rational, scientific principles.[11]

The scientific basis for public health brought with it an expanded role for the physician. Whereas the physician's attention had traditionally been directed to the individual patient, reformers in the Royal Society of Medicine and members of the Health Committee of the National Constituent Assembly envisioned the physician as a civil servant gathering scientific data and performing experiments. And if environmental causes of disease – including social or living conditions – were central to understanding and preventing disease, as eighteenth-century hygienists believed, then the physician would be a sociomedical investigator. But the physician's role did not stop there. He would carry the process one step further, serving the government as a sociomedical expert. In the scientific reform of society, the expert advisor assumed an important place. Once physicians became sociomedical investigators, it followed that their recommendations for public health reform might include not only cleaning up the environment, or sanitary reform, but also improving living conditions, or socioeconomic reform. The fact that poverty was the principal public health problem in eighteenth-century France and that sociomedical investigators associated poverty with disease gave French public health its decidedly social tone.[12]

A major component of public health theory was expertise. Although the physician had traditionally been considered the public health expert, for the new wide-ranging public health, specialists from other areas were needed: pharmacist-chemists to perform laboratory experiments on secret remedies; veterinarians to manage epizootics; and engineers and architects to investigate and solve urban health problems related to the location and construction of buildings, canals, and sources of water. Because of the variety of experts needed, public health was to be a collaborative effort

11 Baker, "Scientism at the End of the Old Régime"; Desaive et al., *Médecins, climat et épidémies*.

12 Rosen, "Mercantilism and Health Policy," p. 210. On poverty and the poor in eighteenth-century France, see Olwen Hufton, *The Poor in Eighteenth-Century France 1750–1789* (Oxford: Clarendon Press, 1974); and Jean Gutton, *La société et les pauvres in Europe, XVIe–XVIIIe siècles* (Paris: Presses Universitaires de France, 1974).

of specialists: scientists, physicians, engineers, and administrators. This notion of broadly based expertise was institutionalized in the Royal Society of Medicine and in the nineteenth-century health councils.

Before and during the Revolution, French reforming physicians incorporated the social contract idea into their theory of public health. The Health Committee of the National Constituent Assembly formally supported the claim that health was a natural right to which all citizens were entitled and asserted that if governments were instituted to protect natural rights, then public health was the duty of the state. The state's duties were broad, providing for citizens' health at all times, not just during medical emergencies. Thus, health was considered a proper area for state intervention, regulation, and control. The notion that health was a natural right included the ideal of equal access (to use a modern expression) to disease prevention and health care. Applying the French ideal of uniformity to public health meant that preventive and therapeutic measures should be uniformly available to all citizens.[13] Equality and uniformity were important components of the Revolutionary idea of public health, and the centralized bureaucracy established during the Revolutionary and Napoleonic eras attempted – but failed – to provide uniform prevention and health care. A good example of this effort was the national vaccination program established by Napoleon and continued by the Restoration regime.

In late-eighteenth-century France, scientists, reforming administrators, and physicians had good pragmatic reasons for promoting public health reform. A deteriorating urban sanitary situation contributed to the emergence of the public health idea. In Paris, for example, some problems demanded the attention of municipal authorities and their expert advisors. The classic examples, investigated by commissions of the Royal Academy of Sciences and the Royal Society of Medicine, were the centuries-old Cemetery of the Innocents (Cimetière des Innocents) in the center of Paris, the Hôtel-Dieu, and the city dump at Montfaucon.[14] In each of these cases, the sanitary situation had become so critical that authorities considered it a serious public health problem. Furthermore, urbanization, the migration of people from the provinces to Paris in the middle to late eighteenth

13 Dora B. Weiner, "Le Droit de l'Homme à la Santé – Une Belle Idée devant l'Assemblée Constituante: 1790–1791," *Clio Medica* 5 (1970): 209–23; Henry Ingrand, *Le Comité de salubrité de l'Assemblée nationale constituante (1790–91)* (Thesis: University of Paris, 1934), pp. 32–104. For the notion of uniformity, see Merritt Roe Smith, "Military Entrepreneurship," in Otto Mayr and Robert C. Post, eds. *Yankee Enterprise: The Rise of the American System of Manufactures* (Washington, DC: Smithsonian Institution Press, 1981), pp. 63–102.

14 On the Cimetière des Innocents, see Caroline and Owen Hannaway, "La Fermeture du Cimetière des Innocents," *Dix-huitième siècle* 9 (1977): 181–91; Tenon, *Mémoires sur les hôpitaux*.

century, exacerbated public health problems associated with street cleaning, garbage disposal, burials, and overcrowded living conditions. A similar situation prevailed in other European cities, where pressure on existing facilities reached the breaking point and traditional methods of management failed. This deteriorating situation, accompanied by a heightened awareness of health and renewed attention to the environmental causes of disease, motivated hygienists to urge public health reform.

Another pragmatic concern was depopulation. France was the first European country to experience a declining birth rate in the late eighteenth century, and from that time public health reformers and statisticians began to debate the relative merits of high versus low birth rates. Two approaches were proposed to increase the population: first, to encourage parents to have more children, and second, to conserve them better by reducing infant and child mortality. Public health reformers took the second approach, pointing out that without adequate means of saving children, bearing more was not only sheer waste but would result in sicker children. The notion that infant hygiene could be practiced not only at the personal level but on a broad scale to reduce infant mortality was an important component of the developing concept of public health. This concern, both humanitarian and populationist, found its expression in the infant welfare movement of the late eighteenth and nineteenth centuries, as well as in advocacy of general public health reform.[15]

A specific motivating factor in the institutionalization of public health was the cattle plague of the early 1770s, the worst of the century. This epizootic was the immediate reason for Turgot's creation of a special consultative commission (Condorcet, Malesherbes, Trudaine de Montigny, Duhamel, Tenon, Vicq d'Azyr) to manage the epidemic. In 1776, after the epidemic had run its course, Turgot established another commission composed of Lassonne, Vicq d'Azyr, and six other specialists from a variety of backgrounds to inquire into the problem of epidemics. In 1778, this commission became the Royal Society of Medicine, discussed earlier.[16]

Although the new interest in public health was not an exclusively French phenomenon, the public health idea was most clearly articulated and institutionalized in France, laying the groundwork for the nineteenth-century public health movement. Several explanations for French leadership exist. First, France was the intellectual leader of Europe, the center of advanced social and scientific thought. Furthermore, France was becoming a modern nation-state possessing the framework of a centralized bureaucracy through which public health reforms could be administered. Finally,

---

15 Marie-France Morel, "Mère, enfant, médecin: La Médicalisation de la petite enfance en France (XVIIe–XIXe siècles)," in Arthur E. Imhof, ed., *Mensch und Gesundheit in der Geschichte* (Husum. Druck: Matthiesen Verlag, 1980), pp. 301–13.
16 Hannaway, "Société Royale de Médecine"; Dakin, *Turgot*, pp. 195–206.

for reasons related to the economic, political, and intellectual situation of Ancien Régime France, the country witnessed a major reform movement in the 1770s and 1780s, one aspect of which was public health reform. When that initiative failed to rectify a deteriorating situation, the resultant Revolution brought with it the vision of a new egalitarian society founded on rational and scientific principles. This vision included the concept of public health as a natural right to be guaranteed by the government and a technocratic ideal, the notion of science in the service of the state, the model for scientists and physicians to serve as expert advisors to the government.[17]

THE PUBLIC HEALTH MOVEMENT

Although there had been much interest in public health since the late eighteenth century, and some reforms had been made and institutions established, by the 1820s the urban health problems of water supply, sewerage, housing, occupational hygiene, and many others had been neither adequately investigated nor solved. In addition, there were urgent new problems created by urbanization and industrialization. In the first half of the nineteenth century, public hygienists investigated the major urban health problems and progressed toward their solution. By the late 1820s, a public health movement composed of physicians, scientists, and administrators began to coalesce.

Nineteenth-century hygienists continued the eighteenth-century public health traditions, with some modifications. For example, whereas the main focus of the founders and members of the Royal Society of Medicine had been epidemic disease, nineteenth-century hygienists were as interested in endemic as epidemic disease, devoting much attention to occupational hygiene. The Royal Society of Medicine (1776–94) was revived as the Royal Academy of Medicine (1820), which became the principal public health advisory body to the national government. Other national academies also debated public health questions. In the 1830s, the Royal Academy of Sciences studied the effectiveness of vaccination, and the Academy of Political and Moral Sciences sponsored a major study of the health of textile workers.

The Paris health council (founded in 1802) filled a new public health role. At first conceived of as a public health advisory board to the prefect of police in Paris, by the 1820s it had also become a model for other cities and departments. Although some hygienists advocated an active role for the national government in public health matters, they still recognized that most public health problems were best managed at the local level. Munici-

---

17 Baker, *Condorcet*, ch. I; Gillispie, *Science and Polity in France*, p. 224. See also Baker, "Scientism at the End of the Old Régime."

pal governments had a long tradition of regulating "nuisances." By the nineteenth century, however, urban health problems had become more urgent as health conditions deteriorated in many towns and cities. Thus permanent health boards staffed by experts seemed to many hygienists and municipal administrators to be the most effective means of first investigating public health problems and then – in conjunction with local authorities – managing them.

A full-fledged public health movement dates from 1829, when a group of hygienists and legal medicine specialists founded the *Annales d'hygiène publique et de médecine légale*. The movement was clustered around this journal and the Paris health council and its offshoots, the provincial health councils. Several developments and events contributed to the emergence of a cohesive public health movement by the 1820s: the reinvigoration of the Paris health council in 1817 under prefect of police Anglès and the founding between 1817 and 1829 of municipal and departmental health councils in Nantes, Lille, Marseilles, Lyon, and Strasbourg, all modeled on the Paris health council; the resuscitation of the Royal Society of Medicine as the Royal Academy of Medicine, founded in 1820 with public health goals; the increasing pace of urbanization in Paris in the 1820s and the inability of the Parisian government to deal effectively with nuisance control, industrial regulation, sewerage, and water supply; the beginning of the public health careers of leading hygienists such as Louis-René Villermé, Alexandre Parent-Duchâtelet, and Louis-François Benoiston de Châteauneuf; the new interest in applying statistics to medicine and public health; and the continued scientific supremacy of Paris and the city's emergence as the medical capital of the Western world.

By the 1820s, urbanization and the beginnings of French industrialization encouraged a heightened interest in public hygiene. The migration of people from the countryside to the cities in search of jobs was characteristic of Paris and the industrializing areas of France – the north and the northeast – where disease became one of the major problems created by rapidly increasing population and facilities inadequate to handle it. After 1830, the population of Paris grew rapidly. Many newcomers had little money and were able to obtain only sporadic employment. Most urban health problems investigated by hygienists were not new, but had become more acute with rising population pressure and a changing climate of opinion that demanded better public health. The Paris cholera epidemic of 1832 and the increasing mortality rate in Paris compared with the rest of the nation pointed up the deplorable state of public health in Paris.[18] Urban

18 Claude Lachaise, "De l'influence de l'entassement de la population sur la mortalité des grandes villes, *Bull. de l'Acad. Roy. de Méd.* 5 (1840–1): 570–80; Louis-François Benoiston de Châteauneuf et al., *Rapport sur la marche et les effets du choléra-morbus dans Paris…*(Paris: Imprimerie royale, 1834). See also François Delaporte, *Disease and Civilization: The Cholera in Paris, 1832* (Cambridge, MA: MIT Press, 1986).

health problems loomed so large that the French public health movement was primarily an urban phenomenon recognized by the hygienists themselves, who asserted that public health reform was fundamental for survival in cities.[19]

Industralization brought public health issues into full relief. Paris had one of the largest working-class populations of any European city in the early nineteenth century, with about 400,000 workers by midcentury. Although a modern factory system developed in the textile industry, most French workers continued to be employed in traditional cottage industries and small workshops. Both handcraft and domestic industries, as well as the new mechanized, factory-based industries, caused public health problems. The social consequences of industrialization were publicized by socialists, humanitarians, and hygienists who vividly described the situation of industrial workers. Both the Birtish and French governments conducted official inquiries into the "condition of the working classes," which became a topic of major concern to public hygienists. As the hygienists saw it, at stake was the health of a large segment of the French population, which was becoming increasingly important both economically and politically.

The application of statistics to medical and public health questions in the 1820s and 1830s contributed to the growth of the French public health movement, for statistical analysis provided what hygienists considered objective scientific proof for their public health theories. Statistical data gave reformers clout. Statistical analysis could be used to measure the health of a group or nation and to assess the effects of health reforms. With statistical data to buttress their beliefs, public hygienists sought to transform public health theories into a body of scientific doctrine in order to establish public hygiene as a scientific discipline. Their efforts in this direction reflected the increasing scientism of the early nineteenth century and attempts to develop a social science or a science of society.

Hygienists' widespread acceptance of an environmentalist approach to disease causation encouraged the growth of the public health movement. The dominant belief among hygienists was that most diseases were not immediately transmissible from a sick to a healthy person by a living organism, but developed because of environmental conditions.[20] Filth and poverty were the two conditions thought most likely to cause disease,

19 Jean-Baptiste Monfalcon and A. P. Isidore de Polinière, *Traité de la salubrité dans les grandes villes* (Paris: Baillière, 1846), pp. 34–40; Alexandre Parent-Duchâtelet, "Essai sur les cloaques ou égouts de la ville de Paris," in *Hygiène publique*, 2 vols. (Paris: Baillière, 1836), 1: 157, 161; Jean-Noël Hallé and P. H. Nysten, "Hygiène," in *Dictionaire des sciences médicales*, ed. Adelon et al., 60 vols. (Paris: C. L. F. Panckoucke, 1812–22), 22: 529, 550.
20 Erwin Ackerknecht, "Anticontagionism between 1821 and 1867,' *Bull. Hist. Med.* 22 (1948): 562–93.

although some hygienists still postulated traditional climatic causes. Thus, hygienists proposed cleaning up the environment, or sanitary reform, and alleviating poverty and its consequences by socioeconomic, administrative, and moral reform. Measures of disease prevention shifted from traditional methods, undertaken only in times of emergency, to the application of sanitary and administrative measures on a permanent basis.

Although the French public health movement was well established by the late 1820s, the cholera epidemic acted as a further stimulus to public health reform. The cholera experience confirmed both social and environmental theories of disease causation. Municipal clean-up campaigns increased awareness at the popular and professional levels of local sanitary conditions. In cities that were spared, such as Lyon, good fortune was attributed to municipal clean-up programs that demonstrated the effectiveness of sanitary reforms. In cities where cholera took many victims – like Paris – fear of the disease and future outbreaks made administrators take sanitary reform seriously. The cholera epidemic moved public health discourse from the theoretical to the practical level.[21]

The public health movement was composed of physicians, pharmacist-chemists, and administrators. The Paris health council and the society of the *Annales d'hygiène publique*, along with other public health institutions, such as provincial health councils and medical societies, provided leadership and organization. Much of the activity of the movement was channeled through the Paris health council. Nearly all the leading hygienists were members of the Paris health council or of one of the provincial health councils.[22] They were also founders, editors, and frequent contributors to the *Annales d'hygiène publique*, the journal that served as the organ of the public health movement.[23] Hygienists published numerous articles and treatises on all aspects of public health, most of which appeared in one

21 Benoiston de Châteauneuf, *Rapport sur la marche et les effets du choléra*; George Sussman, "From Yellow Fever to Cholera: A Study of French Government Policy, Medical Professionalism and Popular Movements in the Epidemic Crises of the Restoration and July Monarchy" (Ph.D. dissertation, Yale University, 1971), pp. 1–213. See also Delaporte, *Disease and Civilization*. Lyon, Archives Municipales de Lyon, I⁵,1, I⁵8, I⁵9 I⁵10.

22 On the Paris health council, see Dora B. Weiner, "Public Health under Napoleon: The Conseil de salubrité de Paris, 1802–1815," *Clio Medica* 9 (1974): 271–84, and Ann Fowler La Berge, "The Paris Health Council, 1802–1848," *Bull. Hist. Med.* 49 (1975): 339–52.

23 Leading hygienists who served as founding editors were Jean-Pierre Barruel, J. P. Joseph d'Arcet, Pierre Kéraudren, Charles C. H. Marc, Alexandre Parent-Duchâtelet, and Louis-René Villermé. Later editors included the leading hygienists J. B. Alphonse Chevallier, Henri Gaultier de Claubry, Adolphe Trébuchet, and Ambroise Tardieu. On the *Annales d'hygiène publique*, see Bernard Lécuyer, "Médecins et observateurs sociaux: les Annales d'hygiène publique et de médecine légale (1820–1850), in *Pour une histoire de la statistique*, s.l.n.d. (Paris: INSEE, 1977) pp. 445–55.

form or another in the *Annales d'hygiène publique*, which provided a forum
and was the main source of publicity for the movement.

The French public health movement was indigenous. Although some
of the early hygienists and reforming administrators were influenced by
the German tradition of the medical police, for example, Prefect Lézay-
Marnésia of the Bas-Rhin, similar ideas had been current in France since
1775.[24] By the 1820s, when the activity of the hygienists began to coalesce
into a public health movement, France had a well-established tradition of
interest in public health dating back some fifty years.

The public health movement was quasi-official, closely tied to the
French government at both the national and municipal levels. The
institutions through which the hygienists functioned were government
sponsored. Health councils were appointed by and under the direct supervision of the prefects (in Paris, the prefect of police), who were in turn
appointed by and immediately responsible to the Minister of the Interior.
The Royal Academy of Medicine, the Academy of Sciences, and the Academy of Political and Moral Sciences came under the immediate jurisdiction
of the national government. The national academies were an important
forum for the debate of public health issues and helped shape national
public health policy. Many leading hygienists were members of the Royal
Academy of Sciences, and a few were active in the Academy of Political
and Moral Sciences.[25] Some of the most important public health treatises
were prize-winning essays in contests sponsored by these academies.[26] For
example, Villermé's *Tableau de l'état physique et moral des ouvriers* was the
result of an official inquiry sponsored by the Academy of Political and
Moral Sciences.[27]

Although the French public health movement was not an official movement, many hygienists functioned in an official capacity. Most held
government positions, or positions dependent on the good will of the
"authority," working at hospitals, in the prison system, on vaccine commissions, and at medical faculties and professional schools. Some hygien-

24 On Lézay-Marnésia, see George Sussman, "Enlightened Health Reform, Profes-
    sional Medicine and Traditional Society: The Cantonal Physicians of the Bas-Rhin,
    1819–1870," *Bull. Mist. Med.* 51 (1977): 565–584.

25 Hygienists in the Royal Academy of Sciences included Jean-Noël Hallé, Etienne
    Pariset, Joseph d'Arcet, Joseph Pelletier, and Antoine-Germain Labarraque, and
    in the Academy of Political and Moral Sciences, Villermé and Benoiston de
    Châteauneuf.

26 One example of a prize-winning essay on an important public health issue is
    Jean-Baptiste Bousquet's essay on vaccination, which won first prize in a contest
    sponsored by the Academy of Sciences. See Jean-Baptiste Bousquet, *Nouveau traité
    de la vaccine et des éruptions varioleuses* (Paris: Baillière, 1848). The first edition of the
    work, published in 1833, was done under the auspices of the vaccine commission
    of the Royal Academy of Medicine.

27 *Tableau de l'état physique et moral des ouvriers employés dans les manufactures de coton,
    de laine et de soie*, 2 vols. (Paris: Jules Renouard, 1840).

ists held administrative posts in the municipal government. Adolphe Trébuchet was head of the sanitary office at the Prefecture of Police in Paris.[28] Two of the mayors of Lyon, physicians Gabriel Prunelle and Jean-François Terme, made important contributions to public health theory and the discipline of public hygiene.[29] Other administrators had a keen interest in public health reform, such as Christian economist Alban de Villeneuve-Bargemont, who, as prefect of the Nord, established the health council of the Nord.[30]

Serving on health councils, holding official posts, and participating in government-sponsored academies, public hygienists were members of the "Establishment." Given the social tone of the public health movement and the fact that some hygienists viewed public health reform as an aspect of socioeconomic reform, one wonders why social theorists and socialists were not attracted to the movement. Some socialists such as Philippe J. B. Buchez, Ulysse Trélat, and François-Vincent Raspail were interested in public health reform and wrote hygienic treatises, but they were not part of the public health movement.[31] Utopian reformers such as Etienne Cabet and Henri de Saint-Simon and his followers were strong advocates of public health reform, but they were never active in the public health movement either.[32] There are two plausible explanations. First, many socialists believed political reform and revolution had to take precedence over other reforms. They assumed that if the political system were changed, then socioeconomic reforms would follow. Most public hygienists, however, were not primarily concerned with political reform, especially after the 1830 revolution. Public hygienists came from a variety of political persuasions, and in theory at least, any type of enlightened government could introduce and administer public health reform. Thus,

---

28 Trébuchet reviewed the reports of the Paris health council for the *Annales d'hygiène publique* and was also the author of *Code administratif des établissemens dangereux, insalubres, ou incommodes*...(Paris: Béchet jeune, 1832).

29 See, for example, C. V. F. Gabriel Prunelle, "De l'action de la médecine sur la population des états," *Revue médicale historique et philosophique* 1 (1820): ix–lxiv, and Jean-François Terme and Jean-Baptiste Monfalcon, *Histoire statistique et moral des enfants trouvés* (Paris: Baillière, 1837).

30 For Alban de Villeneuve-Bargemont the Christian socialist, see *Economie politique chrétienne*, 3 vols. (Paris: Paulin, 1834); on the public health work of Villeneuve-Bargemont, see Ann F. La Berge, "A Restoration Prefect and Public Health: Alban de Villeneuve-Bargemont at Nantes and Lille, 1824–1830," *Proceedings of the Fifth Annual Meeting of the Western Society for French History*, 1977, 5 (1978): 128–137.

31 See, for example, Phillipe J. B. Buchez, *Introduction à l'étude des sciences médicales* (Paris: Eveillard, 1838); Phillipe J. B. Buchez and Ulysse Trélat, *Précis élémentaire d'hygiène* (Paris: Raymond, 1825); see François-Vincent Raspail, *Histoire naturelle de la santé et de la maladie*...2nd ed., 2 vols. (Paris: A. Levavasseur, 1845), and *Manuel annuaire de la santé ou médecine et pharmacie domestique* (Paris: chez l'éditeur de M. Raspail, 1845); see Dora Weiner, *Raspail, Scientist and Reformer* (New York: Columbia University Press, 1968), pp. 270–1.

32 Weiner, *Raspail*, pp. 270–1.

politically oriented reformers were probably not interested in the public health movement, because they saw it as too closely tied to the government. Second, even though some public hygienists advocated social reform, they were still for the most part a professional, Establishment group, too closely linked to authority to attract those of a more revolutionary or even reformist stripe.

Raspail is a good example of a socialist reformer who was passionately interested in public health but who had virtually no connection with the public health movement. Criticizing the Paris health council as inactive and too closely attached to the government, Raspail called for a voluntary, cooperative public health organization and for revolution instead of reform.[33] The French public health movement was quite the opposite of what Raspail wanted. The movement was professional. It was in no sense a voluntary movement, nor was there any interest in making it one. Convinced that effective public health reform had to come from the top, hygienists were more concerned with influencing the authorities and their own professional colleagues than the public. Hygienists emphasized the importance of popular awareness of and participation in a few areas such as vaccination, infant hygiene, personal hygiene, and cholera prevention, but for the most part they focused their attention on a professional and official audience. Most of the achievements of the French public health movement were accomplished without popular participation or awareness, for it was the administrative and professional level that awareness really mattered to the hygienists.

The public health movement was national in scope, although the leadership and organization were Parisian. In other cities, such as Lille and Lyon, hygienists worked for public health reform on health councils, on vaccine commissions, in local medical societies, and in their official posts. The primary public health spokesmen in Lyon, for example, were a small group of physician-hygienists who held key positions in the hospital and municipal administrations. As a result of their work in the local health councils and medical societies, and in municipal and departmental administrations, and because of the influence of their publications, significant public health reforms were made in Lyon between 1815 and 1848.[34]

33 François-Vincent Raspail, *Réforme pénitentiaire. Lettres sur les prisons de Paris*, 2 vols. (Paris: Tamisey and Champion, 1839), 2: 259–90. The definitive work on Raspail is Dora Weiner's *Raspail, Scientist and Reformer*. According to Weiner, Raspail seems to have resisted getting the M.D. degree and becoming part of the medical profession.

34 The most active and influential Lyonnais physician-hygienists were Jean-Baptiste Monfalcon, A. P. Isidore de Polinière, and Jean-François Terme. Others of note included Etienne Sainte-Marie, Ariste Potton, Alexandre Bottex, and Gabriel Prunelle. See Appendix 12 for biographical sketches.

Nevertheless, the community of hygienists who formed the core of the movement was Paris based.

Sociomedical investigation was a central feature of the French public health movement. Because no accurate information was available on many of the public health problems confronting administrators, hygienists considered the collection and publication of accurate public health data a major contribution to the reform effort. Hygienic investigations were descriptive and prescriptive. Prescriptions varied according to the problem. Hygienists often proposed specific solutions to localized problems, which were more easily managed than complex problems affecting a group, a class, or the nation. Investigations of working-class health, for example, produced inquiries like those of Villermé and Eugène Buret, whose proposed reforms were both broad in scope and unattainable, given prevailing political, social, and moral beliefs.[35]

The French public health movement was composed of specialists from many backgrounds. Although a majority of health council members and the editorial board of the *Annales d'hygiène publique* were trained as physicians, a sizable minority were pharmacist-chemists, and membership typically included veterinarians, architects, engineers, and administrators.[36] Of the professional groups that participated in the movement, physicians were dominant. Before the creation of the health councils, local medical societies often served as public health advisory boards to mayors and prefects. Medical societies within the faculties of medicine (such as the Société de l'Ecole de Médecine in Paris) advised the national government on public health concerns until the founding of the Royal Academy of Medicine.

From 1820 to 1840 the French were the European leaders in public health. These decades included the founding of the Royal Academy of Medicine in 1820; the publication of Villermé's statistical work in the 1820s; the publication between 1821 and 1836 of all the hygienic and sociological works of Alexandre Parent-Duchâtelet; the founding of the *Annales d'hygiène publique et de médecine légale* in 1829; the cholera epidemic of 1832–5 and the beginning of the reform of the French quarantine system; and the development by the 1830s of the Paris health council into the preeminent public health authority in France. These decades were the most creative and innovative period of the public health movement, when *hygiène publique* as a professional, scientific discipline was being developed.

35 Villermé, *Tableau*. On the inquiries of Villermé and Buret, see Chapter 5.
36 On the pharmacist-chemists, for example, see Alex Berman, "The Pharmaceutical Component of 19th-Century Health and Hygiene," *Pharmacy in History* (1969): 5–10; on Alphonse Chevallier, one of the leading hygienists, who was a pharmacist-chemist, see Alex Berman, "J. B. A. Chevallier, Pharmacist-Chemist: A Major Figure in 19th-Century French Public Health," *Bull. Hist. Med.* 52 (1978): 200–13.

The second phase of the movement began about 1840 and extended into the 1850s. These were decades of maturity and consolidation. The professional discipline of public hygiene was well defined by this time, with one characteristic of the period being the compilation and publication of all-encompassing works on public health, such as Monfalcon and Polinière's *Traité de la salubrité dans les grandes villes* in 1846 and Ambroise Tardieu's *Dictionnaire de l'hygiène publique* in 1854. This second phase witnessed several important public health events and developments: the passage of the child labor law in 1841; the rejection of social medicine programs by the medical profession in the 1840s; the 1848 public health laws; the second cholera epidemic in 1849; the Melun law of 1850 on unhealthy dwellings; the international hygiene congresses of the 1850s; and finally, the beginning of the second series of the *Annales d'hygiène publique* in 1854. For convenience, but also justifiable in terms of public health developments, 1848 marks an end to this treatment of the public health movement. The second phase coincides with the beginning of the British public health movement, which dated from the late 1830s. By 1848, the organizational, legislative, and administrative success of the British movement, led by Edwin Chadwick, William Farr, and Southwood Smith, began to offer an alternative public health model.[37] Whereas in the 1830s the British had looked to the French for ideas and models, by the 1850s the French were turning to the British.[38] Thus for French leadership in public health we must look to the 1820s and 1830s, when the community of hygienists began to develop.

THE COMMUNITY OF HYGIENISTS

The community of hygienists was that group of physicians, scientists, and administrators who formed the core of the public health movement. The most influential of the French public hygienists were the physicians

---

37 On the nineteenth-century British public health movement, see Edwin Chadwick, *The Sanitary Condition of the Labouring Population of Great Britain*, ed. Michael W. Flinn (Edinburgh: Edinburgh University Press, 1965), esp. Flinn's "Introduction." See also the two biographies of Chadwick: Richard. A. Lewis, *Edwin Chadwick and the Public Health Movement, 1832–1854* (London: Longman, Green, 1952) and Samuel E. Finer, *The Life and Times of Edwin Chadwick* (London: Methuen, 1952); see also John Eyler, *Victorian Social Medicine: The Ideas and Methods of William Farr* (Baltimore: Johns Hopkins University Press, 1979), and Anthony Wohl, *Endangered Lives: Public Health in Victorian Britain* (Cambridge, MA: Harvard University Press, 1983).

38 Antoine Ostrowski, "Etudes d'hygiène publique sur l'Angleterre," *Annales d'hygiène publique* 37 (1847): 5–43; Ambroise Tardieu, "Introduction" to the second edition of *Dictionnaire d'hygiène publique et de salubrité*, 4 vols. (Paris: Baillière, 1862), 1: viii–x.

Alexandre Parent-Duchâtelet and Louis-René Villermé. They were among the founding editors of the *Annales d'hygiène publique et de médecine légale*, to which they were regular and frequent contributors; were members of the Royal Academy of Medicine; and served on the Paris health council. Parent-Duchâtelet received his M.D. from the Paris Faculty in 1814 at the age of twenty-four. Influenced by Jean-Noël Hallé, the father of French hygiene, he devoted himself almost exclusively to public health questions after 1821, although he continued to practice medicine at the Pitié hospital. The result was the publication of a two-volume sociomedical work on prostitution in Paris and twenty-nine articles on public health, most of which first appeared in the *Annales d'hygiène publique* and then after his death were published as a collection entitled *Hygiène publique*. His early studies on ships carrying fertilizer, the Bièvre river, and the sewers of Paris were praised by professional colleagues, and by 1827 he was recognized as one of the leading public hygienists in France. On the death of René Bertin in 1827, Parent-Duchâtelet was one of five contenders for the chair of hygiene at the Paris Faculty of Medicine, but Gabriel Andral was the successful candidate.[39]

Parent-Duchâtelet – whose reputation was international – was the leading French urban and occupational hygienist and the principal hygienist of Paris. His investigations of the sewers of Paris and prostitution were the definitive French works on these subjects. His studies of dock workers, tobacco workers, the horsebutchering industry, hemp retting, and other trades contributed greatly to French leadership in occupational hygiene. Impressed with Parent-Duchâtelet's contributions in this area, Edwin Chadwick called him "the most industrious and able of modern investigators into questions of public health."[40] More than any other individual, Parent-Duchâtelet increased awareness of public health problems in Paris. Parent-Duchâtelet was in great part responsible for transforming the Paris health council into the dominant public health institution in France. From his entry onto the council in 1825 until his death in 1836, his meticulous reports were a principal reason for the high status that institution enjoyed by the mid-1830s. Parent-Duchâtelet was also the major theorist of the new specialty of public hygiene and the principal spokesman for the professionalization of the discipline.

39 On Parent-Duchâtelet, see Ann F. La Berge, "A. J. B. Parent-Duchâtelet: Hygienist of Paris, 1821–1836," *Clio Medica* 12 (1977): 279–301. See Alain Corbin, "Présentation" to Alexandre Parent-Duchâtelet, *La Prostitution à Paris au XIXe siècle*, texte présenté et annoté par Alain Corbin (Paris: Seuil, 1981), pp. 9–42; and Jill Harsin, *Policing Prostitution in Nineteenth-Century Paris* (Princeton NY: Princeton University Press, 1985). Ann F. La Berge, "The Early Nineteenth-Century French Public Health Movement: The Disciplinary Development and Institutionalization of *hygiène publique*," *Bull. Hist. Med.* 58 (1984): 373–5.
40 Chadwick, *Sanitary Report*, ed. Flinn, p. 149.

Louis-René Villermé was Parent-Duchâtelet's friend and colleague. Villermé, who served as an army surgeon during the Napoleonic wars and received his M.D. from the Paris Faculty in 1814, the same year as Parent-Duchâtelet, became interested in public health and social questions by the early 1820s. By the end of the decade, as the author of two major studies on differential mortality, Villermé was the recognized French authority on the influence of standard of living on health. As an investigator of the French prison system in the 1820s, then as a member of the Royal Academy of Medicine, as a founding editor and frequent contributor to the *Annales d'hygiène publique*, and as an associate member of the Paris health council (1831–6), by the 1830s Villermé had established an international reputation as a statistician, social investigator, and public hygienist. The apogee of Villermé's many-faceted career was his two-volume work on the material and moral condition of the French textile workers, the *Tableau de l'état physique et moral des ouvriers employés dans les manufactures de coton, de laine et de soie*, which he began in collaboration with the statistician Benoiston de Châteauneuf in 1834 and published in 1840. Villermé can best be described as a full-time academician, able to devote himself exclusively to sociohygienic investigations and participation in scholarly academies.[41]

Other hygienists who formed the inner circle of the public health movement were Alphonse Chevallier, Jean-Pierre-Joseph d'Arcet, Alphonse Guérard, Charles-Chrétien-Henri Marc, and Adolphe Trébuchet. A central figure in the public health movement was Alphonse Chevallier, a pharmacist-chemist by training and early in his career a research associate of Parent-Duchâtelet. At fourteen he began working in the chemistry laboratory of Nicolas Vauquelin, and at seventeen he became a chemistry aid at the Museum of Natural History. In 1815 he became a pharmacy intern in the hospitals, and after completing his pharmacy studies,

41 The best source is Alphonse Guérard, "Notice sur M. Villermé," *Annales d'hygiène publique* 2e série, 21 (1864): 162–77, which contains a complete bibiography of Villermé's works. Also essential is Coleman, *Death Is a Social Disease: Public Health and Political Economy in Early Industrial France* (Madison: University of Wisconsin Press, 1982). For biographical material on Villermé see also Erwin Ackerknecht, "Villermé and Quetelet," *Bull. Hist. Med.* 26 (1952): 317–29; Pierre Astruc, "Louis-René Villermé, médecin-sociologue (1782–1863)," *Le Progrès médical* (supplément illustré, 1er Oct. 1932), pp. 49–54; Emile Mireaux, "Un chirurgien-sociologue: Louis-René Villermé," *Revue des deux mondes* (15 janv. 1962): 201–12; Marcel Delabroise, *Un médecin-hygiéniste et sociologue: Louis-René Villermé (1782–1863)* (M.D. thesis, University of Paris, 1939). For insights into Villermé's personality, see the correspondence between Villermé and Quetelet: Brussels. Bibliothèque Royale. Académie Royale des Sciences, des Lettres et des Beaux Arts de Belgique. Centre national d'histoire des Sciences. Correspondence Villermé-Quetelet. Cat. 2560 (1826–35) and 2561 (1839–63). I would like to thank Bernard Lécuyer, who graciously permitted me to use his photocopies of the Villermé–Quetelet correspondence.

Chevallier opened his own pharmacy on the Place du Pont St.-Michel, but that venture was short-lived. Subsequently, during the 1820s and 1830s, he devoted himself exclusively to his laboratory on the Quai St.-Michel, becoming – like Parent-Duchâtelet – a full-time researcher and hygienist. Chevallier was elected to the Royal Academy of Medicine in 1824 and to the Paris health council in 1834, and in 1835 he was named adjunct professor at the Pharmacy School. He joined the editorial board of the *Annales d'hygiène publique* in 1832 and published articles in that journal regularly from 1830 to 1870. He collaborated with many other professionals – chemists and physicians – such as Jean-Pierre Barruel, Anselme Payen, Matthew Orfila, and Parent-Duchâtelet. Chevallier's area of expertise was toxicology, or the study of agents such as lead, which when used in containers and counters were hazardous to health. He made major contributions to occupational hygiene, collaborating with Parent-Duchâtelet on several landmark studies and continuing his work in this area long after the latter's death.[42]

Jean-Pierre-Joseph d'Arcet, the son of chemist Jean d'Arcet, played a key role in the public health movement. At the age of nineteen the younger d'Arcet began to devote himself exclusively to the study of chemistry, first under his father and then under Vauquelin, whose special student he became. D'Arcet began his career during the early years of the French industrial revolution, and for more than forty years he took an active part in the development of French national industry, making important contributions to industrial chemistry. He made many of his discoveries during the Napoleonic wars, when the continental blockade forced France to develop its own industries. Like Chevallier, d'Arcet was interested in improving industrial processes to promote workers' health and safety. His contributions to industrial chemistry and its applications were numerous: He improved the safety of certain industrial processes, such as the manufacture of Prussic acid. He collaborated with chemist Louis-Bernard Guyton-Morveau to improve the process of minting coins, and he oversaw the gilding of the Invalides dome. He discovered how to extract gelatin from bones and got involved in the 1830s in the debate within the chemical and medical communities over the use of gelatin as food in hospitals. D'Arcet was convinced of its nutritive value, but others, such as Alfred Donné, then (1831) chief of the clinic at the Charité, and physiologist François Magendie, questioned its use. The baths and fumigating apparati at the St.-Louis hospital were built under d'Arcet's direction, and he helped perfect the testing of river water samples. He introduced gas light-

---

42 T. Gaillard, "Nécrologie. Alphonse Chevallier," *Annales d'hygiène publique* 3e série, 3 (1880): 181–7. See also Alex Berman, "J. B. A. Chevallier." On Vauquelin, see W. A. Smeaton, "Vauquelin, Nicolas Louis," *Dictionary of Scientific Biography* 13: 596–8.

ing in Paris, first installing it at the St.-Louis hospital. D'Arcet participated in many scientific commissions appointed to investigate industrial and public health problems, such as heating and ventilating public buildings and the horsebutchering industry. D'Arcet worked as an assayer at the mint from 1800, and by 1819 was inspector-general and then commissioner-general. He was a member of the Paris health council from 1813, and of the Academy of Sciences from 1821, and was one of the founding editors of and most prolific contributors to the *Annales d'hygiène publique*.[43]

Physician and chemist Alphonse Guérard was destined to hold a key position in the French public health community by midcentury as the editor of the *Annales d'hygiène publique* from 1845 to 1874. But even before assuming editorship of the journal, he made important public health contributions. Guérard began his education at the Ecole Normale but switched to sciences – chemistry and physics – working in the laboratory of Louis-Jacques Thenard at the Collège de France and that of Laugier and Vauquelin at the Jardin des Plantes. His work with Alphonse Chevallier in Vauquelin's laboratory was the beginning of a long friendship and collaboration: on the Paris health council, in the Royal Academy of Medicine, and on the editorial board of the *Annales d'hygiène publique*. He also took courses at the Ecole des Mines, where he studied geology, mineralogy, and mechanics. In 1821, Guérard began his medical studies – seven years after he had left the Ecole Normale. He was too old to enter the competition for the *internat* and the *externat* at the Parisian hospitals but was appointed hospital physician (*médecin des hôpitaux*) in 1828, working until 1845 at St.-Antoine and after 1845 at the Hôtel-Dieu. With his wide-ranging background and education, Guérard had excellent training for a public hygienist – just the kind Parent-Duchâtelet advocated.

Guérard was not successful in the *concours* for the chair of hygiene at the Paris Faculty of medicine, although he put himself up five times in twenty years. With no position at the Faculty, he taught private courses from 1821 to 1836: general chemistry and its applications to medicine and toxicology; medical physics; and finally, hygiene, his science of choice. On the death of René-Nicolas Desgenettes (1837), who held the chair of hygiene at the Paris Faculty from 1830 to 1837, Guérard taught the official hygiene course until a new appointment was made. He was one of the candidates for the position, losing by only one vote to Hippolyte Royer-Collard. In 1852 he competed with Apollinaire Bouchardat for the chair of hygiene and again lost. He was a member of the Paris health council from 1837 and was named to the Royal Academy of Medicine in 1855.

Guérard wrote on all aspects of public hygiene. He was the author of numerous articles, many published in the *Annales d'hygiène publique*, and

43 "Notice sur J. P. J. d'Arcet," *Annales d'hygiène publique* 33 (1845): 5–19.

the two theses he wrote for the *concours* at the Faculty of Medicine were recognized as important hygienic studies. Although hygiene was Guérard's preferred specialty, he also made important contributions to legal medicine. With his colleague Chevallier, he was one of the founders in 1868 of the Society of Legal Medicine, and as editor of the *Annales d'hygiène publique* he established the tie that made that journal the official organ of the Society of Legal Medicine.[44]

Charles-Chrétien-Henri Marc was of the same generation as d'Arcet, Chevallier, and Guérard. He received his M.D. at Erlangen in 1792 and came to Paris in 1795, finally settling there in 1798. With many of the leading Parisian physicians he was one of the founding members of the Société médicale d'émulation, established by Bichat in 1798. Marc first established a manufacture of chemical products, but the business failed, and he then set himself up in private practice. Early in his career he achieved international recognition by writing a popular little book on the advantages of vaccine. The book was translated into several languages, became known all over Europe, and was reprinted in the 1830s under the auspices of the Royal Academy of Medicine as part of the national vaccination program.

In 1811 Marc did a second thesis to get a French medical degree, thereby naturalizing himself among the French medical community. In 1812, when some of the Parisian suburbs were ravaged by intermittent fevers, prefect of the Seine Frochot invited Marc and Etienne Pariset (who would later become permanent secretary of the Royal Academy of Medicine) to serve as epidemic physicians to the affected area. That same year, when the multivolume *Dictionnaire des sciences médicales* was begun, Marc, who was already considered a specialist in public hygiene and legal medicine, wrote more than forty articles for the collection. He was a close friend of Antoine-Augustin Parmentier, one of the founding members of the Paris health council. At Parmentier's request, Marc was appointed to the council in 1816 and quickly became one of the most hard-working and useful members. Shortly after joining, he was put in charge of the service for the drowning and asphyxiated, which the health council oversaw. Marc was called to the Royal Academy of Medicine six weeks after its founding, and in 1833 he was president of that organization. As one of the health council's earliest and most active members, Marc headed the committee of the Royal Academy of Medicine that reported in 1836 on the necessity of establishing health councils throughout the kingdom.

In 1829 Marc was one of the founding editors of the *Annales d'hygiène publique*. He wrote the introduction, in which he expounded upon the

44 T. Gaillard, "M. Alphonse Guérard," *Annales d'hygiène publique* 2e série, 62 (1874): 458–78. On Thenard, see Maurice Crosland, "Thenard, Louis Jacques," *Dictionary of Scientific Biography* 13: 309–14.

goals of public health and legal medicine and gave the journal its professional tone, and was a regular and frequent contributor to the journal. In 1835 he published a major work, *Nouvelles recherches sur les secours à donner aux noyés et aux asphyxiés* and also published on his deathbed his medicolegal testament, *De la folie considérée dans ses rapports avec les questions médico-judiciaires.*[45]

Adolphe Trébuchet (b. 1801), from Nantes (a cousin of Victor Hugo), studied law in Paris. After receiving his law degree in 1824, he took an administrative position at the prefecture of police. He was soon named assistant director of the sanitary office and became the head of that office in 1829, keeping this post until 1858. He was initially a member of the Paris health council because of his position but then was elected a titular member. His publications were among the most important in establishing the discipline of public hygiene: *Code administratif des établissements dangereux, insalubres ou incommodes* (1832); *Jurisprudence de la médecine, de la chirurgie, et de la pharmacie en France* (1834); with Elouin and Labat, *Nouveau dictionnaire de police* (1834); and with Poirat-Duval, a third edition, revised and augmented, of Parent-Duchâtelet's *De la prostitution dans la ville de Paris* (1857). He was also the editor of the reports of the Paris health council, 1849–58 and 1859–62, which, along with earlier reports, formed the most complete collection of information on public and industrial hygiene. From 1848 until his death, he published many articles in the *Annales d'hygiène publique* and became one of its editors in 1840. He was elected to the Academy of Medicine as *associé libre* in 1858.[46]

Many other physicians and scientists, whom we can consider public hygienists, promoted public health through their service on the health councils, as editors of and contributors to the *Annales d'hygiène publique*, and by their research and practical contributions in the field. These included the physicians J. Etienne Esquirol, specialist in legal medicine, psychiatrist, and director of the mental institution of the department of the Seine at Charenton after 1826; Etienne Pariset, epidemiologist, permanent secretary of the Royal Academy of Medicine and spokesman for public health within that organization; Jean-Baptiste Bousquet, the leading French authority on vaccination and director of vaccination for the Royal Academy of Medicine; Pierre-Adolphe Piorry and François Mélier, outspoken spokesmen for public health reform at the Royal Academy of Medicine and both interested in occupational hygiene; occupational hygienist Théophile Roussel; Jean-Noël Hallé, the first holder of the chair of hygiene at the Paris Faculty and Parent-Duchâtelet's mentor; Pierre-François

45 Etienne Pariset, "Eloge de Chr.-H.-Chr. [sic] Marc," *Mém. de l'Acad. Roy. de Méd.* 10 (1843): 29–48.
46 Alphonse Guérard, "Notice biographique sur M. A. Trébuchet," *Annales d'hygiène publique* 2e série, 25 (1866): 5–11.

Kéraudren, inspector-general of the naval health service, Michel Lévy, director of the Val-de-Grâce hospital; and Alphonse Devergie, a founding editor of the *Annales d'hygiène publique* and director of the Morgue after 1830; the veterinarians Jean-Baptiste Huzard senior, inspector-general of the Veterinary School of France at Alfort, and his son, Jean-Baptiste Huzard junior; the statistician and former military surgeon Louis-François Benoiston de Châteauneuf; chemists Jean-Pierre Barruel, Henri Gaultier de Claubry, and Pierre-Joseph Pelletier, who (with Caventou) discovered quinine sulfate; and Antoine-Germain Labarraque, who discovered the disinfectant nature of chloride of lime (eau de Javel).

Numerous other administrators, physicians, and scientists throughout France wrote important treatises and articles on public health and worked for public health reform either at the national or the local level. These included François-Emmanuel Fodéré, specialist in legal medicine and public hygiene, professor at the Faculty of Medicine in Strasbourg; Frédéric-Joseph Bérard and Gabriel Prunelle, public health theorists and professors at the Faculty of Medicine in Montpellier; and the physicians who formed an active local public health movement in Lyon: Jean-Baptiste Monfalcon, A. P. Isidore de Polinière, Etienne Sainte-Marie, and Jean-François Terme. In major cities there was usually a group of physicians, scientists, and administrators who worked for public health reform through their service on the local health councils and medical societies, on vaccine commissions, and in other official posts. Examples of provincial public health activists in addition to those already mentioned are the physicians Hippolyte Combes in Toulouse, Léon Marchant in Bordeaux, Julien Fouré in Nantes, and Jean-Pierre Thouvenin in Lille.

PUBLIC HEALTH THEORY

The public health theories articulated and espoused by the community of hygienists were derived from the eighteenth-century public health idea. Nineteenth-century hygienists clarified, delimited, and defined specific components of public health theory and added to it a particular methodological approach: public hygiene. Developments in the early 1800s, notably urbanization and industrialization, required elaboration and extension of the public health idea. In particular, the beginnings of industrialization and a growing working class posed problems that had to be incorporated in a mature public health theory. In his study of Villermé, William Coleman suggested that nineteenth-century public health theory and the French public health movement were to a great extent shaped by industrialization.[47] For reformers such as Villermé, Monfalcon, and Polinière, the social,

47   Coleman, *Death Is a Social Disease.*

cultural, economic, moral, and public health ramifications of industrialization and the increasing problems associated with a large working
class provided the parameters within which the public health movement
and public health theory developed. For other hygienists like Parent-
Duchâtelet and Chevallier, however, urbanization was more important
than industrialization in developing a theory of public health. These
hygienists focused on urban health problems that had preceded and were
not dependent upon industrialization. Many of these problems dated from
the eighteenth century but were made worse as continued migration from
rural to urban areas increased the pressure on urban systems and facilities
such as water supplies, sewerage systems, and cemeteries.

Influenced by humanitarian ideas, public hygienists urged public health
reforms for the good of society, believing all citizens had a right to health.
Early in his career, Villermé referred to the spirit of the age as one of
reform and the perfecting of institutions, and twenty years later he noted
that humanitarianism had motivated industrialists to clamor for a child
labor law.[48] Fodéré contended that public health was an aspect of social
reform demanded by justice and humanity, and Hallé attributed progress
in naval and colonial hygiene more to humanitarian sentiment than to the
vigilance of the government.[49] Members of the Troyes health council
maintained that a spirit of humanitarianism required society to embrace
the cause of workers.[50] Although eighteenth-century humanitarians and
reformers had been especially concerned about slaves, prisoners, the sick,
and the insane, nineteenth-century hygienists directed their efforts to the
urban poor and workers.[51]

Hygienists argued that health was one of the natural rights that governments were instituted to protect, for it was fundamental to the well-being

48   Louis-René Villermé, *Des prisons telles qu'elles sont et telles qu'elles devraient être*
(Paris: Méquignon-Marvis, 1820), pp. 42, 66–7, 120–1, 177; *Tableau*, 1: 93–108; 2:
360.
49   François E. Fodéré, *Essai historique et moral sur la pauvreté des nations* (Paris: Huzard,
1825), pp. 60, 323–9, 410, 515. Hallé and Nysten, "Hygiène," 22: 549.
50   Pigeotte, Lhoste, and Gréau, "Rapport fait au Conseil de salubrité de Troyes sur les
accidens auxquels sont exposés les ouvriers employés dans les filatures de laine et de
coton," *Annales d'hygiène publique* 12 (1834): 26–30.
51   Richard Shryock, "Medicine and Public Health," in *The Nineteenth Century World:
Readings from the History of Mankind*, ed. Guy Métraux and François Crouzet (New
York: New American Library, 1963), pp. 222–3. See, for example, M. Thouvenel,
Eléments d'hygiène, 2 vols. (Paris: Baillière, 1840), 2: 158–67; Pierre-Adolphe
Piorry, "Extrait du rapport sur les épidémies qui ont régné en France de 1830 à
1836: au nom de la commission des épidémies," *Mém. de l'Acad. Roy. de Méd.* 5
(1836): 19; Pierre-Adolphe Piorry, "Rapport de la commission des épidémies sur
les maladies épidémiques qui ont régné en France en 1836, 1837, et 1838," *Mém. de
l'Acad. Roy. de Méd.* 7 (1838): 141–42; Jean-Baptiste Monfalcon and A. P. Isidore
de Polinière, *Traité de la salubrité dans les grandes villes* (Paris: Baillière, 1846),
pp. 92–3, 131–33.

of society. Some hygienists, motivated by liberalism and favoring the reform of society upon the basis of rational and humanitarian principles, considered public health an integral part of any major reform program. To these reformers, disease – like poverty – was a social evil to be eradicated. They argued that enlightened governments would realize the importance of public health, incorporating it into their reform programs.[52]

Athough hygienists endorsed the responsibility of the state in public health matters, they did not agree on the limits of state involvement. Some, like Villermé, were liberals, favoring only limited state intervention; others, like Parent-Duchâtelet, were statists, looking to the administration to take a leadership role in public health. Most hygienists believed the government had a special obligation to the poor and workers. Fodéré thought a paternalistic government could solve the problems of poverty and health, and occupational hygienist Philibert Patissier argued that it was the government's duty to care for old and infirm workers.[53] Monfalcon and Polinière favored paternalistic legislation and government intervention to improve working-class conditions.[54] Medical reformer Louis F. Delasiauve called for government intervention to preserve the sanitary state of the populace, maintaining that the government had a public health mission.[55] Public health reformer Alban de Villeneuve-Bargemont, prefect of the Loire-Inférieure and later of the Nord, called for government intervention to protect the weak and the poor.[56] Other hygienists did not advocate extensive involvement of the national government in public

52 Piorry, "Rapport de la commission des épidémies," p. 141; L. C. A. Motard, *Essai d'hygiène générale*, 2 vols. (Paris: Pesron, 1841), 1: 193; Fodéré, *Essai sur la pauvreté, passim*; Michel Lévy, *Traité d'hygiène publique et privée*, 2 vols. (Paris: Baillière, 1844), 1: 52; L.F. Delasiauve, *De l'organisation médicale en France sous le triple rapport de la pratique, des établissements de bienfaisance et de l'enseignement* (Paris: Fortin, Masson, 1843), pp. 3–4, 10; Léon Simon in *Résumé complet d'hygiène publique et de médecine légale* (Paris: Bureau de l'Encyclopédie Portative, 1830) gave a clear statement of the importance of public health for the well-being of society on pp. 26–7.

53 Fodéré, *Essai sur la pauvreté, passim*; Philibert Patissier, *Traité des maladies des artisans et de celles qui résultent de diverses professions d'après Ramazzini* (Paris: Baillière, 1822), p. liii.

54 Monfalcon and Polinière, *Traité de la salubrité*, pp. 19–92.

55 Delasiauve, *De l'organisation médicale*, pp. 11–12.

56 Villeneuve-Bargemont, *Economie politique chrétienne*, 1: 27–95. For some other examples of those favoring a paternalistic role, see Philippe J. B. Buchez, *Introduction à l'étude des sciences médicales* (Paris: Eveillard, 1838), p. 246; P. S. Thouvenel, *Eléments d'hygiène*, p. 239; J. J. Virey, *Hygiène philosophique, appliquée à la politique et à la morale* (Paris: Crochard, 1831), p. xvii; Ariste Potton, *De la prostitution et de la syphilis dans les grandes villes et dans la ville de Lyon en particulier* (Paris: Baillière, 1842), pp. 182–3, 235; P. A. Enault, *Choléra morbus. Conseils hygiéniques à suivre pour s'en prévenir* (Paris: Denain, 1831), pp. 26–7; L. F. Lélut, "De la santé du peuple," *Mém. de l'Acad. des Sci. Mor. et Pol.* 7 (1850): 951; Honoré Frégier, *Des classes dangereuses de la population dans les grandes villes et les moyens de les rendre meilleures*, 2 vols. (Paris: Baillière, 1840), 2: 26, 145.

health matters but believed that certain specific problems should be addressed by national legislation. Both Villermé and Parent-Duchâtelet advocated legislative intervention to improve workers' health. Villermé urged the government to undertake prison reform and appoint state inspectors for prisons and hospitals. Although adhering to the principles of liberal political economy, he pointed out the inconveniences of a laissez-faire policy and called for factory legislation. Parent-Duchâtelet urged national legislation to control the public health problems associated with prostitution.[57]

If public health is fundamental to the wealth and well-being of society, then the role of the physician as the preserver and restorer of health is a central component of public health theory. Some hygienists and medical reformers argued that physicians could best serve society as civil servants. Social Catholic reformer Philippe J. B. Buchez advocated a state-supported, nationwide medical service of cantonal physicians to dispense free medical care. Physician L.F. Delasiauve proposed a similar system of civil servants, free medical care, and a nationwide medical service to provide for rural and urban areas. The Royal Academy of Medicine supported a plan similar to that proposed by Delasiauve, but the system was never adopted on a nationwide scale due to opposition from some elements of the medical profession. Such a program was instituted in the Bas-Rhin with the system of cantonal physicians, which would serve as a model for medical reformers throughout the century.[58]

A few theorists went so far as to suggest that public health might become a key aspect of domestic and foreign policy, envisioning a time when the government would call upon physicians as expert advisers. Fodéré emphasized the physician's qualifications for solving social problems because of his intimate acquaintance with them and his humanitarianism. Former surgeon F. V. Charles Menessier saw an important role for the physician as social reformer and legislator, and Pierre-Adolphe Piorry, pathological anatomist and member of the Royal Academy of Medicine, urged physicians to take a more active role in national legislation. Physician Ulysse Trélat made a similar claim, declaring in 1828:

the influence of physicians...should extend to the movement and the progress of society. They have, in effect, a loftier mission than that of concerning themselves

---

57 Villermé, *Les prisons*, pp. 176–7; *Tableau*, 2: 93–108, 355–73; Parent-Duchâtelet, *De la Prostitution dans la ville de Paris*, 2 vols. (Paris: Baillière, 1836), 2: 516–23.
58 Buchez, *Etude des sciences médicales*, pp. 247–8; Delasiauve, *De l'organisation médicale*, pp. 189–203; Isidore Bricheteau, "Rapport de la commission des épidémies," *Mém. de l'Acad. Roy. de Méd.* 9 (1841): 32; George Sussman, "Enlightened Health Reform, Professional Medicine, and Traditional Society: The Cantonal Physicians of the Bas-Rhin, 1819–1870," *Bull. Hist. Med.* 51 (1977): 279–301.

solely with the conservation of individual life: it is to modify and ameliorate collective life also; it is their researches, it is their physiology, it is their public hygiene... which should preside over the perfection of morals and of legislation.[59]

Theories advanced about the physician's role in society derived from humanitarian ideals, the German concept of medical police, and the self-interest of physicians, who were striving to professionalize medicine and establish a monopoly on healing. Two main attitudes prevailed: Some physicians emphasized the growth of the medical profession as a free profession and the development of the private practice of medicine, whereas others asserted that medicine had a social mission and physicians should be civil servants. With both sides claiming public health as their ultimate goal, the discourse between the advocates of liberal and social medicine continued throughout the century.[60]

The fundamental belief of the hygienists was that public health was concomitant with the progress of civilization. Hygienists offered several explanations: Some said improved health resulted from material improvements – a higher standard of living due to increased wealth and more equal distribution of wealth. Most hygienists believed – and presented statistical evidence to prove it – that health and wealth went together, that wealthy societies were healthy societies. Another explanation was increased education, or, as the hygienists called it, "enlightenment." Enlightened individuals, they claimed, realized the importance of health, devoting more attention to personal hygiene. Furthermore, enlightened governments considered public health a state responsibility and enacted public health measures accordingly.[61] Villermé, for example, maintained that

59 Fodéré, *Essai sur la pauvreté*, pp. iii–v; Charles Menessier, *Mission du médecin dans la société* (Montpellier: J. Martel aîné, 1850); Piorry, "Rapport de la commission des épidémies." Ulysse Trélat, *De la constitution du corps des médecins et de l'enseignement médical* (Paris, 1828), p. 64. Cited in Stephen Jacyna, "Medical Science and Moral Science: The Cultural Relations of Physiology in Restoration France," *History of Science* 25 (1987): 117.

60 On the whole question of liberal versus social medicine in nineteenth-century France, see Martha Hildreth, *Doctors, Bureaucrats, and Public Health in France, 1888–1902* (New York: Garland, 1987).

61 For the most optimistic of the theorists, see Philippe Buchez and Ulysse Trélat, *Précis élémentaire d'hygiène* (Paris: Raymond, 1825), pp. 31–3; Alphonse Forcinal, *De l'influence de la civilisation sur l'homme* (Paris: M.D. thesis, 1832); Thouvenel, *Eléments d'hygiène*, 2: 177–8; Etienne Pariset, "Discours prononcé par le secrétaire perpétuel, dans la séance inaugurale, le 6 mai 1824," *Mém. de l'Acad. Roy. de Méd.* 1 (1828): 79–80; Motard, *Essai d'hygiène*, 1: 83; J. F. Rameaux, *Appréciation des progrès de l'hygiène publique depuis le commencement du 19e siècle* (Strasbourg: G. Silbermann, 1839), pp. 18–20; Frédéric-Joseph Bérard, *Discours sur les améliorations progressives de la santé publique* (Paris: Gabon, 1826); Bérard's whole speech is relevant; Lévy, *Traité d'hygiène*, 2: 43–5, 482–3, 520; Louis-André Gosse, *Propositions générales sur les maladies causées par l'exercice des professions* (Paris: M.D. thesis, 1816), p. 7; François Mélier, *Etude sur les subsistances envisagées dans leurs rapports avec les maladies et la mortalité* (Paris: Baillière, 1842), p. 22; Pierre-Adolphe Piorry, *Des habitations et*

good health was dependent on wealth, and that workers' health was improving with industrialization and the progress of civilization. A few hygienists subscribed to this optimistic point of view, but with reservations. Social reformer Eugene Buret questioned whether workers had shared in the progress of civilization, and Fodéré, although generally optimistic, believed he was living in an age of contradictions, observing that industrialization did not seem to benefit society or to coincide with a decrease in poverty or crime or with an improvement in health. Like Fodéré, not all hygienists shared in the prevailing optimism of the age. Julien-Joseph Virey, naturalist, physician, and philosopher, expressed the minority viewpoint, questioning whether public health really was improving with the advance of civilization. On the one hand, he believed that liberty, civilization, and good health were concomitant; but on the other, he feared that civilization made life artificial, and he saw little progress in therapeutic medicine.[62]

Since no specific preventive was known for any disease except smallpox at the time, many hygienists proposed that the progress of civilization was the best prevention against epidemic diseases.[63] Hygienists Jean-Baptiste Bourdon and L. Bourgouin maintained that as civilization advanced, not only were there fewer epidemics and contagious diseases, but as citizens become more enlightened, they realized that fewer diseases are contagious.

de l'influence de leurs dispositions sur l'homme, en santé et en maladie (Paris: Pourchet, 1838), pp. 93–4; Joseph-Henri-Réveillé-Parise, *Physiologie et hygiène des hommes livrés aux travaux de l'esprit*, 4th ed. (Paris: Dentu, 1843), pp. 22, 37; Hallé et Nysten, "Hygiène," pp. 540–6, 550, 604; Parent-Duchâtelet, *De la Prostitution*, 2: 494–6.

62 Villermé, *Tableau*, 1: 366; 2: 25, 297–9, 326, 346; Eugène Buret, *De la misère des classes laborieuses en Angleterre et en France*, 2 vols. (Paris: Renouard, 1840), 1: 357–8; Fodéré, *Essai sur la pauvreté*, pp. ii, 5–17, 57, 243–50, and also *Leçons sur les épidémies et l'hygiène publique*, 4 vols. (Paris: Levrault, 1822–4), 1: 29–30; Virey, *Hygiène philosophique*, 1: vii–xiii, xvii–xxii.

63 Buchez and Trélat, *Précis élémentaire*, p. 31; Forcinal, *De l'influence de la civilisation*, p. 9; "Rapport de la commission chargée de rédiger un projet d'instruction relativement aux épidémies," *Mém. de l'Acad. Roy. de Méd.* 1 (1828): 248; Bricheteau, "Rapport de la commission des épidémies," *Mém. de l'Acad. Roy. de Méd.* 9 (1841): 32; Etienne Pariset, "Mémoire sur les causes de la peste et sur les moyens de la détruire," *Annales d'hygiène publique* 6 (1831): 308–10; L. R. Villermé, "Les épidémies sous les rapports de l'hygiène publique, de la statistique médicale et de l'économie politique," *Annales d'hygiène publique* 9 (1833): 7–18, 55–8; Rameaux, *Progrès de l'hygiène*, p. 19; Bérard, *Les améliorations progressives*, pp. 107–8; Fodéré, *Leçons sur les épidémies*, 1: 247; Menessier, *Mission du médecin*, pp. 47–8; P. A. Enault, *Choléra-morbus*, pp. 9–10; Pariset, Lévy, and Prus saw the progress of civilization as the best preventive against plague. See Lévy, *Traité d'hygiène*, 2: 520, 525; Pariset, "Mémoire sur les causes de la peste," pp. 308–10; René Prus, "Rapport de la peste et des quarantaines," *Bull. l'Acad. Roy. de Méd.* 11 (1846): 688; see also "Rapport de Pariset, Bouillaud, et Renoult sur l'oeuvre de Dr. L. Aubert, *Sur la prophylaxie générale de la peste*," *Bull. de l'Acad. Roy. de Méd.* 6 (1840–1): 795.

For these men, who argued for socioeconomic causes of disease, anticontagionism was a sign of progress.[64]

The existence of a large and growing working class contributed another important component to nineteenth-century public health theory. Lyonnais hygienists made important contributions in this area. Public health theory and reform in Lyon were greatly influenced by the large, vociferous working class, especially after the insurrections of 1831 and 1834, which called attention to the substandard living conditions of workers. Out of both humanitarianism and self-interest, Lyonnais hygienists and social reformers urged improving the living conditions and health of the working classes, emphasizing that moral improvements would result from material improvements.

Lyonnais hygienists believed that the main threats to workers' health came not from occupational hazards but from unhealthy dwellings, insufficient air and water, inadequate sewage disposal, and lack of clean surroundings in which to recuperate from illnesses. Thus they emphasized reforms in these areas. Monfalcon and Polinière believed the fundamental public health reform was improving workers' living conditions:

It is a revolution analogous [to that of the foundlings] that we must obtain in the condition of workers; they have a right to be well fed, well dressed, well lodged; their work should furnish them not only the strict necessity, but a little more. If it is not possible to make all of them rich, we must and can provide them with pure air, pure and abundant water, finally with the conditions of salubrity indispensable to the maintenance of health, without which there is no profitable work.[65]

Thus, without advocating socioeconomic reform, Monfalcon and Polinière urged reform of municipal facilities to benefit the working class. Writing about the nineteenth-century British public health movement, Michael Flinn has suggested that public health in the first half of the century was basically a question of the condition of working-class dwellings. This is an oversimplification, but Monfalcon and Polinière expressed a similar idea, noting that all the causes of unhealthiness came together in the houses of the poor: "True glory for a municipal council is to improve the material condition of workers by putting healthy dwellings at their disposition."[66]

---

64 Jean-Baptiste-Isidore Bourdon, *Mémoire sur la peste, la vérité sur les quarantaines* (Paris: L. Martinet, 1847), pp. 13–16; L. Bourgouin, *Exposition raisonnée des institutions sanitaires depuis leurs origines jusqu'à nos jours* (Paris: Everat, 1829), p. 39.

65 Jean-Baptiste Monfalcon and A. P. Isidore de Polinière, *Traité de la salubrité dans les grandes villes* (Paris: Baillière, 1846), p. 115.

66 M. W. Flinn, "Introduction" to Chadwick, *Sanitary Report*, ed. Flinn, p. 3; Monfalcon and Polinière, *Traité de la salubrité*, p. 38. See also Louis-Auguste Rougier and Alexandre Glénard, *Hygiène de Lyon. Compte-rendu des travaux du Conseil d'hygiène et de salubrité du département du Rhône du 1 janv. 1851 au 31 déc. 1859* (Lyon: Vingtrinier, 1860), pp. 267–73.

Likewise, Monfalcon and Polinière contended that the mission of the health councils was the improvement of the material condition of the working classes and went even further by asserting that the key to better public health for all lay in improving the state of the working class and the poor. The two reformers stressed the interrelatedness of bad health and poverty: Poverty often resulted in bad health; likewise, bad health was a major cause of poverty. They contended that the solution was a policy of enlightened paternalism toward workers. Sharing the attitudes of many hygienists and social reformers, they asserted that government intervention was necessary to protect the laboring classes, to whom the government owed more solicitude than to the rich, because workers were ignorant and apathetic in sanitary matters. It was up to the administration to protect workers' health by passing laws to regulate the construction of houses, for example. The overall goal for these hygienists was not just improved health, however, for like their counterparts elsewhere, Lyonnais physician-hygienists believed that hygiene improved the moral state of workers. Material improvement and better health would result in moral improvement. Monfalcon noted a direct correlation between domestic habits and morals. The health council of the Nord (Lille) agreed that physical and moral improvement of poor workers would result from improved living conditions: "It is thus [by improving the conditions of workers' dwellings] and thus only, that the moralization of the population that has been degraded by misery will become easier and will almost take care of itself, if it is true, as numerous examples demonstrate, that you regenerate the inhabitant by reforming his living quarters."[67]

Hygienists and reformers were motivated to take up the cause of the poor and the workers for economic and nationalistic as well as moral reasons. There was a widespread fear that the health of industrial workers was deteriorating to the point where they would be too weak either to work in factories or serve in the army. Statistics on army recruits showed how bad the health of the poor and workers was in comparison with that of more affluent members of society, and investigators pointed to industrialization as the cause. Hygienists and reformers insisted that public health measures should be instituted to ensure the future vitality of the French populace.[68] Villermé, for example, recommended a law limiting

---

67 Monfalcon and Polinière, *Traité de la salubrité*, pp. 25, 50, 92–3, 120, 140. For a similar point of view, see also Potton, *De la prostitution et de la syphilis*, pp. 183, 235–9; "Assainissement des maisons et des caves servant à l'habitation des indigents," in *Rapport sur les travaux du Conseil central de salubrité du Département du Nord pendant les années 1845 et 1846* (Lille: Ducrocq, 1847), p. 66. Monfalcon noted a direct correlation between domestic habits and morals in *Histoire monumentale de la ville de Lyon*, 9 vols. (Lyon: Bibliothèque de la ville, 1866), 3: 318.

68 Many hygienists as well as other reformers mention this as one of the primary reasons for advocating public health measures. See, for example, Buret, *De la*

working hours for children, noting that prisoners condemned to forced
labor worked twelve hours a day with two hours off for meals and rest,
whereas "free" workers normally worked fifteen to fifteen and one-half
hours.[69]

Hygienists also sought to improve workers' health out of fear and
self-interest, because by the 1830s and 1840s the "laboring and dangerous
classes" were considered both a foyer of infection and the seat of insurrec-
tion and revolution. After the Lyonnais workers' insurrections of 1831 and
1834, Lyonnais hygienists feared further uprisings if measures were not
taken to alleviate workers' low salaries, poor working conditions, and bad
health. Villeneuve-Bargemont saw the signs of social revolution everywhere and argued that if the problems of misery and pauperism (which he
believed to be the underlying cause of disease) were not solved, the class
struggle would worsen. Fodéré, believing poverty was a threat to the
security and tranquillity of the state, maintained that a state with an inadequate distribution of wealth was always on the verge of convulsion.[70]
Such critics argued that the working classes had yet to share in the public
health benefits that accompanied the progress of civilization. Several
theorists – like Villermé – believed that it was a question of time, that
increased wealth would eventually trickle down to workers, raising their
standard of living. Meanwhile, hygienists called for public health and
factory legislation to safeguard workers' health and for increased paternalism by factory owners to promote moral reform among the working
classes.

THE MISSION OF THE HYGIENISTS

The mission of the hygienists was *hygienism*, a term that characterizes the
overarching goals of the nineteenth-century public health movement.
Hygienism became by the end of the century a secular religion, incor-

misère des classes laborieuses, pp. 359–60; Thouvenin, "De l'influence de l'industrie,"
36(1846): 17–18, 32–3, 277 and 37 (1947): 96–101, 110–111; Villermé, *Tableau*, 1:
312–15; 2: 245–7; Villeneuve, rapporteur, "Rapport général sur les épidémies qui
ont régné en France depuis 1771 jusqu'à 1830 exclusivement, et dont les relations
sont parvenus à l'Acadèmie," *Mém. de l'Acad. Roy. de Méd.* 3 (1833): 397–8;
"Réforme industrielle. Enquête. De la condition misérable des hommes, femmes
et enfans dans les manufacturers; des causes de cette misère et des moyens d'y
remédier," *l'Atelier* (2 January 1841): 36; Lévy, *Traité d'hygiène*, 1: 52. See also
Motard, *Essai d'hygiène*, 2: 363, 376–7; Monfalcon and Polinière, *Traité de la
salubrité*, pp. 114, 120.

69   L. R. Villermé, "Sur la durée trop longue du travail des enfans dans beaucoup de
manufactures," *Annales d'hygiène publique* 18 (1837): 168, 175.

70   See Robert Bezucha, *The Lyon Uprising of 1834* (Cambridge, MA: Harvard
University Press, 1974); Villeneuve-Bargemont, *Economie politique chrétienne* 1: 25–
95; Fodéré, *Essai sur la pauvreté*, p. 21;

porating a number of components, including medicalization and moralization. Medicalization meant hygienic imperialism, what Stephen Jacyna has
called "medical expansionism."[71] This was the notion that hygiene and
hygienists should exert their influence on virtually all areas of human
activity – from the personal to the public and political levels. Other principal goals of the hygienists, intimately related to national interests and
including a strong humanitarian component, were lowering the mortality
rate, improving the quality and quantity of life, reducing the incidence of
disease and premature death, increasing the average life expectancy, and
reducing disease-related pain and suffering.

A major element of hygienism was moralization, based on a belief in the
interconnection between the moral and material. Material improvements
would improve the standard of living of the poor and workers – the group
targeted by the hygienists as most in need of reform – and moralization
would enable these people to adopt middle-class values and habits. Moralization was the civilizing mission of physicians, a didacticism dating from
the late eighteenth century – to teach the poor, peasants, and workers, by
example and education how to improve their standard of living, health,
and morals by learning and adopting middle-class habits. The civilizing
mission was basically *embourgeoisement*, a key element of the broader
mission of hygienism. The mission of the hygienists was social, that is,
their civilizing reform efforts were directed principally at the poor and
workers, especially the urban poor. This is not to deny the long-standing
tradition of the epidemic physicians as medical missionaries to the peasants
or, more recently, that of the cantonal physicians, who fulfilled some of
the same functions. But the main focus of hygienism was urban.

Hygienism was still, however, a second-order goal, for behind the
hygiene movement lay the larger vision of the well-ordered society, which
hygienists shared with political leaders, reformers of varying persuasions,
and intellectuals. The well-ordered society was necessary for national
productivity and national security, as well as an end in itself. Although the
ideas of how the well-ordered society would be organized and function
varied depending on one's outlook on life, religious attitudes, and political
persuasion, the dominant forces of conservatism and liberalism both saw
this as a major goal of social and organizational reform. Both conservatives
and liberals grappled with urbanization and industrialization, which challenged the old social order and were conceptualized and debated within the
context of the Revolutionary and Napoleonic experiences. In the 1820s and
1830s, liberals and conservatives both began responding to what would be
referred to by the 1840s as the "social problem," or how best to deal with

71 Stephen Jacyna, "Medical Science and Moral Science," p. 115.

a growing poor and working class in order to maintain the social order necessary for national security.

The two main approaches that characterized the public health movement were liberalism and statism. The leading exponent of liberalism was Villermé, who put much responsibility for hygienism on individuals but who also recognized the need for legislative, administrative, and institutional reform to improve the health of the poor and the workers. The statist approach, best exemplified by Parent-Duchâtelet, placed more emphasis on administrative, institutional, and legislative reform, believing that public health reform went from the top down. The two approaches intersected at many points, however, and it would be a distortion of the hygienic mission to try to characterize the movement by contrasting views or competing ideological camps. The liberal–statist dialectic permeated the public health movement. The difference was one of emphasis, and was neither counterproductive nor divisive. And no doubt, part of the reason for the different approaches had to do with the wide array of problems hygienists investigated. The case of water, so neatly described and analyzed by Jean-Pierre Goubert, illustrates the complementarity of the two approaches. The consensus was that cleanliness was related to morality, general well-being, and public health. Therefore, more water and increased personal use of water were desirable goals. To provide more water was an administrative, organizational, production-oriented problem in which the role of the government was central. Water could be provided by the municipal authorities with public or private financial backing and the assurance that demand for the product existed. Demand had to be created at the individual-private level, where education, attitudes, and habits were critical, because individuals had to be convinced of the benefits of water, had to be taught how and why to utilize it. Water use was cultural and individual, but its provision was municipal and industrial.[72]

Third-order goals concerned the way the broader mission of hygienism was to be achieved, and this was the level at which the community of hygienists focused most of its attention, articulated its goals, and realized considerable success. These were the intermediate and eminently practical goals of legislative and administrative reform to address public health problems and the disciplinary, institutional, and professional goals of the hygienists, which they saw as a precondition for achieving the authority and legitimation necessary to effect policy. Professionalization and disciplinary development accompanied by institutionalization were necessary prerequisites for hygienism.

---

72 Jean-Pierre Goubert, *The Conquest of Water: The Advent of Health in the Industrial Age* (Princeton, NJ: Princeton University Press, 1989).

To achieve these goals, hygienists investigated the major urban health problems and advocated a whole battery of administrative reforms such as housing regulations and improvement of sewerage systems and water supplies. As a result of their sociohygienic studies, they urged legislative reforms: a national public health law instituting a nationwide system of health councils and the reform of the quarantine system. Villermé championed a child labor law and a civil registration act, and Parent-Duchâtelet called for a national law regulating prostitution. These administrative and legislative aims were closely related to the hygienists' goals to develop a discipline of *hygiène publique* and to institutionalize and professionalize it. One of the hygienists' main ambitions was to establish public hygiene as a scientific discipline based on observation, experimentation, and quantification. Just as surgeons and physicians had moved medicine from the library into the hospital, hygienists wanted to move hygiene from the library to the appropriate observation sites: sewers, dumps, factories. The principal theorist of the scientific discipline of public hygiene was Parent-Duchâtelet. In his research and writings he described what he considered to be the scientific methodology of public hygiene and provided a plan for the professionalization of the discipline. He clearly articulated who should be a public hygienist and how he should be trained. Central to the development of public hygiene as a professional scientific discipline were the Paris health council and the *Annales d'hygiène publique*. The health council was the institutional embodiment of the scientific discipline of public hygiene, and by their selection of material the founders and editors of the *Annales d'hygiène publique* defined the limits of the discipline and exemplified the appropriate methodology.

At the beginning of the nineteenth century the domain of public hygiene was very broad. In 1807, when the Paris health council enumerated its tasks, public hygiene included the control of epidemics and the inspection of markets, rivers, cemeteries, slaughterhouses, horsebutchering yards, dumps, public places, occupational hygiene, charlatans, lighting, secret remedies, adulterated drinks and food, epizootics, prisons, and public assistance.[73] By 1829, when a group of public hygienists founded the *Annales d'hygiène publique*, they were able to articulate more precisely the definition and goals of public hygiene. In the introduction to the first volume, Charles Marc described public hygiene as a scientific, professional, administrative discipline, completely distinct from legal medicine. Marc emphasized that public hygiene was more than an administrative discipline, however. It was also a body of doctrine, a scientific discipline.[74]

73 J. G. Victor de Moléon, *Rapports généraux sur les travaux du Conseil de salubrité de la ville de Paris et du département de la Seine, exécutés depuis l'année 1802 jusqu'à l'année 1826* (Paris: Imprimerie municipale, 1828), pp. 102–4.
74 Charles C. H. Marc, "Introduction," *Annales d'hygiène publique* I (1829): ix–xx.

For the founding editors of the journal the subject of hygiene was very broad. The editors clarified the areas of investigation that public hygiene encompassed:

It is [public hygiene] which observes the varieties, the opposition, the influence of climates, and which appreciates their effects; which states and removes the causes contrary to the conservation and well-being of existence; finally, which deals with all the means of public salubrity. It [public hygiene] is concerned with the quality and the properties of foodstuffs and drinks, with the diets of soldiers and sailors. It recognizes the necessity of sanitary laws. Its domain extends to all which concerns endemic diseases, epidemics, epizootics, hospitals, insane asylums, lazarettos, prisons, burials, cemeteries.[75]

For the founders of the *Annales d'hygiène publique* the scope of public hygiene extended even further, into the moral order:

In the investigation of lifestyles, professions, all the nuances of social position, [public hygiene] can, by its association with philosophy and legislation exert a great influence on the development of the human spirit. It can enlighten the moralist and contribute to the noble task of diminishing the number of social infirmities.[76]

Parent-Duchâtelet was very clear about who should be a public hygienist and how he should be trained. Although physicians had traditionally been the public health experts, Parent-Duchâtelet thought that many physicians did not have the qualifications to be public hygienists. His attitude toward physicians deserves discussion, because it has been misunderstood and also because it demonstrates the main cause he championed. His curious and critical attitude toward physicians is clearly expressed in many of his studies.[77] Parent-Duchâtelet was not opposed to physicians and the medical profession as such, but to a certain type of physician – the "library" or bookish physician.[78] He applauded those physicians who applied what he considered the scientific method to medicine and hygiene. Nor did he rule out physicians as hygienists. Because public hygiene was a collaborative effort, physicians willing to practice "scientific" hygiene would make good public hygienists. What he deplored were physicians who parroted the "authorities" without questioning or testing them. He challenged the presumption of some physicians that their medical training qualified them to make pronouncements ex cathedra on any and all aspects

---

75 "Prospectus," *Annales d'hygiène publique* 1 (1829): vi–viii.
76 Ibid.
77 See, for example, "Le rouissage du chanvre considéré sous le rapport de l'hygiène," *Hygiène publique* 2: 479–558; "Mémoire sur les véritables influences que le tabac peut avoir sur la santé des ouvriers," *Hygiène publique* 2: 560; "Mémoire sur les débardeurs de la ville de Paris," *Hygiène publique* 2: 639–41.
78 See Erwin Ackerknecht, *Medicine at the Paris Hospital, 1794–1848* (Baltimore: Johns Hopkins University Press, 1967), pp. xi–xiv.

of public hygiene. Parent-Duchâtelet wanted a radical break with the tradition that the physician was the most qualified person to address public health questions. The nineteenth-century conception of public health was too broad for such a narrow approach. Public hygiene had to be a collaborative effort, and if it was defined this way, then physicians were no more qualified than other specialists.

Although hygiene had traditionally been within the bailiwick of the physician, Parent-Duchâtelet emphasized that the new scientific hygiene required the cooperation of many specialists. He believed that medical education and the practice of medicine did not prepare one to be a public hygienist. Only "those physicians who have made a special study of hygiene and especially public and political hygiene," for example, should be considered qualified to serve on the Paris health council. Even more so than physicians, Parent-Duchâtelet singled out chemists and especially industrial chemists as public hygienists, because "what would many people who have spent their lives in the hospitals and in the exclusive practice of medicine do, when confronted with a steam engine or an industrial procedure?"[79]

In establishing the guidelines for the profession of public hygiene, Parent-Duchâtelet emphasized the proper education for the hygienist. According to him, the medical faculties did not train physicians to be public hygienists. Indeed, the study of public hygiene occupied only a minor place in the medical curriculum of the first half of the nineteenth century, although all three faculties had chairs of hygiene.[80] To receive a medical degree, students had to pass five exams, one of which, number four, included hygiene and legal medicine. Notes from Desgenettes' hygiene course (Desgenettes held the chair of hygiene at the Paris Faculty from 1830 to 1837), for example, indicate that the medical student was not receiving the fundamentals of public hygiene, and he was certainly not

---

79 Parent-Duchâtelet, "Le Conseil de salubrité de la ville de Paris," *Hygiène publique* 1: 6.

80 The chair of hygiene and medical physics (physique médicale) at the Paris Faculty was created in 1794 and was held by Jean-Noël Hallé until his death in 1822. See Ackerknecht, *Paris Hospital*, pp. 149, 156. A chair of hygiene was established at Montpellier in 1826, and that year Frédéric Bérard gave his opening lecture as professor of hygiene. See *Journal des Débats*, 27 October 1826, p. 2; see Bérard's lecture: *Discours sur les améliorations progressives de la santé publique* (Paris: Gabon, 1826). A chair of hygiene was established at the Strasbourg Faculty in 1839. See Jacques Léonard, "Les études médicales en France entre 1815 et 1848," *Revue d'histoire moderne et contemporaine* 13 (1966): 89. One of the contenders was J. F. Rameaux. See Rameaux, *Appréciation des progrès de l'hygiène publique depuis le commencement du 19e siècle* (Strasbourg: Concours, 1839). See also Edwin Lee, *Observations on the principal medical institutions and practice of France, Italy and Germany*, 2nd ed. (London: J. Churchill, 1843), p. 2; see also J. C. Sabatier (d'Orléans), *Recherches historiques sur la Faculté de Médecine de Paris depuis son origine jusqu'à nos jours* (Paris: Deville Cavellin, 1835), p. 245.

being trained in the principles of scientific hygiene.[81] The course outline was in two parts: Part I was medical physics and Part II was hygiene, one section of which dealt with public hygiene. There was quite a difference between what was supposed to be taught and what Desgenettes actually taught. One year, for example, Desgenettes devoted thirty-four out of a total of fifty-two lessons to food. Another year the lessons were devoted to physical and medical geography. Judging from the example of Desgenettes, professors could take considerable leeway. Although medical training was a satisfactory prerequisite to the practice of public hygiene, it alone did not prepare one to be a professional hygienist.

A public hygienist might come from a variety of backgrounds. His academic preparation might be in the medical faculties or professional schools. He could be a physician, a pharmacist-chemist, an engineer, an architect, a veterinarian, or an administrator. Experts were needed from a number of different specialties to investigate and manage complex public health questions. Armed with formal academic preparation, the public hygienist would become a technical expert by on-the-job training. According to Parent-Duchâtelet, the most important training ground for the public hygienist was the health council (*conseil de salubrité*), where he could work with colleagues from a variety of backgrounds to receive the practical training to become a professional expert.[82] The hygienist as a technical expert would function as a professional consultant to the government. There was an established tradition of expert advisors to the French government, and the public hygienist was to continue this tradition. The public hygienist was to be a technocrat.

Related to the disciplinary development of *hygiène publique* was the hygienists' goal of institutionalizing public hygiene. The institution that was to serve this function was the health council. The Paris health council both antedated and was part of the disciplinary development of public hygiene. From its foundation, the Paris health council reflected both the approach to public health inherited from the Enlightenment and Revolutionary periods and the concept of *hygiène publique* as it was being defined by the nineteenth-century hygienists. By the 1830s the Paris health council had become the institutional embodiment of the scientific discipline of *hygiène publique*, a model of how professional technical experts could practice scientific hygiene and function as the public health advisory board to a municipal or departmental government.

81 Baron Desgenettes held the chair of hygiene at the Paris Faculty from 1830 to 1837. He had gained fame as the chief physician of Napoleon's Egyptian army and later had become inspector-general of all military medicine under Napoleon. Paris, Bibliothèque nationale. Nouvelles acquisitions françaises, 20570. Papiers de Baron Desgenettes, 1833. Notes pour servir à un cours d'hygiène.
82 Parent-Duchâtelet, "Le Conseil de salubritè," pp. 8–9.

A main goal of the overall mission of the hygienists was to transform public hygiene from an armchair philosophy to a scientific discipline by applying a scientific methodology including observation, experimentation, and quantification. The principal theorist of the methodology of public hygiene was Parent-Duchâtelet. Both he and Villermé stressed the importance of statistics in making public hygiene scientific.

2

The methodology of public hygiene

French hygienists wanted to make public health a scientific discipline, by which they meant using observation, experimentation, and quantification to study public health problems. Placing problems in historical context also figured prominently in their method. In their methodological approach hygienists were greatly influenced by the empirical tradition of the Enlightenment, eighteenth-century developments in social statistics, and the recent numerical method articulated and practiced by clinician Pierre Louis.[1] Charles Londe expressed the critical spirit hygienists hoped to bring to bear on the study of hygiene: "There is only one way to remove hygiene from every systematic influence: that is to circumscribe it [hygiene] within the rigorous limits of facts and to leave to the facts their natural relationships."[2] Emphasizing a quantitative approach, Villermé expressed a similar idea in his classic study of varying mortality rates in the French departments: "I am going to attempt to bring it [the whole question of the causes of differing mortality] to light by masses of incontestable facts, which for the first time will establish it [the answer] by measurement."[3]

Although a critical approach was not new to scientists, hygienists believed their method constituted a radical break with the way public health problems had traditionally been investigated. As they saw it, traditional Hippocratic hygiene had been scientific, or based on observation. But commentators during the centuries had abandoned the observational method that had characterized classical hygiene. Hygiene had become a sterile list of rules and theories transmitted uncritically from one generation to another. A shift had occurred in the late eighteenth century, hygienists claimed, when French investigators had begun to question

---

1 Martin Staum, *Cabanis: Enlightenment and Medical Philosophy in the French Revolution* (Princeton, NJ: Princeton University Press, 1980), pp. 2–48, 94–121.
2 Charles Londe, quoted in Michel Lévy, *Traité d'hygiène* 2 vols. (Baillière, 1844–5), 1: 46. See Londe's work, *Nouveaux élémens d'hygiène*, 2 vols. (Paris: Baillière, 1827).
3 L. R. Villermé, "Mémoire sur la mortalité dans la classe aiseé et dans la classe indigente," *Mém. de l'Acad. Roy. de Méd.* 1 (1828): 52.

traditional authorities and to encourage an empirical approach to the investigation of public health problems. The hygienist who had best exemplified this critical Enlightenment spirit was physician Jean-Noël Hallé, who did for general hygiene what Parent-Duchâtelet did in the 1820s and 1830s for public hygiene.[4]

PARENT-DUCHÂTELET AND THE SCIENTIFIC DISCIPLINE OF PUBLIC HYGIENE

Among the French hygienists, it was Parent-Duchâtelet who clarified the methodology of public hygiene and emerged as the principal theorist of the scientific discipline of public hygiene. Above all, he promoted an objective, scientific approach both in medicine and in public hygiene. Parent-Duchâtelet's reputation among historians rests primarily on his work on the sewers of Paris and his sociohygienic study of prostitution in Paris. He is remembered for the subject matter he treated and as a precursor of empirical sociology. Although historians have been interested in Parent-Duchâtelet's investigative methods, they have not recognized him as the principal theorist of public hygiene. Even though he made specific public health recommendations such as an expanded sewer system for Paris and a national law to regulate prostitution, his principal goal was to apply the scientific method – as he understood it – to the study of public hygiene.[5]

In his numerous public health investigations Parent-Duchâtelet articulated the scientific methodology of public hygiene.[6] His general approach was skepticism coupled with faith in the empirical method. His work exemplifies the methodology he advocated: collection and analysis of data, firsthand observation, experimentation, and quantification. Parent-Duchâtelet always began the study of a public health problem with a historical investigation, for he believed such problems could only be understood in context. He used official records, archives, and institutional

4 Michel Lévy, *Traité d'hygiène*, 1: 43–4.
5 Alexandre Parent-Duchâtelet, "Essai sur les cloaques ou égouts de la ville de Paris," *Hygiène publique*, 2 vols. (Paris: Baillière, 1836), 1: 156–207; Parent-Duchâtelet, *De la prostitution dans la ville de Paris*, 2 vols. (Paris: Baillière, 1836). Alain Corbin, "Présentation" to Alexandre Parent-Duchâtelet, *La Prostitution à Paris au XIXe siècle*, texte présenté et annoté par Alain Corbin (Paris: Seuil, 1981), pp. 9–47; Jill Harsin, *Policing Prostitution in Nineteenth-Century Paris* (Princeton, NJ: Princeton University Press, 1985), esp. ch. 3; William Coleman, "The Scientific Study of Prostitution," essay prepared for Franco Ricci and Maria Ricci, editors, and based on the talk given in the Jason A. Hannah Lecture series.
6 On Parent-Duchâtelet's methodology and the scientific discipline of public hygiène, see Ann F. La Berge, "The Early Nineteenth-Century French Public Health Movement: The Disciplinary Development and Institutionalization of *hygiène publique*," *Bull. Hist. Med.* 58 (1984): 363–79. On Parent-Duchâtelet's methodology see also Corbin, "Présentation"; Harsin, *Policing Prostitution*; and Coleman, "Scientific Study."

records to understand the historical background of a problem and to acquire numerical data for analysis. Parent-Duchâtelet's use of historical methodology is exemplified in all his public health studies, but especially in his works on the sewers of Paris, the horsebutcher yards, and prostitution.[7] Although understanding a problem's history was the way to begin the study of a public health problem, it was only by firsthand observation, experimentation, and quantification that an investigation would become scientific.

For Parent-Duchâtelet, public hygiene was a science, a branch of scientific medicine. Therefore, he proposed that hygienists borrow the observational methods of physicians. Just as the medical student could not receive all his training in the classroom or the library, but had to go into hospitals to observe patients and diseases, had to study disease at the autopsy table and by application of the numerical method, so the hygienist could not receive all his training from books. His clinical training was to be gotten at the work site: at dumps, in sewers, at factories, and by subjecting numerical data on disease and death to critical analysis. Parent-Duchâtelet explained how scientific hygienists applied physicians' observational methods to public health problems: "We have followed your [the physician's] precepts in the study of hygiene. While you observe your patients at their bedside, we pass days, weeks, months in the horsebutcher yards, where duty leads us, the zeal of science, and above all, our duty as health council members, we who are the guardians of the public health and who appreciate all which can be harmful to health."[8]

The scientific study of some public health problems required experimentation. In his work on the effects of putrid emanations on food and in his study of the alleged harmful effects of hemp retting, Parent-Duchâtelet demonstrated the importance of the experimental method to the scientific hygienist. In both cases, his findings contradicted generally accepted beliefs. For example, most physicians and hygienists believed that putrid emanations from decomposed animal matter altered food substances. To resolve the question scientifically, Parent-Duchâtelet performed a series of twenty-eight experiments, from which he concluded that putrid emanations had no influence on foodstuffs.[9]

---

7 Parent-Duchâtelet, "Essai sur les cloaques ou égouts;" *De la prostitution dans la ville de Paris*; Parent-Duchâtelet, "Les chantiers d'équarrissage de la ville de Paris," *Hygiène publique*, 2: 237–41. For details on these studies, see Chapters 6 and 7.

8 Alexandre Parent-Duchâtelet, "Des obstacles que les préjugés médicaux apportent dans quelques circonstances, à l'assainissement des villes et à l'établissement de certaines manufactures," *Hygiène publique*, 1: 55. (First published in the *Annales d'hygiène publique* in 1835.) Quote, p. 45.

9 Parent-Duchâtelet, "Recherches pour déterminer jusqu'à quel point les émanations putrides provenant de la décomposition des matières animales peuvent contribuer à l'altération des substances alimentaires," *Hygiène publique*, 2: 85–122. (First published in the *Annales d'hygiène publique* in 1831.)

Another public health problem requiring experimentation was hemp retting, a major rural health concern. Hemp was left in streams and ponds to soak; as a result the water appeared dirty, and fetid emanations were given off. Numerous authors had asserted that hemp retting was hazardous to health: It altered drinking water and air and was harmful to fish. The traditional authorities, Ramazzini and Fourcroy, were of this opinion. Many nineteenth-century physicians and hygienists agreed with the authorities, but some dissented. When Parent-Duchâtelet took up the problem, he was confronted with a number of diametrically opposed opinions. "If," as Parent-Duchâtelet said, "questions of salubrity and public hygiene were decided by majority vote, it would be easy, by an arithmetical operation, to discover the truth."[10] But this was not the case, and Parent-Duchâtelet did not have the data on observers and commentators who had voiced differing opinions. Therefore, he could not assess their scientific credentials. He did not know, for example, if the authors were careful observers, if they were operating under the same conditions, or if they had some vested interest in spreading the opinion they advanced. Therefore, Parent-Duchâtelet resolved to do his own experiments. Over a two-year period, he performed fifty experiments on animals and humans to test the claims that had been made. He described how he proceeded:

I first took some hemp…perfectly ripe and completely dried; I cut it into equal fragments three decimeters in length, and standing it upright side by side in a cylindrical vase of the same height, I could exactly fill this vase; having covered all the pieces with ordinary water, I let them macerate for 8, 10 and 15 days at a temperature which varied from 10 to 25 degrees centigrade. By this manner of proceeding I obtained a yellowish, almost brown water, similar in color to a strong tea, which spread for some distance the particular odor of hemp which has been retted.[11]

Believing this water to be similar in every way to water from streams and ponds in which hemp was retted, Parent-Duchâtelet then gave it to a variety of birds and some guinea pigs over a five-month period. He observed that their health did not suffer. He then drank some similarly prepared water himself – a cupful a day for fifteen days – without experiencing the slightest indisposition. Next, he and his colleague, clinician Gabriel Andral, used for experimentation twenty-seven patients at the Pitié hospital, giving them doses of five to six ounces of the water for a period of fifteen days. There were no discernible ill effects. After performing similar experiments to test other claims about the health hazards of hemp retting, Parent-Duchâtelet concluded that many of the assertions were unfounded. He found neither the water nor the air harmful to the health of

10 Parent-Duchâtelet, "Le rouissage du chanvre considéré sous le rapport de l'hygiène," *Hygiène publique*, 2: 479–558, esp. pp. 501–4. Quote, p. 504.
11 Ibid., p. 506.

animals or humans. Parent-Duchâtelet said he hoped his findings would not discourage administrators from providing pure drinking water, a desirable public health provision. His aim, he explained, was not to impede public health progress, but to advance the application of scientific methodology to questions of medicine and hygiene. Addressing physicians, Parent-Duchâtelet put forward his case:

I am speaking to physicians and I want to make them notice how important it is to be well educated in the real action of exterior agents, in order not to make a mistake as to the real cause of certain epidemics and endemics. Isn't it better to ignore the cause of a prevailing disease and to avow this ignorance than to attribute it lightly and without proof to the actions of a body which has contributed nothing to its production? In the latter case one acts always blindly and one gains only useless if not dangerous advice: in the first [case] one remains on the defensive, advises nothing: one looks for and sometimes finds the truth, and if one cannot be useful, at least one can have the satisfaction of not having been pernicious. These ideas which I am developing for the first time have not been furnished to me by my experiments on hemp-retting; they have occupied me for a long time; they have been the subject of grave and serious reflections; they have come to me as a result of observations made during many years.... [12]

Although praised by colleagues and contemporaries, both French and foreign, for his scientific methods and careful research, Parent-Duchâtelet incurred the wrath of critics who accused him of harboring preconceived notions and of acting out of self-interest. Defending himself against such accusations, Parent-Duchâtelet provided a succinct account of his faith in his methodology:

Let me express my complete thoughts: even though I have been accused of only having done research and experiments with preconceived ideas and opinions; even though they [critics] have gone so far as to say that my friend Villermé and I *invent the facts* [his italics] that we report, I know, however, how to be diffident....I know that experiments, or to put it better, the manner of experimenting can sometimes be erroneous. But when you repeat experiments over a period of two years, when you modify them in all manners; when analogous results are reached when done by others; when above all, one has no self-interest at stake in making one opinion prevail over another; we are permitted, I think, to believe in what our senses tell us and to say that our forerunners have been wrong. [13]

In this selection Parent-Duchâtelet expressed his faith in observation and experiment while recognizing that they were subject to error. He also believed in the possibility of an objective observer, because he had great faith in his own observational abilities and detachment. One could say that he had an exalted opinion of his own objectivity. A radical empiricist

12 Ibid., pp. 550–1.
13 Ibid., pp. 555–6.

approach, he thought, would bring public hygienists as close to the truth as possible. Sensory perceptions could be trusted and were a reliable guide to truth. Hygienists could believe what they observed, and if their findings contradicted the authorities, then the latter had to be refuted. Furthermore, Parent-Duchâtelet thought that because of his personal situation and his attitudes, he was capable of proceeding without preconceived notions. Nor did he have any reason to act out of self-interest, he claimed. Characterizing himself as a man "libre et sans place," a man "exempt de préjugés," he consistently maintained that his only interest was in the truth.[14] And the way to arrive at the truth was to bring a critical, positivistic approach to bear on the study of public hygiene. Like his contemporaries – especially Villermé – and sounding like Pierre Louis himself, Parent-Duchâtelet stressed the importance of this method, which he called "statistical," for making public hygiene a positive science:

In collecting and preparing materials I have made the utmost effort to arrive at numerical results on every point; for at the present time a judicious mind is but little satisfied with the expressions *much, often, sometimes, very often* [his italics], etc., which have hitherto been regarded as sufficient even in cases of great consequence. In fact, what is the meaning of the word *much* in these cases? Does it signify ten, twenty, or a hundred? Every assertion of this nature can have no value independent of figures, which alone can admit of comparison; it is only by this method that science can be advanced.... This method, which I term statistical, has been applied for some time to medicine, and has given us a degree of certitude on many points (which makes us predict it will be generally applied).[15]

For Parent-Duchâtelet and Villermé quantification was essential to a critical, positivistic methodology. Indeed, the application of the numerical method to public health questions was the principal novelty in the approach of the public hygienists.

STATISTICS AND PUBLIC HEALTH

The public health movement developed within the context of the *statistics movement* of the 1820s and 1830s.[16] Statistical analysis was an important

---

14 François Valleix, *De la prostitution dans la ville de Paris*...Examen de Valleix (Paris: au Bureau du Journal hebdomadaire, 1836), p. 9.

15 The translation is from an American edition of Parent-Duchâtelet's work. Alexandre Parent-Duchâtelet, *Prostitution in Paris* (Boston: H. C. Brainerd, 1845), pp. 22–3.

16 The term *statistics movement* was used by Erwin Ackerknecht in "Villermé and Quetelet," *Bull. Hist. Med.* 26 (1952): 317–29. This article is based on letters exchanged between the two statisticians and provides some interesting insights into the international correspondence of nineteenth-century statisticians. The nineteenth-century hygienists often used the term *statistics* to refer to what today is called *statistical analysis*. In the nineteenth century the term *statistics* itself was rela-

tool of public hygienists for several reasons. First, public hygienists used statistical analysis to buttress theories about the concomitance of the advance of civilization and the progress of public health. Statistical analysis furnished scientific proof that this theory was correct. Second, hygienists used the numerical method to measure the effects of public health reforms. For example, hygienists compared the decline in morbidity and mortality rates in prisons and hospitals as their sanitary states improved. Third, they used statistical analysis to answer health questions related to the causes of disease and mortality.

Public hygienists believed they could use statistical analysis to measure the progress of civilization and public health. Statisticians such as Adolphe Quetelet, Louis-René Villermé, Louis-François Benoiston de Châteauneuf, Edouard Mallet, and Francis d'Ivernois used mortality rates – which Ivernois called the barometer of a society – the average length of life, and the probable life expectancy to determine the level of civilization. In three letters written to Villermé in the 1830s, Ivernois stressed the importance of using the mortality rate as an indicator of the relative prosperity of a population, arguing that average life expectancy and average longevity were the best means of measuring affluence and material progress. Ivernois asserted that a low mortality rate and a low birth rate were signs of an affluent, advanced society. This theory was contrary to the generally accepted notion that the optimum situation was a low mortality rate and a high birth rate.[17] Indeed, all these statisticians believed that a low comparative

tively new, having first been employed by a German statistician, Gottfried Achenwall, in 1749 to mean "the descriptive analysis of the political, economic, and social organization of states." On the origin of the term see George Rosen, *A History of Public Health* (New York: MD Publications, 1958), p. 175; L. R. Villermé, *Population, Hygiène, Extrait du Journal des cours publics de la ville de Paris* (Paris: Pihan Delaforest, 1828), p. 2. See also Keith Baker, *Condorcet: From Natural Philosophy to Social Mathematics* (Chicago: University of Chicago Press, 1975). In recent years there has been an outpouring of works on the history of statistics and probability. See, for example, Gerd Gigerenzer et al., *The Empire of Chance* (New York: Cambridge University Press, 1989); Lorraine Daston, *Classical Probability in the Enlightenment* (Princeton, NJ: Princeton University Press, 1988); Theodore M. Porter, *The Rise of Statistical Thinking* (Princeton, NJ: Princeton University Press, 1988); William Coleman *Death Is a Social Disease: Public Health and Political Economy in Early Industrial France* (Madison: University of Wisconsin Press, 1982); Ian Hacking, *The Taming of Chance* (Cambridge: Cambridge University Press, 1990); Lorenz Krüger et al., *The Probabilistic Revolution* 2 vols. (Cambridge, MA: MIT Press, 1987).

17   The average length of life (*vie moyenne*) is the average of the total number of years lived by those who died in a given year; the average life expectancy (*vie probable*) is calculated by the list of deaths according to the age of death; the average life expectancy is that age at which half of those born have died, while the other half are still living. The first letter was *Sur la mortalité proportionnelle des populations normandes considérée comme mesure de leur aisance et de leur civilisation* (Geneva: Imprimerie de la Bibliothèque universelle, 1833); the second letter was "Exposé des

mortality rate, a high average longevity rate, and a high probable life expectancy were reliable indicators of public health and civilization. Quetelet pointed out, however, that figures for average length of life and average life expectancy alone were not enough; the composition and age distribution of the population also had to be considered. The measure of years alone, he argued, was insufficient, for years differed in quality. He argued that the ten years between thirty and forty, for example, were more important for the material productivity and vitality of a nation than the ten years between birth and ten.[18] Statistical analysis showed that in advanced countries of Western Europe as time went on, people on the average lived longer, life expectancy increased, and overall mortality decreased. Statistical analysis offered hygienists scientific proof for their belief in the continuing progress of civilization.[19]

Public hygienists also considered the numerical method a scientific way to measure the effects of public health reforms on morbidity and mortality. The effectiveness of sanitary reform in prisons and hospitals could be accurately assessed, they believed, as could declining rates of venereal disease

principales erreurs qui prévalent sur le sujet des populations; graves et nombreuses aberrations des écrivains qui font autorité sur la matière," *Bibliothèque universelle de Genève* 54 (September 1833): 1–50, part I, and 54 (October 1833): 139–78, part II; the third letter was *Sur la mortalité proportionnelle des peuples considérée comme mesure de leur aisance et de leur civilisation. Analyse des quinze registres de l'Etat civil en France. Pour les années 1817–1831* (Paris: Imprimerie de la Bibliothèque universelle, 1834).

18 Adolphe Quetelet, *Sur l'homme et le développement de ses facultés, ou essai de physique sociale* 2 vols. (Paris: Bachelier, 1835), pp. 272–327. For a good biography of the Belgian statistician, see Frank H. Hankins, *Adolphe Quetelet as Statistician. Studies in History, Economics, Public Law*, ed. by the Faculty of Political Science of Columbia University, Vol. 31, No. 4 (New York: Longmans, Green and Co., 1908). See Bernard Lécuyer, "Probability in Vital and Social Statistics: Quetelet, Farr, and the Bertillons," in *The Probabilistic Revolution*, 1: 317–35.

19 See, for example, Quetelet, *Sur l'homme*; the three letters of Ivernois cited in note 17; L. F. Benoiston de Châteauneuf, "Mémoire sur la durée de la vie humaine dans plusieurs des principaux états de l'Europe," *Séances et travaux de l'Académie des Sciences Morales et Politiques* (hereafter cited as *Séances et trav. de l'Acad. des Sci. Mor. et Pol.*) 10 (1846): 31–51; L. F. Benoiston de Châteauneuf, "Institut Royal de France. Académie Royale des Sciences, Note lue à l'Académie des Sciences dans sa séance du 30 janvier 1826, sur les changemens qu'ont subis les lois de la mortalité en Europe, depuis un demi-siècle (1775–1825)," *Moniteur universel*, 6 February, 1826, p. 148; Edouard Mallet, "Recherches historiques et statistiques sur la population de Genève, son mouvement annuel et sa longévité depuis le XVIe siècle jusqu'à nos jours (1549–1833)," *Annales d'hygiène publique* 17 (1837): 5–172; J. H. Fourier, "Notions générales sur la population," *Recherches statistiques sur la ville de Paris et le département de la Seine*, 5 vols. (Paris: Imprimerie Municipale, 1821–9, 1844). 1 (1821): ix–lxviii. Fourier shared many of the ideas of Villermé, Quetelet, and Ivernois regarding population statistics and their significance for providing proof for advancement of civil and public health progress. L. R. Villermé, "De la mortalité dans les divers quartiers de la ville de Paris," *Annales d'hygiène publique* 3 (1830): 294–341; L. R. Villermé, "Mémoire sur la taille de l'homme en France," *Annales d'hygiène publique* 1 (1829): 351–99.

among prostitutes following the application of sanitary measures. The numerical method clearly demonstrated either the efficacy of public health reform or that other causes of disease and mortality had to be isolated.[20] The third main area in which statistical analysis proved useful was the investigation of differential morbidity and mortality. Many treatises written by hygienists and statisticians were attempts to assess to what extent various factors caused disease and mortality among a particular group of people or a given population. Quetelet divided the general causes of mortality into two main areas: natural causes, such as climate, sex, age, time in history, and seasons; and human causes, such as profession, degree of affluence, moral and psychological influences, and educational, political, and religious influences.[21] Hygienists asserted that only if such causes were discovered could adequate preventive measures be taken.

The application of statistics to public health antedated the use of statistics in clinical medicine. As the word itself suggests, *statistics* was an eighteenth-century term that originally denoted an accounting of a state's population and resources to give a precise indication of wealth. Likewise, the concept of statistical probability had its own historic roots, but the work of Condorcet and Laplace placed the notion of a calculus of probability squarely within the concerns of the French scientific community of the early nineteenth century.

Widespread interest within the Parisian medical community in applying statistics to medicine dated from the 1820s with the work of Pierre Louis. Louis's use of his "numerical method" to assess the efficacy of bloodletting showed that the therapy was less successful than had been thought. His work challenged the principal therapy of Broussais's "physiological medicine," which had relied extensively on bloodletting to reduce inflammation, and showed that the numerical method could be a scientific way for physicians to evaluate therapeutic effectiveness. Louis's work and the community of physicians that organized with him the Société médicale d'observation to promote the numerical method opened the way for major discussions on the possible applications of the numerical method in clinical medicine. The institutional structure of Paris medicine provided a setting in which the new method might have wide applicability, since

---

20 See, for example, L. R. Villermé, "Mémoire sur la mortalité dans les prisons," *Annales d'hygiène publique* 1 (1829): 1–100; L. R. Villermé, "Note sur la mortalité parmi les forçats du bagne de Rochefort, sur la fréquence de leurs maladies, et sur la grande tendance que celles-ci ont à se terminer par la mort," *Annales d'hygiène publique* 6 (1831): 113–27; Adolphe Trébuchet in F. S. Ratier, "Mémoire en réponse à cette question: quelles sont les mesures les plus propres à arrêter la propagation de la maladie vénérienne?" *Annales d'hygiène publique* 16 (1836), note 1, p. 282, and note 1, p. 284.
21 Quetelet, *Sur l'homme*, pp. 133–271.

thousands of patients and diseases were readily available for observation and quantification.[22]

Although the application of statistics to public health was widely accepted, the same could not be said of medicine. Throughout the nineteenth century, from Bichat to Bernard, the use of statistics in medicine was highly controversial. The main themes of the controversy were clearly laid out in the debate over medical statistics that took place in 1837 at the Royal Academy of Medicine. In this debate a provincial physician, Risueño d'Amador, professor of general pathology and therapeutics at the medical faculty at Montpellier and a corresponding member of the Academy, read an essay on the calculus of probability applied to medicine. Although he was regarded as a reactionary by most of his colleagues, his main objections were similar to those raised by Bichat, Comte, and Bernard. The main criticism was that statistical probability was an inappropriate tool for the natural and medical sciences, where variation was the norm and variables were too numerous to be controlled. According to critics, the methods of the physical sciences were simply not appropriate for the medical sciences. D'Amador raised many other objections, but in the end he seems to have feared that applying the statistical method to medicine would make medicine impersonal, reduce patients to numbers, and deprive physicians and patients of their individuality.[23]

Louis and his supporters responded by arguing that counting was a traditional method used by all, and that what was being proposed was merely a more systematic method of counting – the numerical method. Louis did not advocate applying the calculus of probabilities to medicine, but counting cases, symptoms, and therapies to arrive at accurate, positive knowledge. In fact, Louis's numerical method and the use of statistical analysis by public hygienists were simple in design and execution. Both attempted to gain more precision in answering medical, social, and public health questions, but neither involved sophisticated mathematical procedures. As Coleman has suggested, the numerical method was simpler and less difficult than the calculus of probabilities. Medical and sociohygienic investigations using statistics, or the numerical method, consisted mainly

22   Pierre Louis, *Recherches sur les effets de la saignée dans quelques maladies inflammatoires* (Paris: Baillière, 1835). Louis had actually done the studies in the 1820s, and some of his work was first published as articles in the *Archives générales de médecine*. On this see Erwin Ackerknecht, *Medicine at the Paris Hospital, 1794–1848* (Baltimore: Johns Hopkins University Press, 1967), p. 104. On Broussais, see the recent book by Michel Valentin, *François Broussais, empereur de la médecine* (Paris: Association des Amis du Musée du Pays de Dinard, 1988), and Erwin Ackerknecht, "Broussais, or a Forgotten Medical Revolution," *Bull. Hist. Med.* 27 (1953): 320–43.

23   *Bull. de l'Acad. Roy. de Méd.* I (1837: 622–806; see also Terence D. Murphy, "Medical Knowledge and Statistical Methods in Early Nineteenth-Century France," *Medical History* 25 (1981): 301–19.

of computing and comparing averages and the use of simple proportions. Users of the numerical method both in medicine and in public health recognized the problems pointed out by mathematicians and critics, such as inadequate sample size and the difficulty of controlling variables, but still felt that statistics was a useful tool in their research arsenal.[24]

L. R. VILLERMÉ AND PUBLIC HEALTH STATISTICS

Villermé was the leading French exponent of public health statistics, along with his friend and colleague Parent-Duchâtelet. Villermé increased the awareness of the statistical method among French hygienists by publicizing the work of European statisticians who were using statistical analysis to answer public health questions. By the late 1820s, Villermé was the recognized French authority on the influence of standard of living on health.[25] The publication in 1823 of the first two volumes of the *Recherches statistiques sur la ville de Paris et le département de la Seine* under the direction of Frédéric Villot and the Prefecture of the Seine provided Villermé with the statistical information he needed to investigate causes of differing mortality among the French and Parisian populations.[26] In two articles

24 *Bull. de l'Acad. Roy. de Méd* 1 (1837): 622–806; Coleman, *Death Is a Social Disease*, pp. 132–7.

25 An excellent treatment of Villermé's statistical work can be found in Coleman, *Death Is a Social Disease*; see also Edmonde Vedrenne-Villeneuve, "L'inégalité sociale devant la mort dans la première moitié du XIXe siècle," *Population* 16 (1961): 665–99. Louis Chevalier attributed much importance to the statistical work of Villermé in *Classes laborieuses et classes dangereuses à Paris pendant la première moitié du 19e siècle* (Paris: Plon, 1958), pp. 410–28. Chevalier said that Villermé's statistical research constituted "the most remarkable document [of the age] on misery" (p. 157). There is a good brief discussion of Villermé's statistical work in Bernard Lécuyer and Anthony Oberschall, "Sociology: The Early History of Social Research," *International Encyclopedia of Social Sciences*, ed. David L. Sills, v. 15 (1968), pp. 45–7. On Villermé's investigations see also Bernard Lécuyer, "Démographie, statistique et hygiène publique sous la monarchie censitaire," *Annales de démographie historique* (1977): 215–45.

26 Four volumes of the *Recherches statistiques sur la ville de Paris et le département de la Seine* were published under the prefecture of Chabrol from 1821 to 1829: 1 (1821), 2 (1823), 3 (1826), 4 (1829). Frédéric Villot, head of the statistical office at the Prefecture of the Seine, did most of the compilations. Leading statistician Jean-Baptiste Fourier, who was appointed by Chabrol as mathematician at the Statistical Bureau of the Department of the Seine, wrote introductory essays to each of the volumes. On Fourier and these introductory essays see Porter, *The Rise of Statistical Thinking*, pp. 97–102, and Coleman, *Death Is a Social Disease*, p. 143. A fifth volume of the series was not published until 1844 during the prefecture of Rambuteau. For a brief history of the statistical office, see Coleman, *Death Is a Social Disease*, pp. 141–8. In addition to statistical data gathered from the *Recherches statistiques*, Villermè used data gathered from prisons and other institutions, documents made available to him by the Prefecture of the Seine, monthly mortality records kept by the mayor of the ninth arrondissement, tables sent to him by the hospital administration, and statistics on population movement in France furnished by the Minister of the Interior.

published during the 1820s Villermé developed his thesis on the relationship of poverty, disease, and mortality: that socioeconomic factors, that is, the environment created by affluence or poverty, were the primary determinants of differing mortality rates among the Parisian and French populations.[27]

Today this idea is commonplace, but in the early nineteenth century several competing theories were advanced to explain differences in morbidity and mortality. Hygienists had traditionally attributed differences in disease and death rates to climatic and topographical factors such as proximity to rivers, elevation, prevailing winds, humidity, temperature, and access to fresh air and sunlight. In medical topographies and hygiene manuals published in the late eighteenth and early nineteenth centuries, certain areas of a city were considered healthy and others unhealthy based on these factors.[28] Since the late eighteenth century, however, some hygienists had begun to shift their explanations of disease causation from climatic to social causes. By the 1820s there were two principal and opposing theories regarding the influence of poverty and affluence on morbidity and mortality. The more widely accepted theory was that as civilization advanced, public health improved. As a people became more civilized, they became wealthier, and wealth resulted in better health. Thus disease and death rates were greater among uncivilized than civilized people and greater among the poor than the affluent classes. The opposing theory, based on the idea that civilization is a generally corrupting influence, stated that wealth contributed to early death because of laziness, luxury, passions, and excesses detrimental to health. Villermé wanted to find out if statistical data could determine the probable causes of differing mortality rates among the French population because, although many had opinions on the subject, few had offered any proof. As Villermé said, "I am going to attempt to bring it [the whole question] to light by masses of incontestable facts, which for the first time will establish it [the answer] by measurement."[29]

In his first study Villermé sought to resolve the controversy over whether the rich were healthier and lived longer than the poor.[30] Com-

---

27 "Mémoire sur la mortalité en France;" "De la mortalité dans les divers quartiers de la ville de Paris."

28 The best example from the period is Claude Lachaise, *Topographie médicale de Paris* (Paris: Baillière, 1822). On Lachaise, see Chevalier, *Classes laborieuses*, pp. 172–4.

29 Villermé discussed the two theories in "Mémoire sur la mortalité," pp. 51–2. Quote, p. 52.

30 "Mémoire sur la mortalité en France." This study had first been presented to the Royal Academy of Sciences in 1824 and the Royal Academy of Medicine in 1826. On November 29, 1824, Villermé read an essay to the Royal Academy of Sciences entitled "Sur la mortalité en France dans la classe aisée comparée à celle qui a lieu parmi les indigens." See *Journal des Débats*, December 10, 1824, p. 3. In 1826, Villermé was chairman of a statistical commission within the Royal Academy of

paring a wealthy arrondissement of Paris, the first, with a poor one, the twelfth, Villermé found that in the former the mortality rate for at-home deaths was only 1/58.24, whereas in the latter it was 1/42.63. These figures did not include deaths in institutions such as hospitals, hospices, and prisons. If institutional deaths were added, the differences were even more striking, for hospitals and hospices were patronized primarily by the poor. For example, as Villermé demonstrated, the at-home mortality rate for the twelfth arrondissement was 1/43, whereas the total mortality rate including institutional deaths was 1/24. Focusing on an even smaller area, he chose two wards of the ninth arrondissement for which he had specific figures, the Ile St.-Louis, a wealthy quarter, and the Arsenal, a poor quarter. On the Ile St,-Louis the mortality rate was 1/46.4, whereas in the Arsenal it was 1/38.36. Narrowing down the sampling even further, Villermé chose a crowded street, the Rue de la Mortellerie, where the poverty-stricken inhabitants lived in deplorable conditions, and compared it with the four quais of the Ile St.-Louis, where the apartments were large and spacious and the inhabitants materially well off. The rate of at-home deaths on the Rue de la Mortellerie was 1/32.68, whereas for the four quais of the Ile St.-Louis it was 1/52.40. Then, using property taxes as an indication of relative wealth or poverty, Villermé drew up a table ranking the arrondissements from the wealthiest to the poorest. He correlated these figures with the ratio of at-home deaths and found that, with one exception, the wealthiest arrondissements had the lowest rates of at-home death and vice versa (Table 1). He then turned to the departments for further observations. Comparing the mortality rates of departments that could be classified as rich or poor, he found the average mortality of the rich departments to be 1/46.31, whereas that of the poor ones was 1/33.72 (Table 2).[31] Villermé concluded in this first study that mortality and the average length of life in France were directly related to the degree of affluence or poverty. The difference was so great that in some rich departments the mortality rate for all deaths was as low as 1/50, whereas in the twelfth arrondissement of Paris the mortality rate was more than twice as high, or 1/24.21.

In the second study Villermé sought to isolate specific causes for

Medicine that presented a report on the same question. See *Journal des Débats*, August 23, 1826, pp. 3–4. See the report: Villermé, "Rapport lu à l'Académie royale de Médecine, au nom de la Commission de statistique, sur une série de tableaux relatifs au mouvement de la population dans les douze arrondissemens municipaux de la ville de Paris, pendant les cinq années 1817, 1818, 1819, 1820 et 1821," *Archives générales de médecine* 10 (1826): 216–47.

31 Departments were classified as rich or poor depending on revenue, taxes, and division of wealth. Villot did the calculations for Villermé, using Chaptal's *De l'industrie françoise*, 2 vols. (Paris: A.-A. Renouard, 1819), the 1820 budget, and the most recent official population figures. See "Mémoire sur la mortalité," p. 70.

Table 1. *Correlation of wealth and mortality rates in the twelve arrondissements of Paris; Arrondissements ranked from wealthiest to poorest based on property taxes*

Arrondissement	Untaxed property, or percentage of poor families	At-home mortality 1817–21
2ᵉ	07	1 out of 62
3ᵉ	11	60
1ᵉʳ	11	58
4ᵉ	15	58
11ᵉ	19	51
6ᵉ	21	54
5ᵉ	22	53
7ᵉ	22	52
10ᵉ	23	50
9ᵉ	31	44
8ᵉ	32	43
12ᵉ	38	43

Source: From "Mémoire sur la mortalité en France," p. 63. Mortality figures are from tables 1817–21 in *Recherches statistiques*.

differing mortality rates.[32] Systematically, he examined and refuted all traditional causes advanced by hygienists to account for the healthfulness, or *salubrité*, of an area. He checked the distance from, and proximity to, the river as a possible factor but could establish no constant correlation. He then considered various topographical and climatic conditions that might affect mortality rates, such as elevation, type of soil, and exposure to wind, but these factors too seemed to exert no appreciable influence. Nor did the width of streets, the height of houses, the number of gardens and squares, the direction of streets and winds, the availability of sunlight, or the purity of the water appear to have any direct influence on mortality rates.

32 "De la mortalité dans les divers quartiers de la ville de Paris." For this article Villermé also had access to the 1822–6 mortality statistics, in addition to those for 1817–21, which he had used in the first article. The material for this article came from the *Recherches statistiques sur la ville de Paris*, under the direction of Villot, head of the Bureau of Archives and Statistics of the Department of the Seine. In 1825 Villot addressed to the Royal Academy of Medicine a series of tables in manuscript on the movement of population in Paris from 1817 to 1821. The Academy designated a commission to make a report on Villot's work, with Villermé being named reporter. Other members of the commission were Desgenettes, Desmarest, Esquirol, J. B. Fourier, Jacquemin, and Yvain. Villermé enlarged the work to include the years 1822–6, taken out of the recently published Volume 4 of the *Recherches statistiques*. See Villermé, "De la mortalité dans les divers quartiers," p. 294, and "Rapport lu à l'Académie," pp. 216–47.

Table 2. *List of rich and poor departments of France*

Department	Average annual mortality for five years
Mortality of the rich departments of France, 1817–21	
Calvados	1 out of 50.70
Côte d'Or	43.83
Eure	43.87
Eure-et-Loir	43.46
Gironde	44.05
Loire-Inférieure	45.33
Lot-et-Garonne	46.68
Maine-et-Loire	45.23
Manche	48.58
Orne	50.70
Pas-de-Calais	44.35
Sarthe	50.65
Deux-Sèvres	48.28
Average for all rich departments	46.31
Mortality of the poor departments of France, 1817–21	
Hautes-Alpes	1 out of 34.93
Cher	36.25
Corrèze	37.99
Côtes-du-Nord	33.50
Finistère	26.26
Ille-et-Vilaine	34.72
Indre	37.87
Landes	36.12
Lozère	37.19
Loire	34.05
Haute-Loire	38.46
Morbihan	31.24
Nièvre	35.89
Haute-Vienne	35.25
Average for all poor departments	33.72

Source: Tables V and VI at the end of "Mémoire sur la mortalité," pp. 91–2. Certain rich and poor departments were not included because of special circumstances affecting mortality. See "De la mortalité," pp. 88, 90.

Villermé's findings flatly contradicted traditional theories: The arrondissement that should have had the lowest mortality rate, according to the climatic theory, in actuality had the next to the highest. And the arrondissement that had the least favorable climatic and salubrious conditions had

Table 3. *Proportion of surface area occupied by buildings in twelve*
arrondissements of Paris: arrondissements ranked from least crowded to
most crowded

Arrondissement	Percentage of surface area occupied by buildings
5ᵉ	46
8ᵉ	46
10ᵉ	53
3ᵉ	55
11ᵉ	55
1ᵉ	57
4ᵉ	59
9ᵉ	60
6ᵉ	62
12ᵉ	64
2ᵉ	75
7ᵉ	82

Ranked according to mortality rates from lowest to highest: 2ᵉ, 3ᵉ, 1ᵉ and 4ᵉ, 6ᵉ, 5ᵉ, 7ᵉ, 11ᵉ, 10ᵉ, 9ᵉ, 8ᵉ and 12ᵉ

Source: "De la mortalité dans les divers quartiers de la ville de Paris," p. 305.

the lowest mortality rate. Based on this research, Villermé could find no explanation for the great differences in mortality rates from one arrondissement to another in geographical location, in climatic conditions, or in what hygienists regarded as a healthful situation. He then examined another traditional theory that related crowded conditions and high population density to mortality. Mortality rates were higher in cities than in small towns and in the countryside, and hygienists had therefore postulated that houses crowded together and narrow streets caused disease, for humans crowded together vitiated the breathing air. Using documents from arrondissement surveys done by the Prefecture of the Seine, Villermé calculated the amount of surface area covered by buildings in each arrondissement. The greater the proportion of surface area covered by buildings, the less space there was available for gardens, squares, trees, and wide streets – those conditions that allowed for fresh air and sunlight and were considered health-promoting. The figures suggested that in Paris the width of streets and the number of squares, gardens, and trees did not contribute as much as had been thought to the healthfulness of an area. The arrondissements with the highest mortality rates were among those with the most open space, and vice versa (Table 3). Villermé then checked to see if high population density was related to high mortality rates, but he found no

Table 4. *Population density of twelve arrondissements of Paris, ranked from least densely populated to most densely populated*

Arrondissement	Average amount of surface area occupied by each individual, in square meters
1er	64.51
8^e	46.83
12^e	36.98
10^e	46.24^a
2^e	25.87
11^e	21.87
5^e	18.65
9^e	16.47
3^e	15.31
6^e	12.74
7^e	10.61
4^e	6.56

Ranked according to mortality rates from lowest to highest: 2e, 3e, 1er and 4e, 6e, 5e, 7e, 11e, 10e, 9e, 8e and 12^e

^{a} This is obviously an error; it probably should be 36.24.
Source: "De la mortalité dans les divers quartiers de la ville de Paris," p. 306.

consistent correlation. For example, the fourth arrondissement, which had the highest population density in the city, had one of the lowest mortality rates. Conversely, some of the least densely populated arrondissements had the highest mortality rates (Table 4). Some hygienists confused population density and overcrowded conditions. Villemé made a distinction, maintaining that high population density per se was not necessarily a cause of disease and death unless accompanied by poverty. Overcrowded conditions connoted poverty; high population density alone did not. This same distinction was later made in the 1834 report by the cholera commission. Villermé's findings suggested that in Paris, population density did not explain varying mortality rates.

Finally, Villermé examined the effect of cleanliness, adequate clothing and shelter, and good food and drink on mortality rates. As all these factors were related to a certain degree of affluence, Villermé postulated that a comparison of the wealth of the population of a given area would be a way to measure the influence of these factors on health and mortality. Property tax records provided a general indication of living standards, for the poor paid no taxes. Using the property tax records for each arrondissement, Villermé found that as the proportion of poor in an arrondissement increased, so did the mortality rates. Conversely, the wealthiest arrondissements had the lowest mortality rates (Table 5). The final, somewhat

Table 5. *Correlation of wealth and mortality rates in twelve arrondissements of Paris. Arrondissements ranked from wealthiest to poorest based on property taxes*

Arrondissement	Untaxed Property, or percentages of poor families	At-home mortality 1817–21	1822–6
2ᵉ	07	1 out of 62	71
3ᵉ	11	60	67
1ᵉʳ	11	58	66
4ᵉ	15	58	62
11ᵉ	19	51	61
6ᵉ	21	54	58
5ᵉ	22	53	64
7ᵉ	22	52	59
10ᵉ	23	50	49
9ᵉ	31	44	50
8ᵉ	32	43	46
12ᵉ	38	43	44

Source: "De la mortalité dans les divers quartiers," pp. 296–7, 310. Typographical errors on p. 310 have been corrected, based on other tables in Villermé's articles.

revolutionary, conclusion that Villermé reached in the second study was that climatic and topographical factors, which hygienists and physicians had said exerted a great influence on health, could not explain the marked difference in mortality rates from one area of the city to another, the effect of these causes being masked by the affluence or misery of the population.

Villermé added to these two studies his other research on prison mortality, the height of Frenchmen, and the average duration of illnesses at different ages, as well as the research of his colleague, Benoiston de Châteauneuf, and concluded that the health of the poor was always precarious, that they were shorter in stature, and that their mortality was excessive in comparison with the health, physical development, and mortality of people in the comfortable and wealthy classes. Affluence and the material conditions it provided were truly the first among health conditions, he asserted. Villermé provided statistical documentation for what many French hygienists and social investigators had been predisposed to believe, namely, that the poor were sicklier and died earlier than the comfortable classes.[33]

33 "Mémoire sur la mortalité dans les prisons"; "Mémoire sur la taille de l'homme en France," *Annales d'hygiène publique* 1 (1829): 351–99; "Sur la durée moyenne des maladies aux différens âges," *Annales d'hygiène publique* 2 (1829): 241–66. See Benoiston de Châteauneuf's tables at the end of Villermé's "Mémoire sur la mortalité," pp. 95–8. Louis-François Benoiston de Châteauneuf (1776–1856), a former army surgeon, was a leading statistician-hygienist in the 1820s and 1830s.

By 1831, the results of Villermé's statistical investigations were well known to hygienists, physicians, and government officials both in France and abroad. Villermé had reported on his research to the Royal Academy of Sciences in 1824 and the Royal Academy of Medicine in 1826. His colleague, Benoiston de Châteauneuf, whose investigations complemented his own, had presented a report to the Royal Academy of Sciences in 1830. Several articles by both men had been published in the *Annales d'hygiène publique*. There was also substantial coverage of Villermé's research in other journals and in the major Parisian newspapers. The Paris health council incorporated the Villermé thesis into its 1829 report, noting that epidemics nearly always took a higher toll of lives among the poor than the rich and that misery was the main cause of disease.[34]

Thus by 1831, when cholera was moving westward across Europe and when French hygienists and the government began to consider preventive measures, many French hygienists and physicians subscribed to the Villermé hypothesis, maintaining that mortality and morbidity were higher among the poor than the affluent. A sampling of M.D. theses, pamphlets, and articles published on cholera reveals that it was a widely held belief that the disease would take more lives among the poor than among the comfortable classes.[35] Commissions sent by the French government to Eastern Europe and England to investigate the cause and course of

34 Villermé's "De la mortalité dans les divers quartiers de la ville de Paris" had appeared in the *Annales d'hygiène publique* in 1830. His "Rapport lu à l'Académie royale de Médecine" had been published in the *Archives générales de médecine* in 1826. See also Benoiston de Châteauneuf, "De la durée de la vie chez le riche et chez le pauvre," *Annales d'hygiène publique* 3 (1830): 5–51, a copy of a report sent to the Royal Academy of Sciences: Benoiston de Châteauneuf, "Note lu à l'Académie des Sciences, sur les changemens qu'ont subis les lois de la mortalité." See also Chevalier, *Classes laborieuses*, pp. 32–8, for a discussion of the dissemination of statistical information. *Rapports généraux des travaux du Conseil de salubrité pendant les années 1829 à 1839 inclusivement* (Paris: Imprimerie municipale, 1840), 1829: 22–3, 34. The editors of the 1829 report had the benefit of hindsight, for the report was not written until 1833, at which time the cholera epidemic had provided a test case.

35 A vast number of articles, pamphlets, and theses were published on cholera. See, for example, François Leuret, "Mémoire sur l'épidémie, désignée sous le nom de choléra-morbus," *Annales d'hygiène publique* 6 (1831): 313, 384, 432; Henri Scoutetten, *A Medical and Topographical History of the Cholera-Morbus, including the Mode of Prevention and Treatment*, trans. A. Sidney Doane (Boston: Carter and Hendee, 1832), pp. 21–2, 53, 71, 81; François Boisseau, *Traité du choléra-morbus considéré sous le rapport médical et administratif* (Paris: Baillière, 1832), pp. 162, 165, 191; Adolphe Valérian, *Considérations générales sur le choléra-morbus épidémique, suivies de quelques conseils hygiéniques adressés à mes concitoyens* (Montpellier: M.D. thesis, 1832), p. 44; B. Saturnin Lataste, *Aperçu sur le choléra épidémique* (Montpellier: M.D. thesis, 1832), p. 16; F. Fougnot, *Dissertation sur le choléra-morbus épidémique* (Paris: M.D. thesis, 1832), p. 9; L. F. Trolliet, A. P. Isidore de Polinière, and Alexandre Bottex, *Rapport sur le choléra-morbus de Paris* (Lyon: Babeuf, 1832), pp. 22–3. See the recent works on cholera in France: François Delaporte, *Disease and Civilization: The Cholera in Paris, 1832* (Cambridge, MA: MIT Press, 1986); Patrice Bourdelais and Jean-Yves Raulot, *Une Peur bleue: Histoire du choléra en France, 1832–1854* (Paris: Payot, 1987).

the disease returned reports that pointed to poverty and unsanitary conditions as the main predisposing causes.[36] Before cholera invaded France, for public health and political reasons, hygienists and physicians had been careful to point out that the disease cut across class lines, taking its victims indiscriminately, but hygienists generally believed that the poor would suffer the most. François Leuret reported that the wealthy in Berlin and Vienna had not been spared. But after the epidemic had run its course in Paris, statistical data showed that the poor had suffered more than the comfortable and wealthy classes.[37]

The Paris cholera epidemic offered a good opportunity to test the Villermé hypothesis. When cholera invaded the city in the spring of 1832, the municipal administration began keeping accurate mortality records, which, after the epidemic was over, could be used for a scientific investigation of the disease and how it had chosen its victims. At the request of the prefect of police, a commission of the Paris health council prepared a report on preventive measures and instructions in case the disease invaded the city. The commission recommended, among other things, that all physicians, surgeons, and health officials should keep an exact record of the sick they cared for – their names, sex, professions, and addresses – as well as clinical observations.[38] In Paris, an analysis of cholera mortality statistics showed higher mortality among the poor. In 1832, after the worst of the epidemic was over, Villermé was appointed to a commission, along with Benoiston de Châteauneuf, Parent-Duchâtelet, and others, to prepare a report. The commission published its official report in 1834. Although the report did not endorse the Villermé hypothesis, it did lend further support to it. Having examined all possible causes to explain varying mortality rates from one area of Paris to another, the commission concluded that in most cases, but not all, mortality was higher in poor, overcrowded areas. The commission made a distinction between overcrowding and high population density. Overcrowding connoted poor living condi-

36 George Sussman, "From Yellow Fever to Cholera: A Study of French Government Policy, Medical Professionalism and Popular Movements in the Epidemic Crises of the Restoration and the July Monarchy" (Ph.D. dissertation, Yale University, 1971), pp. 215–16; Erwin Ackerknecht, "Anticontagionism between 1821 and 1856," *Bull. Hist. Med.* 22 (1948): 576–7; Scoutetten, *A Medical and Topographical History of the Cholera-Morbus.* Scoutetten had been sent by the government to Berlin to observe the cholera.

37 See, for example, Leuret, "Mémoire sur l'épidémie" pp. 313–14; Lataste, *Aperçu sur le choléra,* p. 16. Villermé referred to both points of view in "Des épidémies sous les rapports de l'hygiène publique, de la statistique médicale et de l'économie politique," *Annales d'hygiène publique* 9 (1833): 7. Villermé maintained (p. 55) that the poor suffered the most not only during the cholera epidemic but during all epidemics.

38 *Rapports généraux des travaux du Conseil de salubrité pendant les années 1829 à 1839 inclusivement* (Paris: Imprimerie municipale, 1840), 1830–4, p. 79. See also the *Moniteur universel* for 1832, in which mortality statistics were published daily.

tions and was found to be a contributing cause of disease. High population density did not necessarily connote poverty. Even before the publication of the official report, Villermé had demonstrated his hypothesis in an article on the incidence of cholera in the furnished lodgings (*maisons garnies*) of Paris. Villermé found that in the lodgings of the wealthy and middle class (hotels, pensions) the disease had taken very few victims, whereas in the lodgings of the poor and the dregs of society (cheap boarding houses) the proportionate number of victims was much higher.[39]

As a result of statistical studies carried out independently during the 1830s and 1840s, other statisticians and hygienists, both French and foreign, arrived at conclusions similar to those of Villermé and the cholera commission. Comparing the mortality rates of a poor control group and a rich one, Benoiston de Châteauneuf found that the mortality rates of the poor were significantly higher than those of the rich; in some age brackets the rates were almost twice as high, leading him to conclude that longevity was closely related to wealth.[40] Foreign statisticians whose works were

39 Benoiston de Châteauneuf et al., *Rapport sur la marche et les effets du choléra-morbus dans Paris et les communes rurales du département de la Seine* (Paris: Imprimerie royale, 1834). Other members of the commission were Alphonse Chevallier, chemist and member of the Paris health council; Devaux, auditor to the Conseil d'Etat; Millot, of the Ecole Polytechnique; Petit, a physician and member of the Paris health council; Pontonnier, head of the First Division at the Prefecture of the Seine; Adolphe Trébuchet, head of the sanitary office at the Prefecture of Police; and Frédéric Villot, head of the statistical office at the Prefecture of the Seine. An abridged English translation of the work is, *Report on the Cholera in Paris* (New York: Samuel S. and William Wood, 1849), translated and printed on the recommendation of the Board of Health and the Academy of Medicine of the City of New York. *Report on the Cholera*, pp. 72, 164; Sussman has an interesting discussion on the findings and conclusions of the commission in "From Yellow Fever to Cholera," pp. 329–47. On the report on the cholera commission, see also Delaporte, *Cholera in Paris*. See Villermé, "Note sur les ravages du choléra-morbus dans les maisons garnies de Paris, depuis le 29 mars jusqu'au 1er août 1832, et sur les causes qui paraissent avoir favorisé le développement de la maladie dans un grand nombre de maisons," *Annales d'hygiène publique* 11 (1834): 385–410.

40 "De la durée de la vie chez le riche et chez le pauvre," *Annales d'hygiène publique* 3 (1830): 5–15. The article had originally been an essay sent to the Royal Academy of Sciences. In a report read to the Academy of Political and Moral Sciences on July 25, 1840, entitled "Sur la durée de la vie chez les savants et les gens de lettres," he related profession and longevity rather than wealth and longevity. See *Mém. de l'Acad. des Sci. Mor. et Pol.* 3 (1841): 627–53. Benoiston de Châteauneuf published many articles in the *Annales d'hygiène publique*. Along with Villermé, he was a member of the Academy of Political and Moral Sciences and collaborated with Villermé on the inquiry that resulted in the *Tableau de l'état physique et moral des ouvriers*. See *Mém. de l'Acad. des Sci. Mor. et Pol.* 2 (1839): li–lxiii. Villermé and Benoiston de Châteauneuf also collaborated on other works at the request of the Academy of Political and Moral Sciences. For example, see Benoiston de Châteauneuf and Villermé, "Rapport d'un voyage fait dans les cinq départements de la Bretagne, pendant les années 1840, 1841, d'après les ordres de l'Académie des Sciences morales et politiques," *Mém. de l'Acad. des Sci. Mor. et Pol.* 4 (1844): 635–782. Villermé used the work of Benoiston de Châteauneuf, citing him as a source and adding some of his tables as an appendix to his article on mortality in Paris.

published in the *Annales d'hygiène publique* and whose investigations were therefore well known to the French hygienists, such as Johann Ludwig Casper of Berlin and Edouard Mallet, Francis d'Ivernois, H. C. Lombard, and Marc d'Espine, all of Geneva, also investigated the causes of varying mortality rates. Acknowledging the pioneering work of Villermé, they elaborated on some of his findings and examined ramifications of his hypothesis. They all reached conclusions that stressed the influence of affluence and misery on mortality rates. Casper investigated the influence of civil state on longevity. Finding that married people lived longer than single ones, he postulated that the married were probably wealthier, and suggested that it was level of affluence rather than civil state that was the determining factor. Mallet, who studied the Genevan population from the sixteenth to the nineteenth centuries, and Lombard, who examined the influence of profession on longevity, reached conclusions similar to those of Villermé. Lombard's data indicated that the affluence associated with varying professions was the major determining factor, with the difference in longevity between the poor and affluent classes of workers being seven and one-half years, or one-eighth of the total life span.[41]

Analysis of population statistics led Sir Francis d'Ivernois to accept wholeheartedly the Villermé hypothesis. Ivernois modified Villermé's argument, emphasizing that it was *nonmisery* that prolonged life, rather than affluence (the absence of poverty rather than the presence of wealth).

41 Johann Ludwig Casper, "De l'influence du mariage sur la durée de la vie humaine," *Annales d'hygiène publique* 14 (1835): 227–39. Edouard Mallet, "Recherches historiques et statistiques sur la population de Genève, son mouvement annuel et sa longévité depuis le XVIe siècle jusqu'à nos jours (1549–1833)," *Annales d'hygiène publique* 17 (1837): 5–172. Geneva had been an important center for statistical studies since the eighteenth century. In the early nineteenth century there were at least four major statisticians in Geneva, all of whose works were regularly published in the *Annales d'hygiène publique*: H. C. Lombard, Marc d'Espine, Edouard Mallet, and Sir Francis d'Ivernois. Geneva was a good place for statistical studies, for mortality records according to age had been kept since 1560, and probable life expectancies and average length of life had been figured out by statisticians since the sixteenth century (Cramer: 1560–1770; Joly and Odier: 1771–1813; Mallet: 1814–33). Marc d'Espine also believed that the city was convenient for statistical studies, as it was composed of what he called "a complete and natural population." This material on Geneva comes from Marc d'Espine, "Notice statistique sur les lois de mortalité et de survivance aux divers âges de la vie humaine, sur la vie moyenne et la vie probable d'après les 10,203 décès qui ont eu lieu dans le canton de Genève pendant les 8 années de 1838 à 1845," *Annales d'hygiène publique* 38 (1847): 289–322. Sir Francis d'Ivernois did not share this opinion, however. He believed that peculiar circumstances prevailed in Geneva that made it a bad place to use as an example, and that statistical generalizations derived from using Geneva as a base were likely to be inaccurate. See "Exposé des principales erreurs qui prévalent sur le sujet des populations," the "Second Letter to Dr. Villermé." H. C. Lombard, "De l'influence des professions sur la durée de la vie," *Annales d'hygiène publique* 14 (1835): 88–131. Lombard referred specifically to Villermé's research, stating that by using a different method, Villermé had earlier reached the same conclusions. See p. 104.

Ivernois showed how the infant mortality rate was a sure guide to the misery or affluence of a civilization, maintaining that the most affluent countries had fewer babies and conserved them better, whereas poorer countries had higher birth and infant mortality rates. Ivernois concurred with Laplace that the prosperity of a nation could be judged by an analysis of its population. Ivernois's optimism about increasing longevity, probable life expectancy, and declining mortality rates was guarded, however. Emphasizing the influence of affluence on mortality, he suggested that this favorable situation was probably limited to affluent urban populations, and that lower mortality rates among the poorer classes and rural inhabitants were probably due to a decrease in famines and plagues rather than an improved standard of living.[42]

Marc d'Espine's research on the Genevan population from 1838 to 1843 also confirmed Villermé's findings. Establishing two control groups of rich and poor from the statistical records of citizens who had died, Espine found the average age of death among the rich to have been 53.2. years, whereas among the poor it was only 40.8, with the average for the population as a whole for those years being 42.2. He concluded that misery shortened life by two years, while affluence prolonged it by eleven years.[43]

Additional research by Villermé in the 1830s on morbidity and mortality rates among the working classes further strengthened his hypothesis. In several articles and finally in his major work on French textile workers, the *Tableau de l'état physique et moral des ouvriers...*, Villermé confirmed his earlier conclusions and proved by additional statistical evidence that the original hypothesis held true under a variety of circumstances. Opposing the views of many social investigators who believed that industrialization per se was a cause of the unhealthiness and high mortality of workers, Villermé concluded that the real plagues of the working class were low

---

42 See the second letter to Villermé, "Exposé des principales erreurs qui prévalent sur le sujet des populations." Perhaps the most interesting of the Genevan statisticians, Ivernois had been in exile in England from 1792 to 1814. See Ackerknecht, "Villermé and Quetelet," p. 325. He and Villermé carried on an active correspondence during the 1830s, Ivernois's principal ideas being succinctly expressed in three letters written to Villermé in 1833 and 1834, all of which were analyzed in the bibliographical section of the *Annales d'hygiène publique*. For reviews of the first two letters, see "Bibliographie," *Annales d'hygiène publique* 12 (1834): 200–3; for a review of the third letter, see "Bibliographie," *Annales d'hygiène publique* 13 (1835): 519. First letter to Villermé, *Sur la mortalité proportionnelle des populations normandes*. Third letter to Villermé, *Sur la mortalité proportionnelle des peuples*.

43 Marc d'Espine, "Influence de l'aisance et de la misère sur la mortalité. Recherches critiques et statistiques," *Annales d'hygiène publique* 37 (1847): 323–57, and continued in 38 (1847): 5–32. Villermé reported on Espine's work at the Academy of Political and Moral Sciences, praising his public health work in Geneva and his research on the correlation of wealth and mortality. See *Séances et trav. de l'Acad. des Sci. Mor. et Pol.* 12 (1847): 242–8. Espine spoke favorably of Villermé's work, stating that Villermé had given a truly scientific basis to the question and his research had solved the problem in a general sense (pp. 323–6).

wages and long working hours, which predisposed them to disease and death.[44]

In his application of statistical analysis to public health and social questions, Villermé stands out as a primary exponent of the scientific methodology that characterized the French public health movement. By quantitative documentation he proved – according to the standards of the age – the validity of the long-held belief that the poor suffered more from disease and died earlier than the rest of the population. Villermé's methodology is, however, open to criticism. Like most of his contemporaries, he relied on official sources, primarily data gathered by the municipal authorities and published in the *Recherches statistiques sur la ville de Paris.* He had no control group, but instead used fluctuating populations (in a department, arrondissement, or quarter). Furthermore, some of the mortality statistics he used were not compiled by age distribution. Villermé was aware of these difficulties and lamented the incompleteness of French official statistics, which did not furnish age, sex, or occupation.[45] Finally, Villermé's samplings were too small to be valid. But Villermé must be judged according to early-nineteenth-century standards and the standards of his profession. Even though the gathering of statistical information antedated 1800, by the 1820s methods of statistical analysis were not widely understood. There were no general agreement in scientific circles on the value of statistics or even on its definition, much less on the way data should be gathered and interpreted.[46] Villermé's methodology constituted a radical departure from the treatment traditionally given public health questions. By using statistical data to support their theories, Villermé, Parent-Duchâtelet, and other hygienists contributed to the transformation of public hygiene from an armchair philosophy to a scientific discipline.[47]

44 "Sur la population de la Grande-Bretagne," *Annales d'hygiène publique* 12 (1834): 217–71; "Nouveaux détails concernant l'influence du développement excessif des manufactures sur la population en Angleterre," *Annales d'hygiène publique* 13 (1835): 344–53; "Sur la durée trop longue du travail des enfans dans beaucoup de manufactures," *Annales d'hygiène publique* 18 (1837): 164–76; *Tableau de l'état physique et moral des ouvriers employés dans les manufacturers de coton, de laine et de soie,* 2 vols. (Paris: Jules Renouard, 1840).

45 *Séances et trav. de l'Acad. des Sci. Mor. et Pol.* 7 (1845): 7–10.

46 The science of statistics was still in its infancy. In 1832 the *Journal des Débats* lambasted the Royal Academy of Sciences for the obscure and vague definition members gave for the new term: "statistics describes the climate, territory, and political and natural divisions." The *Journal des Débats* preferred to define statistics as the "descriptive part of political economy." See *Journal des Débats*, April 15, 1832, p. 4.

47 See Vedrenne-Villeneuve, "L'inégalité sociale devant la mort," pp. 679–90. Parent-Duchâtelet discussed these "armchair philosophers" in "Mémoire sur les véritables influences que le tabac peut avoir sur la santé des ouvriers," *Hygiène publique*, 2: 560. See pp. 564–7 for a discussion of authors whom Parent accused of accepting old theories without testing them. See also Parent-Duchâtelet, "Mémoire sur les débardeurs de la ville de Paris," *Hygiène publique*, 2: 614–18, 640.

Villermé's studies on differing mortality rates had a great impact on public health theory both in France and abroad. His findings furnished what was considered to be scientific proof for the dominant belief of the French hygienists: that public health improvements were concomitant with the advance of civilization. Villermé illustrated this theory in an article on epidemics written after the Paris cholera epidemic, contending that as civilization advanced, both the frequency and the intensity of epidemics decreased, and when an epidemic did occur, the poor classes, those who had benefited least from the progress of civilization, suffered the most. Villermé had shown in his earlier study on mortality in Paris that the Parisian poor in the 1820s were dying at the same rate as the whole Parisian population in the fourteenth century. This comparison suggested that although the proportional mortality of the affluent had declined significantly through the centuries, whole segments of the population had been exempt from the progress of civilization. Only as affluence became more widespread, Villermé asserted, would these elements of society realize decreasing mortality rates.[48] Villermé's studies on differing mortality rates also provided scientific evidence for the belief of many hygienists that diseases had social as well as biological and chemical causes. Villermé's research established a statistical basis for the so-called social theory of epidemiology, an important component of the prevailing environmental theory of disease causation. His research confirmed the beliefs of many hygienists, physicians, and social reformers, who maintained that social problems were at the root of many diseases. Villermé's statistical investigations also had an impact on public health theory outside of France. British hygienists such as Southwood Smith and Edwin Chadwick and Rudolf Virchow in Germany were influenced by Villermé's statistical work, accepting his data as proof of the social causes of disease and differing mortality, and incorporating his thesis into their own public health theories.[49]

48 "Des épidémies sous les rapports de l'hygiène publique," *Annales d'hygiène publique* 9 (1833): 5–18, 55–8; "De la mortalité dans les divers quartiers de la ville de Paris," pp. 335–7; It was not a question of medical advances resulting in lower mortality rates. At this time, even vaccination did not seem to have an appreciable influence on mortality rates. See Villermé, "Des épidémies," pp. 36–42. It was not until late in the nineteenth century that medical developments seemed to influence mortality rates. Most authors ascribe decreasing mortality rates before the late nineteenth century to material improvements, such as better diet. On this question see Thomas McKeown, *The Modern Rise of Population* (New York: Academic Press, 1976). On the social theory of epidemiology see George Rosen, "What Is Social Medicine? A Genetic Analysis of the Concept," *Bull. Hist. Med.* 21 (1947): 674–733.

49 Ann F. La Berge, "Edwin Chadwick and the French Connection," *Bull. Hist. Med.* 62(1988): 23–41; Erwin Ackerknecht, *Rudolf Virchow: Doctor, Statesman, Anthropologist* (Madison: University of Wisconsin Press, 1953), pp. 46, 128. See also George Rosen, "What Is Social Medicine?" pp. 676–7, 684.

The wide dissemination and rapid acceptance by leading French hygienists of research like that of Villermé helped give the public health movement its decidedly social tone. Later research proved the validity of the theories held by the nineteenth-century social epidemiologists. Writing in the 1890s, for example, statistician Jacques Bertillon pointed out that infant mortality rates were almost three times as high in the poor as in the wealthy arrondissements of Paris. For the years 1893–7 in a wealthy arrondissement, the eighth, the infant mortality rate was 108.5/1000, whereas for the poor fourteenth, the figure was 309.6/1000. Unable to identify specific disease-causing organisms, nineteenth-century hygienists emphasized the social and material environments in which disease developed and advocated both sanitary and social reform as the most effective public health measures.[50]

Among the French hygienists, Villermé was the leading spokesman for statistics and public health. He corresponded with leading foreign statisticians such as Quetelet and Ivernois and publicized their work in France. Quetelet and Villermé carried on an active correspondence, dating from the 1820s, when Quetelet visited Paris and made the acquaintance of Fourier, Villermé, and other statisticians.[51] As an editor of the *Annales d'hygiène publique*, Villermé promoted statistics as a tool for public hygienists and ensured the publicity of statistics by publishing articles by French and other European statisticians. The works of Casper, Espine, Mallet, Lombard, Ivernois, Quetelet, and Benoiston de Châteauneuf all appeared in the journal. By 1835, when Quetelet's pathbreaking work *Sur l'homme et le développement de ses facultés ou essai de physique sociale* was published, much of the material had already appeared as articles in the *Annales d'hygiène publique*. New books on statistics were reviewed in the bibliographical section, and occasionally letters exchanged between Villermé and other statisticians were published. By publicizing statistical work being done in Prussia, Belgium, Geneva, and Great Britain, Villermè

50 On the relationship between standard of living and disease, see Thomas McKeown and C. R. Lowe, *An Introduction to Social Medicine* (London: Blackwell Scientific Publications, 1974), pp. 67–70. The whole work is pertinent. Bertillon, cited in Ann-Louise Shapiro, *Housing the Poor of Paris, 1852–1902* (Madison: University of Wisconsin Press, 1985), p. 184.

51 The correspondence of Villermé and Sir Francis d'Ivernois has already been mentioned. We know that Ivernois wrote three long letters to Villermé, because they were all published either in pamphlet form or as articles in journals. In addition, they were reported on in the *Annales d'hygiène publique*. Yet unfortunately, no letters from Villermé have been discovered, nor did Villermé mention any. It is possible that additional correspondence between them took place, but I have found neither the correspondence nor any reference to it. See the correspondence between Villermé and Quetelet; also see Ackerknecht, "Villermé and Quetelet"; for articles by Quetelet that appeared in the *Annales d'hygiène publique*, see 3 (1830): 24–36; 7 (1832): 361–8; 9 (1833): 303–36; 10 (1833): 5–27; 12 (1834): 294–311; for a report in the Royal Academy of Medicine of Quetelet's work by Villermé, see "Bibliographie," *Annales d'hygiène publique* 8 (1832): 459–66.

and the other editors of the journal hoped to improve the accuracy of French statistics and make them more useful to public hygienists. For example, censuses taken in other countries were reported on, giving Villermé a chance to comment on the insufficiency of official French statistics. The *Annales d'hygiène publique,* under the editorship of Villermé and his hygienist colleagues, served as the forum for the exchange of statistical knowledge applied to public health questions.

In addition, through reports of Villermé and others at the Royal Academy of Medicine, the Royal Academy of Sciences, and the Academy of Political and Moral Sciences, French physicians and public hygienists became acquainted with statistical work being done elsewhere in Europe on population and public health. For example, Villermé reported on censuses taken in Sardinia and Prussia to the Academy of Political and Moral Sciences, stressing the superiority of Sardinian and Prussian official statistics to French official statistics, which were known to be incomplete.[52] The founders of the Academy of Political and Moral Sciences recognized the importance of statistics, devoting one of the sections of the academy to political economy and statistics. This was the section to which Villermé belonged. Other renowned statisticians and political economists were elected to the academy: Benoiston de Châteauneuf was admitted as an *académicien libre*; Thomas Malthus was a foreign associate; and Quetelet was a corresponding member. The Royal Academy of Medicine, of which Villermé was a member, also debated statistical topics. An 1826 statistical commission from the Royal Academy of Medicine, of which Villermé was chairman, did much of the initial research on Parisian mortality rates, using data from the *Recherches statistiques sur la ville de Paris.* The commission arrived at the tentative conclusion, which Villermé would later elaborate on elsewhere, that poverty was the primary cause of bad health and high mortality in Paris.[53]

OFFICIAL STATISTICAL PUBLICATIONS

By the 1830s, French public hygienists recognized the importance of statistical analysis for investigating public health problems. It had also become

52 *Séances et trav. de l'Acad. des Sci. Mor. et Pol.* 9 (1846): 470–72; Villermé read a report on *Recensement des états prussiens en 1843* by M. W. Dieterici, director of the Bureau of Statistics in Berlin; "'Recensement de la population sarde pour l'année 1838,' Rapport verbal fait à l'Académie des Sciences Morales et Politiques, dans sa séance du 6 juin 1840," *Annales d'hygiène publique* 24 (1840): 241–64. The title of the Sardinian work was *Informazioni statistiche, etc. Censimento della popolazione* (Turin, 1839).

53 After its reorganization in 1829, the Academy was divided into eleven sections; section 8 was devoted to public hygiene, legal medicine, and medical police; in this section there were six titular members and four adjuncts. See *Mém. de l'Acad. Roy. de Méd.* 2 (1833): 61–5; Villermé, "Rapport lu à l'Académie Royale de Médecine au nom de la commission de statistique."

apparent to the national government, the Parisian administration, and the medical profession that statistical analysis was a method that could serve them well. Indeed, the gathering of statistical information by governments was not new, for monarchs had found it advantageous to have an exact accounting of their population and resources, the collection of such information in France dating from the seventeenth and eighteenth centuries. As early as the reign of Louis XIV, the French government had displayed an interest in keeping accurate population statistics, since population was considered a sign of wealth and power. Specific regulations related to the compilation of statistical information for Paris dated from 1670, when Colbert ordered that each month an extract of the civil registers should be compiled, giving births, deaths, marriages, and the number of hospital admissions. These figures were to be published annually, along with remarks on diseases observed during the year. The regulations went into effect in 1708.[54] The first attempt at a systematic assessment of the French population dated from 1697, when the central authority ordered Intendants to prepare reports on their areas of jurisdiction, including detailed historical, political, economic, and demographic descriptions. These reports, submitted from 1697 to 1700, served as the basis for most eighteenth-century French population studies. The most important of these studies was Montyon's *Recherches et considérations sur la population de la France*, published in 1778 under the name of Moheau and considered the first real population treatise in the French language.[55] In 1796 the government began publishing an annual statistical report, the *Annuaire* of the Bureau of Longitude, which contained – along with much other statistical information – birth and death statistics.

Between 1815 and 1848 two major official statistical collections were undertaken in France. The *Recherches statistiques sur la ville de Paris*, begun in the 1820s, was a project of the two prefects of the Seine, Gilbert Chabrol and Claude Rambuteau. The first four volumes were published between 1821 and 1829 when Chabrol was prefect of the Seine, and Volume 5 was published in 1844 under the prefecture of Rambuteau. Frédéric Villot, archivist and head of the statistical office at the prefecture of the Seine, was in charge of researching, coordinating, and tabulating the statistical information in the collection, and Jean-Baptiste Fourier, the leading French statistician, authored the introductory essays to Volumes 1 to 4, discussing the theory of probability and the methodology involved in

54 Paul E. Vincent, "French Demography in the Eighteenth Century," *Population Studies* I (1947–8): 44–59; on Montyon see also William Coleman, "Inventing Demography: Montyon on Hygiene and the State," in *Transformation and Tradition in the Sciences: Essays in Honor of I. Bernard Cohen*, ed. Everett Mendelsohn (New York: Cambridge University Press, 1984), pp. 215–35.
55 "Statistique. Mouvement de la population de la ville de Paris. Rapport fait à M. le préfet de la Seine, sur le recensement de 1846," *Annales d'hygiène publique* 39 (1848): 200.

gathering and interpreting statistics.[56] Although the collection contained statistical information on all aspects of Parisian life, the population statistics most interested the public hygienists.

The first two volumes of the *Statistique générale de la France*, a multi-volume statistical collection undertaken by the national government, were published in 1835. By 1852, thirteen volumes had appeared. Although many topics were covered, population was the major interest of hygienists. Volume 3, published in 1837, contained population statistics for the nation.[57] Alexandre Moreau de Jonnès, head of the statistical office of the Ministry of Commerce, was named director of the collection.

There was no direct relationship between the official French statistical collections and the public health movement. The collections were not undertaken for public health reasons, nor were the projects initiated at the instigation of public hygienists. However, statisticians and hygienists used the collections and acted as critics of official French statistics. Since population statistics were an important part of all three collections, it is at first glance curious that prominent statistician-hygienists like Benoiston de Châteauneuf and Villermé, both good friends of the government, were not more actively involved in the collection and publication of French official statistics. A brief discussion of the three collections will readily explain why this was the case. The *Annuaire* of the Bureau de Longitude antedated the French public health movement. It was eighteenth century in outlook, not having benefited from the advances made in statistical analysis by the French in the early nineteenth century. For example, as Villermé pointed out, the *Annuaire* presumed that the population was stationary and used the outmoded mortality table of Etienne Duvillard, which dated from the eighteenth century. The *Recherches statistiques sur la ville de Paris* antedated the statistical work of Villermé, who was in the early 1820s best known as a prison reformer.[58] When the collection was begun, one of the most

56 Hankins, *Adolphe Quetelet*, pp. 49–50; Villermé, "Des épidémies," p. 13. See in Volume 1, for example, the article by Fourier, "Notions générales sur la population," *Recherches statistiques* 1 (1821): ix–lxviii.

57 *Statistique générale de la France*, 34 vols. (Paris: Imprimerie royale, 1835–73). The other topics covered in the collection were territory, argriculture, mines, industry, commerce, navigation, colonies, interior administration, finance, military force, marine, justice, and public instruction. The title of Volume 3 was *Territoire et population*. The first two volumes are entitled *Documents statistiques sur la France*. For the first *Statistique générale*, undertaken during the Napoleonic era, see Marie-Noëlle Bourguet, "Décrire, Compter, Calculer: The Debate Over Statistics during the Napoleonic Period," in *The Probabilistic Revolution*, ed. Lorenz Kruger, Lorraine Daston, and Michael Heidelberger, 2 vols. (Cambridge, MA: MIT Press, 1987), 1: 305–16, and her book: *Déchiffrer la France: La statistique départementale à l'époque napoléonienne* (Paris: Editions des Archives Contemporaines, 1988).

58 Etienne Duvillard was an eighteenth-century mathematician who set up a mortality table and a mortality law still being used in France in the first half of the nineteenth century. See, for example, Villermé, "Sur la durée moyenne des maladies aux différens âges," *Annales d'hygiène publique* 2 (1829): 249–50; *Les prisons telles qu'elles sont et telles qu'elles devraient être* (Paris: Méquignon-Marvis, 1820).

prominent French statisticians, whose reputation was international, was Fourier, permanent secretary of the Royal Academy of Sciences from 1822 to 1830. Fourier, appointed to the Bureau of Statistics of the department of the Seine in 1815 by his personal friend Chabrol, oversaw the publication of the first four volumes of the *Recherches statistiques* and contributed an introductory article to each volume. Benoiston de Châteauneuf, who had already acquired a reputation in statistical circles following the publication in 1820 of his work on the consumption of foodstuffs in Paris, collaborated on the collection. He prepared one of the statistical tables for Volume 1. However, since most of the tables are without attribution, the extent of his participation cannot be determined. It is probable that Villot did most of the compilation and tabulation.[59]

By 1834, at the time of the inception of the *Statistique générale de la France*, Villermé's reputation as a public hygienist and statistician was secured, as was Benoiston de Châteauneuf's, whose statistical investigations after 1820 were along the same lines as those of Villermé. Benoiston de Châteauneuf had also done statistical research under the auspices of the Royal Academy of Sciences, and both men were members of the Academy of Political and Moral Sciences. It was then possible, given their professional qualifications, that either of these men might have been chosen to direct the program of collecting and publishing French national statistics.

Instead, Thiers chose Moreau de Jonnès. Although Villermé and Ivernois did not consider Moreau de Jonnès a competent statistician, he had been working in the field since his entry into the national administration in 1817. Moreau de Jonnès, a former naval officer, had a long-standing interest in statistics, and when Adolphe Thiers became Minister of Commerce in 1834, he put Moreau de Jonnès in charge of the statistical office. In 1816 Moreau de Jonnès had been named a corresponding member of the Royal Academy of Sciences following the publication of his essays on the geography, topography, and natural history of Martinique. In the 1820s he achieved a certain notoriety in public health circles as a champion of the government's contagionist policy vis-à-vis yellow fever and was a member of the Superior Health Council. In any case, the *Statistique générale* was not intended to concentrate on population statistics or health statistics, the areas in which Benoiston de Châteauneuf and Villermé had done most of

59 I. Grattan-Guinness, *Joseph Fourier, 1768–1830* (Cambridge, MA: MIT Press, 1972), pp. 456–7, 486–93. The articles by Fourier were "Notions générales sur la population," 1 (1821): lx–lxxviii; "Mémoire sur la population de la ville de Paris depuis la fin du XVIIe siècle," 2 (1823): xiii–xxviii; "Mémoire sur les résultats moyens déduits d'un grand nombre d'observations," 3 (1826): ix–xxxc; "Second mémoire sur les résultats moyens et les erreurs de mesures," 4 (1829): ix–xlviii. One table labeled as being compiled by Benoiston de Châteauneuf was the Table of Deaths Caused by Lung Disease, 1816–1819, which appeared in Volume 1. Benoiston de Châteauneuf, *Recherches sur les consommations de tout genre de la ville de Paris en 1817*, 2 vols. (Paris: Cosson, 1820–1). On Benoiston de Châteauneuf, see Coleman, *Death Is a Social Disease*, pp. 297–8.

their work, but was to be a general accounting of the nation's resources, a type of project being pursued in this era by many European state and municipal governments. Furthermore, in 1834, Villermé, in collaboration with Benoiston de Châteauneuf, embarked on another government project, the investigation of the condition of French textile workers, under the auspices of the Academy of Political and Moral Sciences.[60]

Hygienists used official statistical collections in spite of shortcomings, because they needed statistical data to test their theories and to gauge public health progress. They were therefore in a position, along with foreign hygienists and statisticians, to criticize the weaknesses of French official statistics and to show how they could be properly compiled to be more useful to researchers. The *Recherches statistiques* supplied more useful information for public hygienists than either the *Annuaire* or the *Statistique générale*. Hygienists praised the *Recherches statistiques* for its professional tone and scientific methodology. The most advanced methods available at the time were used in gathering and compiling material for the *Recherches statistiques*, and competent professionals were employed. Villermé expressed confidence in the collection, attesting to the authenticity and exactitude of the first two volumes, and he and Parent-Duchâtelet made extensive use of the collection in their research.[61] Another strength of the *Recherches statistiques* was that it furnished complete population statistics – in contrast to the *Annuaire* and the *Statistique générale*. The *Recherches statistiques* supplied the age, sex, and civil state of the Parisian population, and from this material it was possible to draw a population profile. In the mortality tables the collection provided both the number of deceased and age at time of death. Statistician-hygienists could therefore use the *Recherches statistiques* to compute average longevity rates as well as average probable life expectancies. The *Recherches statistiques* did have its faults, however. Villermé criticized the methodology, and Parent-Duchâtelet disputed some of the data. But as Chabrol had made clear in his introduction to Volume 1, the administration's goal in undertaking the collection was to acquire general knowledge of the population, not to produce a rigorous scientific document.[62]

60 Pierre Larousse, *Grand dictionnaire universel du XIXe siècle*, 17 vols. (Paris: Larousse and Boyer, 1866–90) 2: 556. In 1847 Moreau de Jonnès was named a *membre libre* of the Academy of Political and Moral Sciences. For an interesting discussion of Moreau de Jonnès, see Bourdelais and Raulot, *Histoire du choléra*, pp. 47, 67–8, 79, 160–1; *Tableau statistique du commerce de la France en 1824* (Paris: Rignoux, 1826); *Statistique de l'Espagne* (Paris: Cosson, 1834). The result was the *Tableau de l'état physique et moral des ouvriers employés dans les manufactures de coton, de laine et de soie*.

61 Villermé, "Rapport lu à l'Académie Royale de Médecine au nom de la commission de statistique," p. 216; Villermé, "Mémoire sur la mortalité en France," passim; Villermé, "De la mortalité dans les divers quartiers," pp. 294–5.

62 Villermé, "Mémoire sur la distribution de la population française," *Annales d'hygiène publique* 17 (1837): 266; Parent-Duchâtelet, "Les chantiers d'équarrissage de la ville de Paris," *Hygiène publique* 2: 160–1; Chabrol, "Extrait d'un rapport fait

Compared to the *Recherches statistiques* the two other collections were of limited value to hygienists, for they did not supply the age of the deceased, and therefore their figures could not be used to estimate probable life expectancies and average longevity rates. Nor did the *Statistique générale* give a profile of the whole population by age. The *Annuaire* furnished population figures according to age, but Villermé asserted that the information was not accurate because it assumed a stationary population. Because of the inadequacies of the *Annuaire* and the *Statistique générale*, Villermé and Ivernois maintained that French official statistics were some of the most backward in Europe, for they did not furnish adequate information on the population and scientific methods were not used in gathering data. Villermé pointed out how backward and inadequate French collections were compared with those of Belgium. Physician-hygienist François Mélier complained in a meeting of the Royal Academy of Medicine that the *Statistique générale* was unprofessional and unscientific. Pointing out serious omissions, Mélier contended that had the Royal Academy of Medicine or professional statisticians been consulted, they could have shown the administration how to compile accurate statistical tables.[63]

Had Mélier's suggestion been taken, the *Statistique générale* might have compared more favorably with the *Recherches statistiques* and other national collections. Yet there were problems. Although reasonably adequate population statistics existed for Paris, none were available for the whole nation. This gap could possibly have been filled had the methodology used in Paris been more closely followed. But, practically speaking, gathering accurate figures was almost impossible, for in many areas of France no reliable birth and death records were available. In addition, the problems involved in taking an accurate national census were legion. Villermé's solution for improving French official statistics was to follow the British model. He called for legislative intervention to bring about reform in collecting and recording statistical information. In both the United States and Great Britain, laws had been passed to provide for the gathering and collecting of population statistics. Villermé was especially impressed with the 1837

à son excellence, le Ministre de l'Intérieur par M. le Comte de Chabrol, Conseiller d'Etat, Préfet du Département de la Seine, le 3 juillet 1818," *Recherches statistiques* 1 (1821): lxxxiv.

63 "Mémoire sur la distribution de la population française," p. 266; *Séances et trav. de l'Acad. des Sci. Mor. et Pol.* 7 (1845): 7–10; "Quelques remarques sur les statistiques; propositions à ce sujet," *Bull. de l'Acad. Roy. de Méd.* 9 (1843–4): 700–5. On Mélier, see William Coleman, "Medicine against Malthus: François Mélier on the Relation between Subsistence and Morality (1843), *"Bull. Hist. Med.* 54 (1980): 23–42. See also William Coleman, *Yellow Fever in the North: The Methods of Early Epidemiology* (Madison: University of Wisconsin Press, 1987), pp. 59–138, for a discussion of Mélier's role in investigating the yellow fever epidemic in St.-Nazaire in 1861.

British Registration Act and urged the passage of a similar French law. He believed that were a law passed, prescribing the procedure and the exact day the census was to be taken, census takers might arrive at precise results.[64]

Although French hygienists lacked a good set of official national population statistics, they utilized data from other sources in order to quantify their research. These included statistical collections prepared in cities and departments, army recruitment figures, civil registers, and prison, hospital, and welfare records. Statistical information obtained from all these sources was of central importance to the public health movement, for such figures pointed out more accurately and clearly than words the factors that influenced mortality and morbidity. Statistical analysis was essential for the hygienists' claim to objectivity and scientific methodology.

In addition to gathering statistical information, the national government implemented a number of public health policies related to vaccination, health care, and epidemic control, all of which antedated the public health movement and provided the context in which the movement developed.

64   *Séances et trav. de l'Acad. des Sci. Mor. et Pol.* 7 (1845): 7–10; Villermé, "Mémoire sur la distribution de la population française," pp. 267–80. On statistics and public health in Britain, see John M. Eyler, *Victorian Social Medicine: The Ideas and Methods of William Farr* (Baltimore: Johns Hopkins, University Press, 1979). For earlier statistical work in Britain, see Ulrich Troehler, "Quantification in British Medicine and Surgery, 1750–1830, with Special Reference to Its Introduction into Therapeutics" (Ph.D. dissertation, University of London, 1978).

3

The context of public hygiene: National public health policy

The public health movement developed within the context of Restoration initiatives, policies, and institutions that reflected and built upon traditional public health concerns – epidemic prevention and control – as well as the public health idea inherited from the Enlightenment and Revolutionary eras. Hygienists believed that the scope of public health was all-encompassing; nothing was unrelated to the preservation of health. The Restoration government, however, took a more focused view, concentrating on a few specific problems and working through a limited number of institutions. Public health institutions and policies emanating from the Restoration government included the Royal Academy of Medicine, which advised the government on public health matters and helped shape national public health policy; the sanitary administration, created by the 1822 sanitary law, whose purpose was to prevent the importation of contagious epidemic diseases; and national health care policies and programs including *officiers de santé* and the *médecins des épidémies*, and the national vaccination program with its depositories (*dépôts de vaccine*) and committees.

THE ROYAL ACADEMY OF MEDICINE AND PUBLIC HEALTH

The Royal Academy of Medicine continued the policies and programs of the Royal Society of Medicine, advising the government on major public health questions. The Royal Society of Medicine was founded in 1776 as a governmental commission to deal with the problems of epidemics and epizootics, and during the late 1770s and 1780s it acted as a national clearinghouse, receiving information from its provincial correspondents and intendants and dispatching members to give assistance to areas invaded by epidemics.[1] The institution was founded with public health goals, the idea

---

1 The discussion of the Royal Society of Medicine is based on the following sources: Caroline Hannaway, "The Société Royale de Médecine and Epidemics in the Ancien Régime, *Bull. Hist. Med.* 46 (1972): 257–73; Charles C. Gillispie, *Science and Polity in France at the End of the Old Regime* (Princeton, NJ: Princeton Univer-

being that close collaboration between the Royal Society and the royal power would result in an effective national public health service. In one sense the Society's outlook regarding public health was traditional: Its principal aim was to protect the nation from epidemics, and to this end an epidemic service was created throughout the kingdom. But the program of the Society was also all-encompassing and forward-looking in its approach. Permanent inquiries were to be conducted into the sanitary state of the kingdom based on an active correspondence between provincial physicians and the Society; the Society would distribute instructions on the best methods of preventing and combatting diseases to its provincial correspondents; in each area a local epidemic service would be organized, and new remedies would be sent to the Society for examination. Imbued with the rational philosophy and the didactic impulse of the eighteenth century, the physicians of the Royal Society of Medicine wanted not only to minister to the immediate health needs of French citizens but also to spread enlightened ideas, which they believed went hand in hand.[2] Their mission was to preach the gospel of hygienism, which was becoming an important civilizing force. The members also investigated specific urban health problems, such as whether cemeteries should be moved out of the center of cities and how to provide cities with safe, abundant drinking water. The work of the Royal Society exemplified what became the dominant nineteenth-century French approach to public health: to engage specialists from a variety of backgrounds to investigate scientifically the causes of disease.

The Royal Society of Medicine was suppressed during the radical phase of the Revolution in 1794, but the theories its members espoused determined the course French public health would take. Between the abolition of the Royal Society in 1794 and the founding of the Royal Academy in 1820, the national government looked to the medical faculties for public health advice. Between 1794 and 1820, two institutions served as public health advisory boards to the national government: the Société de l'Ecole de Médecine and the Paris Faculty of Medicine. Observing the need for a consultative body, the Minister of the Interior formed in 1800 (an VIII) within the Ecole de Santé, as the Paris Faculty was called at the time, an

sity Press, 1980), pp. 186–256; Jean-Paul Desaive, Jean-Pierre Goubert, et al., *Médecins, climat et épidémies à la fin du XVIIIe siècle* (Paris: Mouton, 1972). The principal source on the Royal Society of Medicine is Caroline Hannaway. "Medicine, Public Welfare and the State in Eighteenth-Century France: The Société Royale de Médecine of Paris (1776–1793)" (Ph.D. dissertation, Johns Hopkins University, 1974).

2   Harvey Mitchell, "Rationality and Control in French Eighteenth Century Medical Views of the Peasantry," *Comparative Studies in Society and History* 21 (1979): 100–1; George Rosen, "Mercantilism and Health Policy in Eighteenth-Century French Thought," *From Medical Police to Social Medicine: Essays on the History of Health Care* (New York: Science History Publications, 1974), p. 216.

academic society, the Société de l'Ecole de Médecine, to undertake research related to medical topography and to give advice on public health and medical matters. By 1804 the Society had sixty titular members, twenty-seven of whom were professors at the Ecole de Santé. The Society functioned in an advisory capacity until 1821, when it was dissolved, its functions being assumed by the Royal Academy of Medicine. The Paris Faculty of Medicine also acted as an advisory board on public health matters from 1808 until the founding of the Royal Academy of Medicine and the Superior Health Council (1822). Two examples of its work are documented: In 1817 the Minister of the Interior asked the Faculty's opinion on the contagiousness of yellow fever and what measures should be applied, and in 1819–20 he sought an investigation and a report from the Faculty on the health and safety of importing a fertilizer known as *poudrette*.[3]

The Royal Academy of Medicine took over the advisory functions that had been performed by other groups in the intervening years and continued the traditions of the Royal Society of Medicine. The ordinance establishing the Royal Academy of Medicine stated that the institution was especially created to advise the government on all public health matters: "This Academy will be especially instituted to respond to the requests of the Government on all which is related to public health and principally on epidemics, diseases particular to certain countries, epizootics, different cases of legal medicine, the propagation of vaccine, the examination of new remedies, natural or artificial waters...."[4]

3 J. C. Sabatier (d'Orléans), *Recherches historiques sur la Faculté de Médécine de Paris depuis son origine jusqu'à nos jours* (Paris: Deville Cavellin, 1835), pp. 116–18. A.N., F⁸9, "Rapport en réponse à la demande du Ministre de l'Intérieur, relativement à la nécessité de prévenir l'introduction de la Fièvre jaune par la voie des communications commerciales, séance du 28 août 1817; A.N., F⁸77 Seine, Rapport sur l'importation de la poudrette dans les colonies, séance du 2 déc. 1819, Extrait du Registre des Délibérations de l'Assemblée des Professeurs de la Faculté de Médecine de Paris. Sailors had gotton sick, and the Minister of the Marine had asked the Minister of the Interior for advice. He had turned the problem over to the Faculty of Medicine. Parent-Duchâtelet did a report on the same problem and presented it to the Royal Academy of Medicine in 1821. See "Recherches pour découvrir la cause et la nature d'accidens très graves développés en mer à bord d'un bâtiment chargé de poudrette," *Hygiène publique*, 2 vols. (Paris: Baillière, 1836), 2: 257–85.
4 *Mém. de l'Acad. Roy. de Méd.* 1 (1828): 2; see the article by Vaillard, "Role de l'Académie de Médecine dans l'évolution de l'hygiène publique," *Bull. de l'Acad. Nationale de Méd.* 84 (1920): 403–10. On the immediate background and the founding of the Royal Academy of Medicine, see George Weisz, "Constructing the Medical Elite in France: The Creation of the Royal Academy of Medicine, 1814–1820," *Medical History* 30 (1986): 419–43. See also by George Weisz, who is working on a major study of the Royal Academy of Medicine, "The Medical Elite in France in the Early 19th Century." *Minerva* 25 (1987): 150–70. Public health was by no means the only function of the Royal Academy of Medicine. See John Lesch, "The Paris Academy of Medicine and Experimental Science," in *The Investigative*

A royal ordinance of 1822 named physician Etienne Pariset permanent secretary and Baron Portal, the king's first physician, honorary president. In his inaugural address Pariset expounded on the public health goals of the Academy and spoke eloquently about the importance of public health for the welfare of society. Noting the relationship between medicine and political economy, Pariset expressed the prevailing opinion among hygienists that public health was the result of a more perfect civilization, since sick people made bad laws, and vice versa. After enumerating ways in which hygienists could concentrate their efforts, such as improving hospitals, prisons, and public baths and providing pure water, Pariset concluded by saying: "This small number of examples gives us enough of a glimpse of what a limitless field we would have to survey if we followed step by step all the details of civil, military, and naval hygiene, details of which not a single one, however, ought to be neglected by us, because there is not a single one of them whose perfection is not necessary for the perfection of everything."[5]

The Academy was organized into temporary and permanent commissions that handled communications with the government and judged essays submitted for consideration. Temporary commissions were established to examine questions that did not fall within the categories of the permanent commissions, and the latter, each composed of six or nine members, prepared annual reports on their particular areas, which were submitted to the Minister of the Interior. The epidemic, the mineral water, and the secret remedy commissions – all permanent – were re-creations of groups established within the Royal Society of Medicine, and the vaccine commission was new. Each commission functioned as the national administration in its area and reported to the Minister of the Interior (after 1830, the Minister of Commerce), the official in charge of public health at the national level.[6]

The epidemic commission coordinated the work of the epidemic physicians and prepared general reports on epidemics in France based on

Tradition: Experimental Physiology in Nineteenth-Century Medicine, ed. William Coleman and Frederic L. Holmes (Los Angeles: University of California Press, 1988), pp. 100–38.

5 Pariset was at the time a physician at Bicêtre, a large Parisian hospital. *Mém. de l'Acad. Roy. de Méd.* 1 (1828): 16–17, 29. On the death of Pariset in 1847, Fr. Dubois d'Amiens replaced him as permanent secretary. See Fr. Dubois, "Eloge de Pariset," *Mém. de l'Acad. Roy. de Méd.* 13 (1847): XLII–LXX. On Pariset, see George Sussman, "Etienne Pariset: A Medical Career in Government Under the Restoration," *Journal of the History of Medicine and Allied Sciences* 26 (1971): 52–74; *Mém. de l'Acad. Roy. de Méd.* 1 (1828): 57–106. Quote, pp. 94–5. On Pariset's role as preparer and presenter of eulogies for members of the Royal Academy of Medicine, see also George Weisz, "The Self-Made Mandarin: The Eloges of the French Academy of Medicine, 1824–47," *History of Science* 26 (1988): 13–39.

6 *Mém. de l'Acad. Roy. de Méd.* 2 (1833): 67–8; 3 (1833): 380; 4 (1835): 30.

individual summaries sent in by epidemic physicians. These documents, approved by the Royal Academy of Medicine, were then sent to the Minister of the Interior, typically prefaced with a policy statement by the commission. The commission's first major report covered the sixty-year period from 1771 to 1830. Using information gathered by the Royal Society of Medicine and the Société de Médecine de la Faculté, as well as data furnished by epidemic physicians, the commission compiled a list of 900 epidemics (excluding smallpox, which was handled by the vaccine commission) gathered from 1,160 different reports dealing with 1,370 communes, 179 arrondissements, and 72 departments. In subsequent reports prepared at varying intervals throughout the first half of the century, the commission made recommendations on how to reduce the incidence and severity of epidemics and improve public health in the countryside.[7]

The epidemic commission emphasized that rural health care had been neglected, noting that most hygienic improvements had occurred in cities and that epidemics were still commonplace in the countryside. Commission members argued that reform could not be left in the hands of administrators without public health expertise and urged physicians to take an interest in rural health reform. Therefore, the commission recommended a nationwide system of cantonal physicians – a medical civil service – to help prevent epidemics. The members were realistic, however, in recognizing that physicians alone could not solve the problem of epidemics in rural France, for they believed the major causes of disease and epidemics in the countryside were unhealthy dwellings and vitiated air, conditions that would not be solved by physicians but that required fundamental changes in rural habits and practices.[8]

The mineral water commission was the central coordinating body for mineral water establishments and their personnel. The commission ex-

7 The Royal Society of Medicine had a vast project of compiling a medical topography for all of France, but the Revolution interrupted its work and the project was never completed; see Hannaway, "Société royale de Médecine." See the report of the epidemic commission: Villeneuve, chairman, "Rapport général sur les épidémies qui ont regné en France, depuis 1771 jusqu'à 1830 exclusivement, et dont les relations sont parvenues à l'Académie," *Mém. de l'Acad. Roy. de Méd.* 3 (1833): 377–429. Members of the epidemic commission in 1833 were Martin-Solon, Mestivier, Villermé, Thillaye, and Villeneuve (chairman). Pierre-Adolphe Piorry, chairman, "Rapport sur les épidémies qui ont regnés en France de 1830 à 1836" (Extrait), in *Mém. de l'Acad. Roy. de Méd.* 6 (1837): 1–24; Pierre-Adolphe Piorry, chairman, "Rapport de la commission des épidémies sur les maladies épidémiques qui ont regnés en France en 1836, 1837 et 1838," *Mém. de l'Acad. Roy. de Méd.* 7 (1838): 141–156; Isidore Bricheteau, "Rapport de la commission des épidémies pour l'année 1839 et une partie de 1840," *Mém. de l'Acad. Roy. de Méd.* 9 (1841): 31–64; Henri Gaultier de Claubry, "Rapport sur les épidémies qui ont regnés en France de 1841 à 1846 fait au nom de la commission des épidémies," *Mém. de l'Acad. Roy. de Méd.* 14 (1849): 1–188.
8 Piorry, "Rapport...1836, 1837 et 1838," p. 144; Bricheteau, "Rapport," pp. 32–4.

amined documents submitted by physician-inspectors of these establishments, whose job required them to compile statistics, propose reforms, and assess the therapeutic use of mineral waters. Mineral water sources belonged to the state, department, commune, or charitable institution or to individuals. A royal ordinance of 1823 regulated natural mineral water sources and the manufacture of artificial mineral water. According to the ordinance, anyone wishing to administer mineral waters as treatment or sell them (except in pharmacies) had to be authorized by government medical inspectors. The stated mission of these inspectors was to oversee the conservation of mineral water sources and to improve them, and, in the case of artificial mineral water, to ensure that it conformed to the approved formula and was neither altered nor adulterated. Inside mineral water establishments, inspectors exercised surveillance over the distribution of waters and their therapeutic use. Inspectors prepared annual reports on their observations for the mineral water commission, which forwarded them to the Minister of the Interior. These documents reveal the inspectors' concern about quality of water and variations in water, as well as methods of treatment and length of cures.[9]

The role of the secret remedy commission was based on an 1810 decree providing that any new or perfected remedy should first be examined by a delegated medical commission to guarantee its merits and novelty. Beginning its work in 1824, the secret remedy commission had more day-to-day tasks than the other commissions, since it was responsible for making monthly reports to the Academy on formulas and remedies submitted to it. The Royal Society of Medicine had also policed the trade of proprietary remedies and determined scientifically their therapeutic value. Between 1779 and 1789 the secret remedy commission had examined 442 remedies, of which only 100 received permission for sale. From 1825 to 1833 the commission of the Royal Academy of Medicine handed down a decision on sixty secret remedies, fifty-seven of which were rejected, either because they were not new or because they lacked therapeutic value. The Academy, however, had no power to forbid the use of remedies, only to judge

---

9 F. V. Mérat, "Rapport fait à l'Académie royale de Médécine sur les eaux minérales de France pendant les années 1834, 1835 et 1836 au nom de la commission des eaux minérales," *Mém de l'Acad. Roy. de Méd.* 7 (1838): 45–108; For all legislation relating to mineral waters see Maxime Durand-Fardel et al., *Dictionnaire général des eaux minérales et d'hydrologie médicale*, 2 vols. (Paris: Baillière, 1860); see the review of the book by Maxime Vernois in *Annales d'hygiène publique* 2e série, 14 (1860): 473–8. The salaries of the medical inspectors were paid by the mineral water establishments. They varied depending upon the classification of the mineral water source. Sources were classified according to the rental proceeds of the establishment. See the recent article by George Weisz, "Water Cure and Science: The French Academy of Medicine and Mineral Water in the Nineteenth Century," *Bull. Hist. Med.* 64 (1990): 393–416.

them when the Minister of the Interior asked for an opinion. The commission found that most of the supposedly new remedies were old, well-known formulas.[10]

Questions of professional monopoly versus free trade came to a head in the Academy's debate over patents for secret remedies. The administration handed out patents for remedies that, according to the secret remedy commission, contravened the 1803 laws regulating the practice of medicine and pharmacy. The commission maintained that government policy aided charlatans and was a public health threat, for by granting the patent the government seemed to have authorized the product, whereas in fact it had only recognized the inventor's right to sell it. According to the commission, it was the inventor's responsibility to prove the product's worth and defend it against counterfeiters. The secret remedy commission argued that the 1803 laws did not allow secret remedies to be patented, since patents were issued only for legal products. Free trade did not apply to medicine, the commission contended, arguing that the preparation and distribution of medicines should be restricted to physicians, surgeons, health officers, and pharmacists. Wanting to extend its authority to include food and cosmetics, the commission proposed that the government issue patents for these products only after members had certified their harmlessness. The government was inconsistent in this area, sometimes submitting such products to the commission and sometimes not, usually abiding by the commission's decision and occasionally overriding the decision and issuing patents for products judged harmful by the commission.[11]

The permanent vaccine commission of the Royal Academy of Medicine was the successor of the Central Vaccine Commission (established in 1803). After 1824 the duties of the vaccine commission included compiling statistics on smallpox in France, preparing an annual report on the progress of vaccine, recommending ways to eliminate obstacles to vaccine, and identifying the most zealous vaccinators and distributing prizes to them.

10 Etienne Pariset, "Compte-rendu des travaux de l'Académie pendant l'année 1833," *Mém. de l'Acad. Roy. de Méd.* 4 (1835): 30–1; Caroline Hannaway, "The Regulation of Remedies in Eighteenth-Century France," paper delivered at the 28th International Congress for the History of Medicine, Paris, August 1982. See also Matthew Ramsey, "Traditional Medicine and Medical Enlightenment: The Regulation of Secret Remedies in the Ancien Régime," *Historical Reflexions/Réflexions historiques* 9 (1982): 215–32. See also Matthew Ramsey, *Professional and Popular Medicine in France, 1770–1830: The Social World of Medical Practice* (New York: Cambridge University Press, 1988); Itard, "Rapport général sur les remèdes secrets," *Mém. de l'Acad. Roy. de Méd.* 2 (1833): 24–31.

11 Nicolas Adelon, chairman, "Projet de lettre à M. le Ministre des Travaux Publics et du Commerce, touchant la concession de brevets d'invention pour remèdes," *Bull. de l'Acad. Roy. de Méd.* 2 (1837–8): 157–64.

The vaccine commission was at the helm of the government's vaccination campaign, to be discussed in detail later.[12]

The Royal Academy of Medicine, limited to an advisory and administrative capacity, had no legislative functions. The government submitted questions to the Academy, which a commission, permanent or temporary, studied and reported on to the whole Academy. The report was then discussed and voted on as presented or amended, and the final majority opinion became the Academy's position on the issue. Not all members were satisfied with the Academy's advisory role. Pathological anatomist Pierre-Adolphe Piorry, for example, urged the Academy to act as a pressure group and to lobby for public health legislation. Since physicians were the experts, they should advise the government: "It is up to [the Academy] to provoke legislation and to request protective measures....It is not up to physicians to make the health laws; but it is up to them to demonstrate the utility of the laws and to solicit them."[13]

The government was responsive to the Academy's opinion and usually tailored its actions accordingly. A good example was the case of Nicolas Chervin's attack on the national sanitary legislation following publication of the results of the investigating team (which included Chervin) that went to Gibraltar in 1828 to observe the yellow fever epidemic there and returned an anticontagionist report. The opinion of the Academy, influenced by Chervin's report, resulted in a drastic reduction of the sanitary administration. By the 1830s the Royal Academy of Medicine had become the principal advisory body to the national government in public health matters and was rapidly becoming one of the most prestigious medical assemblies in the world. Speaking of the significance of the 1846 plague commission report, René Prus, the reporter, emphasized the importance of the Academy to the national government. "You will show, gentlemen, that the government is right in considering you the most competent body with regard to the great questions of public health."[14]

SANITARY POLICY AND SANITARY ADMINISTRATION

The traditional area of public health concern was contagious and epidemic diseases, and for centuries governments had enacted public health measures in response to plague and leprosy. The last great European plague epidemic occurred in Marseilles in 1720, and in order to combat it, the

12 Pariset, "Compte-rendu...1833," pp. 32, 49–50.
13 *Mém. de l'Acad. Roy. de Méd.* 3 (1833): 393. Quote is from 6 (1837): 16.
14 Ackerknecht, *Medicine at the Paris Hospital*, pp. 116–17; quote is from *Bull. de l'Acad. Roy. de Méd.* 11 (1846): 870.

government revived the Marseilles Intendancy of Health and invoked the traditional means of fighting epidemics: quarantines, lazarettos, *cordons sanitaires*, and sequestration. Following the epidemic, sanitary institutions were established to prevent the importation of plague by examining ships entering the harbor, enforcing quarantines, maintaining lazarettos, and supervising personnel who inspected goods and performed fumigations. These institutions were located in the Mediterranean ports of Toulon and Marseilles, where ships from the Near East and Africa – where plague was endemic – arrived.[15]

In the early nineteenth century *la police du port*, the policy and administration of preventing the importation of contagious diseases by sea, or *la police sanitaire* (as it was called after the passage of the 1822 sanitary law), was directed at plague, yellow fever, and cholera. Before 1819 the sanitary administration of the Mediterranean ports was directed at plague alone. Although yellow fever epidemics had occurred sporadically in areas of North America since the late eighteenth century and in Spain in the early years of the nineteenth, the threat did not appear imminent for France until yellow fever broke out, first in Cadiz in 1819, then in Barcelona in 1821.

The Spanish yellow fever epidemics motivated the French government to pass a national sanitary law. The 1822 law created a national administration to prevent the importation of plague, cholera, and yellow fever and provided for implementation of the law by existing institutions – health intendancies, health commissions, prefects, and mayors. The government also founded (by an ordinance of September 3, 1822), under the aegis of the Minister of the Interior (the official in charge of public health under the Restoration regime), the Superior Health Council (*Conseil supérieur de santé*) in charge of a national public health surveillance and enforcement of the 1822 law. In instituting the Superior Health Council, the government reinforced a traditional approach to public health, identifying it with preventing the importation of contagious diseases. This approach and the narrowly defined function of the Superior Health Council contrasted to the new, all-encompassing public health idea being espoused by the Paris health council and the Royal Academy of Medicine.[16]

15 On the 1720 plague epidemic see Charles Carrière, Marcel Cordurié, and Ferréol Rébuffat, *Marseille, ville morte. La peste de 1720* (Marseilles: Garcon, 1968): material on the Marseilles sanitary intendancy (*la police du port*) in A.N., $F^8$22–37, mostly dealing with the Napoleonic era and the Restoration.

16 As both Sussman and Ackerknecht have given the details of the Restoration sanitary policy and the anticontagionist–contagionist controversy over yellow fever, I will present the story in its broadest outlines here. See George Sussman, "From Yellow Fever to Cholera: A Study of French Government Policy, Medical Professionalism, and Popular Movements in the Epidemic Crises of the Restoration and July Monarchy" (Ph.D. dissertation, Yale University, 1972, pp. 1–213); Erwin Ackerknecht, "Anticontagionism Between 1821 and 1867," *Bull. Hist. Med.*, 22 (1948): 562–93. Members of the commission sent to Cadiz were the physicians

The medical basis of the Restoration sanitary policy was the epidemio-logical theory of "contagionism," which had the support of only a minority of French physicians and hygienists. Contagionists believed that diseases were immediately transmissible from one person to another by contact and by an organism known as a *contagium animatum*, or an animal-cule, a living entity that carried disease. The contagionist view had prevailed in Western Europe since the sixteenth century, and sanitary institutions and policies were founded upon the principle. The main disease in question until the eighteenth century was plague, which many physicians considered contagious, but the contagiousness of other diseases remained unexamined. By the early nineteenth century, most French physicians rejected contagionism as a scientific explanation for the cause of many diseases, especially the "fevers" – yellow fever, cholera, and plague. French hygienist Etienne Pariset, statistician Alexandre Moreau de Jonnès, and Marseillais physician L. J. M. Robert – all convinced contagionists – were notable exceptions. Etienne Pariset, the permanent secretary of the Royal Academy of Medicine and a member of the Paris health council, remained one of the most dedicated to the theory of contagion. A member of the government commissions sent to Spain in 1819 and 1821 to decide on the contagion or noncontagion of yellow fever, he and other members returned the contagionist report that motivated the government to institute the sanitary legislation of 1822. In 1829, Pariset was a member of a gov-ernment commission sent to Egypt to study the plague, which many hygienists, including Pariset, thought to be contagious. Alexandre Moreau de Jonnès, a government spokesman for contagion, in addition to being

Etienne Pariset and Mazet; to Barcelona the Minister of the Interior sent Pariset, Mazet, Bally, François, and Rochoux; the Minister of War sent Audouard. This material is in Ackerknecht, "Anticontagionssm," pp. 571–2, and Sussman, "From Yellow Fever to Cholera," pp. 17, 131–3. For members of the Central Sanitary Commission, see Appendix 2. The sanitary administration in Marseilles served as the model for the other intendancies set up as part of the nationwide sanitary program established by the 1822 law. See, e.g., A.N., F^{8}29, Intendans de la santé publique au Ministre de l'Intérieur, September 15, and 19, 1820. The Minister of the Interior relied on the advice of two members of the Marseilles intendancy, Etienne Majestre and Bruno Rostand, who went to Paris to give advice on the proposed law. They were also members of the Central Sanitary Commission. See the *Moniteur universel*, September 30, 1821, pp. 1373–4, royal ordinance giving preventive measures against the importation of yellow fever from Spain, and December 25, 1821, pp. 1729–30, Ch. Dep. séance du 24 déc. On p. 1730 is a complete draft of the law. For the complete text of the law, see Louis-Joseph-Marie Robert, *Guide sanitaire des gouvernemens européens*, 2 vols. (Paris: Crevot, 1826), 2: 845–85. See also *Recueil des textes officiels concernant la protection de la santé publique (1790–1935)*, 9 vols. (Paris: Ministère de la santé publique, 1957), 1: 243–8 for laws and ordinances of March and August 1822 relative to the sanitary police. See also *Moniteur*, August 11, 1822, pp. 1189–91. On the development of the *Conseil supérieur de santé*, see Sussman, "From Yellow Fever to Cholera," pp. 7, 23, 35–6, 214–15; *Moniteur*, September 3, 1822, pp. 1289 and 1294. For members of the Superior Health Council, see Appendix 2.

the head of the statistical section in the Ministry of Commerce in the 1830s and in charge of the publication of the *Statistique générale de la France*, also sat on the Superior Health Council. Pariset was also a member. Robert was a physician at the lazaretto of Marseilles and a member of the Bouches-du-Rhône health council.[17]

The "enlightened" and predominant theory among many French physicians by the 1820s was anticontagionism, a neo-Hippocratic environmental, atmospheric explanation of disease causation. Anticontagionists subscribed to a miasmatic or infectionist theory of disease, believing that disease was spread by chemical miasms emanating from unclean conditions such as rotting organic matter and stagnant water. According to this theory, air rather than personal contact was the medium by which disease was spread. Anticontagionists believed most, but not all, diseases to be infectious, that is, contracted by means of being in a particular locality where the air was vitiated by deleterious miasms. Many hygienists could best be described as "contingent contagionists," recognizing the contagiousness of some diseases – smallpox and syphilis, for example – but maintaining that many diseases that had long been thought to be contagious were not.

Anticontagionists "proved" by observation and experiment that cholera, yellow fever, and plague were not immediately contagious and questioned the contagiousness of other diseases. In 1828 the Royal Academy of Medicine, influenced by the research of Nicolas Chervin, a physician who devoted his life to the study of yellow fever and proof of its noncontagion, returned an anticontagionist verdict with regard to yellow fever. Shortly thereafter, an investigation team sent to Gibraltar to observe the yellow fever epidemic returned an anticontagionist report, since they found no evidence to justify the transmissibility of the disease from person to person. The physicians sent to Gibralter were the clinicians Pierre Louis, Armand Trousseau, and Nicolas Chervin. The last dominated the commis-

17 Ackerknecht, "Anticontagionism"; George Rosen, *A History of Public Health* (New York: MD Publications, 1958), pp. 182–91, 277–93; Charles-Edward-Amory Winslow, *Man and Epidemics* (Princeton, NJ: Princeton University Press, 1952), pp. 7–17; see Pariset, *Observations sur la fièvre jaune faites à Cadix en 1819* (Paris: Audot, 1820), and "Mémoire sur les causes de la peste"; on Pariset, see George Sussman, "Etienne Pariset"; see also Fr. Dubois, "'Eloge de E. Pariset,' lu dans la séance publique annuelle du 14 déc. 1847," *Mém. de l'Acad. Roy. de Méd* 13 (1847): xlii–lxx, which also includes a list of all the published works of Pariset. See, for example, Alexandre Moreau de Jonnès, *Rapport au Conseil supérieur de santé sur le choléra-morbus pestilentiel* (Paris: Cosson, 1831); for material on the Central Sanitary Commission and the Superior Health Council, see p. 157 of Moreau de Jonnès's work; on this, see also Sussman, "From Yellow Fever to Cholera," pp. 35–6; for a listing of the members of the *Conseil supérieur de santé* in any given year, consult the appropriate volume of the *Almanach Royal*. For another contagionist view, see also Robert, *Guide sanitaire*. See also Robert, *Guide sanitaire* 2: 845–85, for a complete copy of the sanitary law of 1822.

sion and used the investigation to support his anticontagionist position. Curiously, the report, published in 1830, contained no conclusion on the cause or transmission of yellow fever or on what public health measures should be taken. The Gibraltar epidemic followed the major discussion on yellow fever in the Royal Academy of Medicine on Chervin's documentation on yellow fever in the Americas. Chervin made public the lessons of the Gibraltar experience, claiming that the causes of the disease were local, not imported. Heavy night air seemed to be especially dangerous. Chervin argued that the causes of yellow fever were atmospheric, and to avoid the disease one had only to leave the infected area.[18]

Anticontagionists opposed the government's 1822 sanitary policy from its inception. Chervin spearheaded attacks of the sanitary legislation, and his efforts and the prevailing opinion among the medical profession led the Royal Academy of Medicine to adopt an 1828 report that supported the noncontagion of yellow fever. As a result, the government began to disband its sanitary administration, and the chambers refused to vote money for the program. The national sanitary administration was severely damaged following the opposition of the majority of the medical profession and the anticontagionist stance of the Royal Academy of Medicine. A scaled-down sanitary administration continued to function throughout the period, however, with further modifications occurring in response to the anticontagionist opinion of the medical profession vis-à-vis cholera in the 1830s and plague in the 1840s.[19]

Government commissions sent to Poland and Russia to study cholera before the 1832 Paris epidemic produced anticontagionist reports, and the commission established in Paris to report on cholera likewise did not find it to be contagious. The Prus plague report (1846) of the Royal Academy of Medicine was also anticontagionist. Hygienists advanced varying hypotheses of disease causation, since they could not pinpoint the actual causes of diseases. Confirming their hypotheses would provide a basis for public health measures and an alternative to the government's sanitary policy, which most hygienists believed to be outdated, ineffective, and reactionary.[20]

18 On the Gibraltar epidemic, see William Coleman, *Yellow Fever in the North: The Methods of Early Epidemiology* (Madison: University of Wisconsin Press, 1987), pp. 21–31.

19 For example, the 1822 expenditures for the sanitary establishments were 869,476 francs; by 1830, only 135,844 francs had been spent; by 1831, the expenditure was reduced further to 96,755 francs. See *Documents statistiques sur la France publiés* par le Ministre du Commerce, 1 (1835): 148–9. The full collection is *Statistique générale de la France*, 34 vols. (Paris: Imprimerie royale, etc., 1835–73).

20 See Ackerknecht, "Anticontagionism"; for a discussion of the controversy over yellow fever, see the works of Chervin, who during the 1820s combatted the contagionist theories of Pariset and the various government commissions: *Examen des principes de l'administration en matière sanitaire* (Paris: Didot, 1827); *Examen critique*

After 1828, the Superior Health Council was almost inactive, having lost its raison d'etre. Representative of an older approach to public health, the council was for all practical purposes divorced from the public health movement. Nevertheless, it continued to operate throughout the first half of the century, the government occasionally asking its opinion on public health matters. Its importance as a public health advisory board was eclipsed, however, by the Royal Academy of Medicine and the Paris health council. As part of the public health reforms of 1848 (August 10, 1848), the Superior Health Council was replaced by the Consultative Committee on Public Hygiene (*Comité consultatif d'hygiène publique*), which was established under the authority of the Minister of Agriculture and Commerce, who now held national responsibility for public health. Appointed to the committee were François Magendie, Louis Aubert-Roche, François Mélier, Hippolyte Royer-Collard, and Villermé. Magendie, experimental physiologist and pharmacologist, had gone to Sunderland, England, in 1832 to investigate cholera and had returned with anticontagionist conclusions. Louis Aubert-Roche, one of the organizers of the Egyptian health service after 1825, believed plague to be noncontagious. A specialist in colonial hygiene, he would later organize the health services for the Suez Canal Company. Mélier, one of the leading public health spokesmen in the Royal Academy of Medicine, was, along with Royer-Collard, a member of the Prus commission. In 1851 Mélier became General Inspector of Sanitary Services for the French government. Royer-Collard held the chair of hygiene at the Paris Faculty of Medicine from 1837 to 1850 and was appointed to the committee by virtue of his position. Until the end of the century the Committee's duties remained essentially the same as those of the Superior Health Council, but by the last decades of the nineteenth century the Committee had become important as a national public health advisory board, responsible for directing national health policy.[21]

des prétendues preuves de contagion de la fièvre jaune observée en Espagne (Paris: Baillière, 1828); *Petition adressée à la Chambre des Députés relative à la question de la contagion et aux mesures sanitaires* (Paris: Pinard, 1833); for the report of the Royal Academy of Medicine, see *Rapport lu à l'Académie Royale de Médecine, dans les séances des 15 mai et 19 juin 1827, au nom de la commission chargée d'examiner les documents de M. Chervin concernant la fièvre jaune* (Paris: Didot, 1828); for biographical material on Chervin and a complete list of his publications, see Fr. Dubois, "Notice historique sur M. Chervin," *Mém. de l'Acad. Roy. de Méd.* 12 (1846): xxxvii–lix; for the anticontagionist point of view taken by the Paris cholera commission, see Louis-François Benoiston de Châteauneuf, *Report on the Cholera in Paris* (New York: S. S. and W. Wood, 1849); for the Prus commission report on the noncontagion of plague adopted by the Royal Academy of Medicine in 1846, see René Prus, chairman, "Rapport de la peste et des quarantaines," *Bull. de l'Acad. Roy. de Méd.* 11 (1846): 545–934.

21   *Recueil des textes officiels*, 2: 230. For the fate of the *Comité consultatif* in the late nineteenth century, see Martha Hildreth, *Doctors, Bureaucrats and Public Health in France, 1888–1902* (New York: Garland, 1987).

THEORIES OF DISEASE CAUSATION AND THE PUBLIC HEALTH MOVEMENT

In his now classic article "Anticontagionism between 1821 and 1867" (1948), Erwin Ackerknecht interpreted early-nineteenth-century theories of disease causation within the broader political context, associating anticontagionism with liberalism and contagionism with reaction and government bureaucracy. Ackerknecht related the ascendancy of anticontagionism to the rise of liberalism (the July Monarchy) and its decline in the 1860s to the age of reaction. Margaret Pelling (1978) challenged this interpretation, in light of the British experience, as simplistic and inaccurate, arguing that neither physicians nor disease theories could be so neatly fitted into two distinct and opposing camps. Roger Cooter, in a 1982 article, sought to take the analysis one step further by incorporating Pelling's critique and providing a new way of conceptualizing anticontagionism.[22]

Cooter developed the argument that anticontagionism was favored by those seeking to assert expertise and authority. If the cause of disease was found in the atmosphere, then disease arose from impersonal forces and blame could not be placed on particular individuals. Because atmospheric causes explained everything, they explained nothing. Furthermore, air could not be easily objectified. It was not an entity that lent itself to scientific study. The atmosphere was hard to study, because the investigator could not constrain it. Cooter suggests that the incomprehensibility of dealing with this notion of disease causation opened the way for expert interpretation.[23]

In his recent book *Yellow Fever in the North*, William Coleman discussed these different interpretations of the contagionist – anticontagionist debate and related them to the broader theme of the development of the science of epidemiology. For us, the question is: How important was this debate to the public health movement? Although the debate was central to the national government's sanitary policy, it was peripheral to the public health movement.

The anticontagionist–contagionist debate did not figure prominently in the discourse of the community of hygienists. With the exception of

---

22 Coleman, *Yellow Fever in the North*, pp. 187–94. Margaret Pelling, *Cholera, Fever, and English Medicine: 1825–1865* (Oxford: Oxford University Press, 1978), pp. 295–310. Roger Cooter, "Anticontagionism and History's Medical Record," in *The Problem of Medical Knowledge*, ed. P. Wright and A. Treacher (Edinburgh: Edinburgh University Press, 1983), pp. 87–108. James Riley pointed out for the eighteenth century that an environmental theory of disease causation, although anticontagionist, incorporated many elements of contagion theory. See James Riley, *The Eighteenth-Century Campaign to Avoid Disease* (New York: St. Martin's 1987).

23 Cooter, "Anticontagionism and History's Medical Record."

cholera, public hygienists were not primarily concerned with epidemic diseases. Instead they focused on endemic and occupational diseases – the diseases of poverty. As William Coleman has pointed out, for the hygienists, death was indeed a social disease. Furthermore, public hygienists cannot be neatly divided into Ackerknecht's two opposing camps, and so Pelling's analysis of British physicians applies to the French situation as well. Hygienists generally held disease-specific etiological notions. At a time when therapeutic skepticism characterized the Paris clinical school, hygienists were also etiological skeptics. There was a consensus on the causes of some diseases: Hygienists readily accepted the contagiousness of smallpox and venereal diseases, but other diseases – especially fevers – were problematic. Because the available evidence was contradictory and inconclusive (the Gibraltar commission reached no conclusions, for example), hygienists resisted adhering to any system. Most were neither declared anticontagionists, like Chervin, nor confirmed contagionists, like Moreau de Jonnès.

Public hygienists focused their attention primarily on social causes of disease, a point emphasized by Ackerknecht himself. Leading hygienists and statisticians like Villermé, Parent-Duchâtelet, Chevallier, and Benoiston de Châteauneuf found in numerous wide-ranging studies that the variable that was most closely correlated with incidence of disease and premature death was poverty – a salary inadequate to supply basic needs. Thus the community of hygienists advanced an alternative view of disease causation, a social theory of epidemiology.

Some anticontagionist-environmental theories struck Villermé and Parent-Duchâtelet as especially ill-conceived and not based on scientific investigation. In his studies of varying mortality in Paris, Villermé found no evidence to support the traditional environmental-climatic etiology and argued instead for a social theory of disease causation. Parent-Duchâtelet questioned the atmospheric-miasmatic theory. In his studies of the Bièvre River and the Parisian horsebutcher yards, he found no support for the miasmatic-anticontagionist theory. Parent-Duchâtelet took a sociohistorical viewpoint in his occupational studies of stevedores, sewer workers, and prostitutes, investigating historical context, socioeconomic conditions, and lifestyles in order to determine disease causation and to deny unsupportable causes advanced by other investigators.[24]

The community of hygienists focused much of their effort on urban and occupational diseases, areas of sociohygienic investigation in which the anticontagionist-contagionist controversy did not form part of their theoretical framework. In their studies of occupations and industrialization, for

24 For Villermé's studies, see Chapter 2. For Parent-Duchâtelet's studies, see Chapter 6.

example, hygienists found that the main causes of disease were related to level of income and concomitant living conditions. Once again, socio-hygienic inquiry upheld a social theory of epidemiology.

Hygienists were only peripherally concerned with two of the three diseases debated in the Royal Academy of Medicine. Plague and yellow fever occupied little of their attention. In the case of cholera, public hygienists serving on the commission that wrote the report on cholera in Paris (which included Benoiston de Châteauneuf, Villermé, and Parent-Duchâtelet) concluded, not surprisingly, by arguing for a social theory of disease causation. Indeed, the Paris cholera epidemic seemed to offer scientific confirmation of the social theory.[25]

This analysis does not imply blanket rejection of contagionist or anti-contagionist theories by the hygienists. One could argue that since the social theory was not contagionist, it was anticontagionist or environment-alist. But that was not the way anticontagionism was normally construed, and the social theory was really competing with the atmospheric/sanitary/filth theory. It is more accurate to see the social theory as an alternative theory that did not deny or exclude the contagiousness of certain diseases or the possibility of atmospheric causation, but that moved the analysis to a different level by arguing that the broader framework in which disease, whether contagious or infectious, operated was social.

There is another problem with trying to apply the Ackerknecht model to the public hygienists. Not only do the contagionist-anticontagionist camps not work, but the political labels "liberal," "reactionary," and "government bureaucracy" are not helpful either. Hygienists were of varying political persuasions. For example, Villermé was a liberal but Parent-Duchâtelet was a statist. Both subscribed to the social theory of epidemiology; neither was a confirmed contagionist or anticontagionist. The social theory transcended political allegiances, as did public hygiene itself.[26]

In the final analysis, both Pelling's and Cooter's analyses tell us more about the community of hygienists than Ackerknecht's. Cooter has pro-vided a richer texture for our understanding of environmental-atmospheric causes of disease. His analysis applies to the public health movement in the sense that the difficulty of grappling with atmospheric causes, of doing scientific studies, and of reaching conclusions surely encouraged hygienists to search out more easily manageable and quantifiable variables. Since hygienists wanted to promote themselves as experts in the new discipline of public hygiene, their ability to deal with these slippery questions, to provide scientific and statistical studies, enhanced their reputations and contributed to the prestige that public hygiene enjoyed.

HEALTH CARE POLICIES AND PROGRAMS

Eighteenth-century reformers, physicians, and the government had proposed medical and public health reforms to provide health care to all. Their goal was to provide medical care for the sick and to prevent epidemics and illnesses by sanitary measures, education, and vaccination. Public health assumed an important place in the Revolutionary reform programs. In 1790, physician Ignace Guillotin presided over a special Health Committee within the Constituent Assembly, consisting of thirty-four members, including seventeen physicians. The committee proposed a nationwide public health organization of arrondissement health councils (boards of health) invested with their own power to police medicine, pharmacy, and public health, and also endorsed a plan for a nationwide system of cantonal physicians – or a medical civil service. Committee members may have borrowed this idea from some of the German states, where such an institution had existed since the fifteenth century. According to the committee's plan, cantonal physicians would replace the epidemic service, which under the Ancient Régime had been managed by royal intendants acting through special physicians charged with preventing and controlling epidemics, and later by the Royal Society of Medicine. Cantonal physicians were also to be public health doctors, conducting hygienic inquiries, preparing medical topographies, investigating epidemics, taking care of the poor, providing maternal and child protection, performing inoculations, and keeping statistical records. In short, the Health Committee proposed a comprehensive system of public health and social medicine.[27]

The Health Committee's program was not realized during the Revolution. The Legislative Assembly merged the Health and Mendicity committees to form the Committee of Public Assistance, and although one section was designated for public health, the committee's main concern was a general welfare program. Yet, the legacy of the Health Committee was great. Both the health councils and the system of cantonal physicians were established in the early nineteenth century, though not on so broad a scale as envisaged and with some modifications. The Health Committee articulated the principles on which national public health policy and the public health movement would be founded: an idea of public health

27   The discussion of public health during the Revolution is based on the following sources: Dora B. Weiner, "Le Droit de l'homme à la santé – une belle idée devant l'Assemblée Constituante: 1790–91," *Clio Medica* 5 (1970): 209–23; Henry Ingrand, "Le Comité de salubrité de l'Assemblée nationale constituante (1790–91," (Thesis, University of Paris, 1934).

grounded in the belief that health was a natural right to which all citizens were entitled and that it was the state's responsibility to protect the public health.

The Health Committee's program for a medical civil service was partially realized under Napoleon, but not in the manner the committee had proposed. Instead, two positions, health officer (*officier de santé*) and epidemic physician, were established throughout the nation. In 1803, the Napoleonic government established a secondary grade of medical personnel, the health officers, who provide medical care in rural areas, where it was difficult to attract physicians. Additionally, health officers offered an alternative to charlatans and other illegal healers, whose craft was widely perceived by physicians and administrators to be a threat to public health and the legitimate practice of medicine. Health officers, who were never popular with physicians, continued to function throughout the nineteenth century, performing a much needed service in some areas.[28]

Epidemic physicians provided health services during medical emergencies. Napoleon attempted to standardize the eighteenth-century network of epidemic physicians by creating a nationwide institution, and decreed in 1805 that an epidemic physician would be appointed in each arrondissement. Once an epidemic was reported, an epidemic physician was sent to the afflicted area to treat the sick, prescribe medicines, distribute food, and give instructions to local medical personnel. Like the epidemic physicians from the Royal Society of Medicine, the nineteenth-century epidemic physicians also had a civilizing mission. It was their express duty to spread "enlightenment," or personal hygiene practices, to the rural population. With the health officers and epidemic physicians Napoleon tried – but ultimately failed – to institutionalize the notion of equal access to health care. The Health Committee's program of cantonal physicians was established in one department, the Bas-Rhin. In 1810 Prefect Adrien Lézay-Marnésia instituted a departmentwide system of salaried cantonal physicians to provide preventive and therapeutic medicine to rural inhabitants and to carry out the departmental vaccine program. The program was successful, especially with vaccination, and by the 1830s became a model for medical reformers who advocated the bureaucratization of medicine, or a medical civil service.[29]

The governments of the Restoration and the July Monarchy continued

---

28   Pierre Huard, "L'officiat de santé (1794–1892)," *Concours médical* 83 (1961): 3231–9. On illegal healers see Matthew Ramsey, "Medical Power and Popular Medicine: Illegal Healers in Nineteenth-Century France," *J. Soc. Hist.* 10 (1976–7): 560–87, and Ramsey, *Professional and Popular Medicine*.

29   On the epidemic physicians see Evelyn Ackerman, *Health Care in the Parisian Countryside, 1800–1914* (New Brunswick, NJ: Rutgers University Press, 1990), ch. 3; Huard, "L'officiat de santé"; George Sussman, "Enlightened Health Reform, Professional Medicine and Traditional Society: The Cantonal Physicians of the Bas-Rhin, 1810–1870," *Bull. Hist. Med.* 51 (1977): 656–84.

the programs established during the Ancien Régime and the Revolutionary and Napoleonic eras: epidemic physicians, health officers, and physicians attached to vaccine depositories and mineral water establishments. The cantonal physicians' program was never enacted on a national scale, however. In spite of continued interest in a medical civil service, the governments of the Restoration and the July Monarchy initiated no new national health program. Nor did epidemic physicians become the standardized institution intended by the original decree. Although many departments had one epidemic physician per arrondissement, some departments, such as the Gironde, had only one for the whole department, whereas others, such as the Aube, never had any epidemic physicians at all. Until 1852 in the Aube, health council members performed the duties of epidemic physicians. Typically, however, epidemic physicians were the leading doctors in an area; during the early years of the Restoration they made seasonal rounds, giving vaccinations and dispensing advice and medicine.[30]

Health officers were unpopular with physicians, who considered them a threat to public health and their own practices. Claiming they provided inferior medical care, in the 1840s physicians tried, but failed, to eliminate the health officers, so that there would be only one grade of medical practitioner. The cantonal physicians were better received, at least by reforming physicians and social reformers. In the Bas-Rhin and Haut-Rhin, these publicly salaried rural practitioners superseded the epidemic physicians in importance and were responsible for the success of the vaccination program. They gave free medical care to the poor, performed vaccinations – their principal duty – prepared reports on the local sanitary situation, and provided medical topographies. Thus, by contrast with the epidemic physicians, they were on duty all the time, not just during medical emergencies.[31]

30 Dr. Léon Marchant occupied this post during the 1830s and 1840s. He was secretary of the health council of the Gironde and edited its annual reports during these years. A.D., Aube, M 1615. A. Vauthier, *Rapport général sur les travaux du Conseil d'hygiène de Troyes...1830...1867* (Troyes: Dufour-Bouquot, 1867), p. 61. Health council correspondents were supposed to function as epidemic physicians. See *Recueil des principaux travaux des conseils de salubrité du département de l'Aube* (Troyes: Cardon, 1835), pp. 1–4. Until 1819 epidemic physicians furnished free medicine to the poor, but that year the Minister of the Interior suppressed the medicine chests (*caisses de médicaments*) and ended this aspect of the service, to the chagrin of some epidemic physicians. See A.N., F⁸57, prefect of the Loire-Inférieure to Minister of the Interior, January 27, 1819.

31 See, for example, the vaccination records of Drs. Bessard and Gautron; A.N., F⁸57, Bessard, epidemic physician to subprefect, November 10, 1819; A.N., F⁸57, Gautron, epidemic physician to subprefect, November 27, 1819. On epidemic physicians, see Ackerman, *Health Care in the Parisian Countryside*, pp. 60–65; Sussman, "The Glut of Doctors in Mid-Nineteenth-Century France," *Comparative Studies in Society and History* 19 (1977): 292–3; Sussman, "Cantonal Physicians," p. 684.

THE VACCINATION PROGRAM

The Napoleonic government launched a major campaign to propagate vaccination, following its introduction into France in 1799–1800, for physicians believed vaccination was a sure preventive against smallpox.[32] The Central Vaccine Committee, established in 1803 under the auspices of the Minister of the Interior and under the leadership of the Duc de la Rochefoucauld and Michel-Auguste Thouret, functioned for twenty years as the national coordinating agency for the government's vaccination program. The Duc de la Rochefoucauld remained the honorary and perpetual president of the Committee until 1823, when it was abolished, to be merged with the Royal Academy of Medicine.[33] From 1823, the vaccine commission of the Royal Academy of Medicine took over the duties of the Central Vaccine Committee. One of the major duties, first of the Central Vaccine Committee and later of the vaccine commission, was to collect statistical data sent in from the departments on the number of vaccinations performed relative to births, smallpox cases, smallpox deaths, and disfigurements. Prefects sent quarterly reports to the Minister of the Interior, who forwarded them to the Central Vaccine Committee or the vaccine commission, which then compiled them and issued an annual report on the progress of vaccination in France. An imperial decree of 1809 established

32 One source claims that vaccination was introduced into the Bas-Rhin as early as 1799. Another source gives 1800 as the date. On the introduction of vaccine into the Bas-Rhin in 1799, see the interesting report on the history of vaccination by Franc Reisseissen (who was a physician at the Strasbourg orphan home and one of the vaccinating doctors attached to the vaccine depository), "Rapport à Monsieur le préfet du département du Bas-Rhin sur les vaccinations pratiquées dans le département pendant l'an 1811," in A.N., F⁸120. Jean-Baptiste Bousquet, on the other hand, reported that in 1798 Jenner made his discovery of vaccination public, and by 1800 vaccination was introduced into France by an English doctor, William Woodville, whose treatise on vaccination was published in France in 1800. See Jean-Baptiste Bousquet, "Eloge d'Edouard Jenner," *Bull. de l'Acad. Roy. de Méd.* 13 (1847): xxxvii–xxxviii. Bousquet was the leading French authority on vaccine during the period. He was also editor of the *Bulletin de l'Académie Royale de Médecine* from 1836 to 1850. On the introduction of vaccine into France, see also R. G. Dunbar, "The Introduction of the Practice of Vaccination into Napoleonic France," *Bull. Hist. Med.* 10 (1941): 635–50. For a detailed discussion of vaccination in Napoleonic and Restoration France, see Yves-Marie Bercé, *Le chaudron et la lancette: Croyances populaires et médecine préventive (1798–1830)* (Paris: Presses de la Renaissance, 1984). See also Pierre Darmon, *La Longue Traque de la variole: Les pionniers de la médecine préventive* (Paris: Perrin, 1986).

33 Bousquet, "Eloge." Members of the Central Vaccine Committee were Pinel, Thouret, Leroux, Parfait, Mongenot, Guilletin, Doussin-Debreuil, Marin, and Sulmade. See Bousquet, *Nouveau traité de la vaccine et des éruptions varioleuses* (Paris: Baillière, 1848), p. XI. See also the earlier work: *Traité de la vaccine et des éruptions varioleuses ou varioliformes...*(Paris: Baillière, 1833). Members of the vaccine commission of the Royal Academy of Medicine in 1836 were Girard, Cornac, Jadelot, Danyou, Sulmade, and Eméry (chairman). See *Bull. de l'Acad. Roy. de Méd.* 1 (1836): 808–22. See also *Journal des Débats*, November 14, 1824, p. 263.

twenty-five depositories for the conservation of vaccine (*dépôts de conservation de vaccine*) throughout France, with a physician in charge of each, and established vaccine committees in twenty-five cities where none existed. These committees typically included the prefect, mayor, and eminent physicians and surgeons.[34]

The national government encouraged vaccination by making it available free to those who could not afford to pay and by bestowing annual awards on medical personnel who vaccinated the largest number of people or who made significant research contributions. Cash prizes and gold and silver medals were awarded. In 1832, for example, of the prize recipients 3 shared the first prize of 1,500 francs, 4 got gold medals, and 100 received silver medals.[35] The government tried to educate citizens about the benefits of vaccine by publishing a manual, *La Vaccine soumise aux simples lumières de la raison*, written by Charles Marc in simple language so that it would be accessible to all. It was first published in 1809 and reprinted in 1836 under the auspices of the Royal Academy of Medicine. The book consists of discussions on vaccination among a curé, a physician, and several villagers. The villagers present all the usual prejudices against vaccination

34 See, for example, the reports of the Royal Academy of Medicine such as Jean-Baptiste Bousquet, *Rapport présenté à M. le Ministre de l'Agriculture et du Commerce, par l'Académie royale de médecine, sur les vaccinations pratiquées en France pendant l'année 1844, 1847, 1856, 1858–1859*, 4 vols. (Paris: Imprimerie royale, 1846–60. See reports in *Bull. de l'Acad. Roy. de Méd.* for 1835 in 1 (1836–7): 808–22; for 1839 in 6 (1840–1): 671–82; for 1840 in 7 (1841–2): 699–706. After 1830 the annual reports were addressed to the Minister of Commerce, to whom public health was delegated under the July Monarchy. Decree of March 16, 1809. In 1803, when the Central Vaccine Committee was set up in Paris, the prefect of the Gironde established a vaccine committee in Bordeaux, as well as committees in the subprefectures. See A.N., F^{8}110, "Rapport sur les vaccinations faites dans le département de la Gironde, le 2e jour complémentaire de l'an 13." A departmental vaccine committee was set up in 1808 in the Aube. See A.N., F^{8}102, Arrêté concernant la réorganisation du Comité de Vaccine, et les renseignemens à lui fournir par les officiers de santé. Préfecture de l'Aube, 29 oct. 1808. See also Circulaire pour la propagation de la vaccine, 18 nov. 1808. The vaccine committee in Strasbourg dated from 1801. See F^{8}120, Reisseissen, "Rapport." For Marseilles, see A.N., F^{8}103, Minister of the Interior to Prefect, October 8, 1812. The vaccine committee of Lyon dated from 1803. See A.N., F^{8}121, Histoire de l'établissement de la Vaccine à Lyon et dans le département du Rhône (1807). A.N., F^{8}110, Affiche. Extrait des registres des arrêtés de la préfecture de la Gironde, 4 août 1810.

35 Money for vaccinations came from the general councils of the departments, which in 1840, for example, voted 179,293 francs for vaccinations, or an average of 34 centimes for each child vaccinated. See *Bull. de l'Acad. Roy. de Méd.* 7 (1841–2): 705; see, for example, for 1839, *Bull. de l'Acad. Roy. de Méd.* 6 (1840–1: 1023–9. For awards given by the Central Vaccine Committee see *Journal des Débats*, March 18, 1817. For information on prizes and medals, see *Mémoires de l'Acad. Roy. de Méd.* 4 (1835): 49–50.

from both a religious and a medical point of view; then the curé and the physician show them how their opinions are faulty. At the end of the book, the villagers, having been convinced of the benefits of vaccination, decide to have their children vaccinated.[36]

From 1800 to 1820 national and local administrations made great efforts to convince or compel parents to have their children vaccinated. Free vaccinations were available at hospices and hospitals, or sometimes in other locales. In Bordeaux, for example, vaccinations were performed at the local medical society because of the popular fear of hospitals. The prefect explained:

But a repugnance greater than this obstacle [the inconvenient location of the foundling hospital] shared by both rich and poor, would prevent all classes from vaccinations performed at this hospital. The public would presume that the vaccine...was taken from foundlings, and as they know that those who find asylum there are ordinarily the fruit of licentiousness and they suppose, with reason, infected...with a venereal virus or some other organic vice, they would fear that the germ of such would be transmitted with the vaccine....In general, in Bordeaux, we approach hospitals with the greatest repugnance.[37]

Private physicians in cities and towns also performed vaccinations as part of their regular practice, and in the countryside epidemic physicians and health officers made regular vaccination rounds. Mayors seconded their efforts by posting notices about the arrival of vaccinating physicians and encouraging all to take advantage. From the pulpit, local curés exhorted the faithful to avail themselves of vaccine. In many areas the lower, un-educated classes, both urban and rural, displayed great resistance to vaccination. Some parents, for example, blamed all subsequent children's illnesses on vaccine. Many rural folk saw smallpox as a necessary purifica-tion, dangerous to avoid. Others thought vaccination could cause other diseases and might transmit the bad dispositions of the child who furnished the vaccine to the one who received it. Sometimes an epidemic increased resistance to vaccination if any who had been vaccinated got the disease. The correspondent of the Nantes health council from St.-Philibert noted that during the 1827 smallpox epidemic, inhabitants paid more attention to the ten vaccinated people who contracted the disease than to the several thousand who were spared. Authorities used various methods to try to overcome the resistance and apathy of the lower classes. In Nancy, for

36   *Ouvrage destiné aux pères et mères de famille des villes et des campagnes*, 2nd ed. (Paris, Baillière, 1836).
37   A.N., F⁸110, prefect of the Gironde to the Minister of the Interior, May 28, 1810.

example, the prefect, in the hope of frightening parents into having their children vaccinated, had a man who had lost his sight from smallpox paraded through the streets. In Nantes during the 1809 smallpox epidemic, daily notices were posted announcing the names of the dead – mostly children – and their ages and urging citizens to be vaccinated.[38]

More forceful measures were also used: In some localities unvaccinated workers were not hired; unvaccinated children were not allowed to enter schools; and their parents were disqualified from welfare benefits and denied entry to hospices and hospitals. These stringent measures were not always enforced, however, since teachers and employers often failed to cooperate.[39] More important, in 1821 Baron Capelle, Secretary-General of the Ministry of the Interior, expressed his disfavor with discrimination against the unvaccinated, believing draconian measures were no longer needed. It was a real constraint, Capelle noted, to place unfortunate people in a position of renouncing their welfare or submitting to an operation they regarded as dangerous and illicit. Capelle further commented that such constraints were not in keeping with the principles of good government. From the 1820s, the administration moved from constraint to persuasion, encouraging physicians by paying bonuses for each vaccination performed and awarding prizes for the best vaccinators. In the Loire-Inférieure from 1820 to 1823, a thirty-centime bonus was given from departmental funds to vaccinators for each free vaccination performed. Free vaccinations were given to indigents. In Paris, parents were paid a bonus of five francs for each child vaccinated, the equivalent of one or two days' wages for the average male worker.[40]

The goal of the national government was to have all the infants of an arrondissement or department vaccinated. Success varied. Vaccination figures, often incomplete and not standardized, were received quarterly by the Minister of the Interior/Commerce. They still serve as a general

---

38 A.N., F⁸110, Vaccine committee to prefect, Compte rendu 1815. See also Bercé, *Le chaudron et la lancette*, pp. 151–66; *Rapport général sur les travaux du conseil de salubrité de Nantes pendant l'année 1826* (Nantes: Mellinet-Malassis, 1827), p. 38; *Rapport sur les travaux du conseil de salubrité de Nantes pendant l'année 1827* (Nantes: Mellinet-Malassis, 1827), p. 94; *Journal des Débats*, September 25, 1825, p. 3; A.N., F⁸113, Affiche 1809. Département de la Loire-Inférieure, liste des individus morts de la petite vérole en 1809.

39 In the Meurthe, parents who refused were not allowed to send their children to school. See *Journal des Débats*, September 25, 1818. For Troyes, see A.N., F⁸102, Circulaire 18 novembre 1808; arrêté pour la propagation de la vaccine, 18 novembre 1808. For Paris, see A.N., F⁸124, arrêté préfectoral, 22 novembre 1817. For Bordeaux, see A.N., F⁸110, arrêté, 7 décembre 1809. For Lille, see A.N., F⁸118, Extrait des registres des actes de la préfecture du Nord, Lille, le 28 mars 1816. For Strasbourg, see A.N., F⁸120, Reisseissen, "Rapport."

40 A.N., F⁸124, Circular no. 38 to prefects from Baron Capelle, Secretary-General of the Ministry of the Interior, September 4, 1821. See A.N., F⁸113, prefect of the Loire-Inférieure to Minister of the Interior, April 30, 1822. A.N., F⁸124, prefect of the Seine Chabrol to Minister of the Interior, December 18, 1817.

comparative indicator to measure the program's progress. In fact, the government's goal was unrealistic, since it did not take into account the infant mortality rate; one of every four or five babies died during the first year of life. Babies and children too weak or sick to take vaccine were ignored, and older children and adults were not factored in. Nonetheless, some outstanding vaccinators met the government's goal. M. Deshayes, health officer in Chapelle-Cassemer (Loire-Inférieure) who vaccinated all the children in his area, did such a thorough job in ten years that the only vaccinations left to be done were on those born each year.[41]

The Bas-Rhin had an impressive vaccination record, attributable by local authorities to its system of cantonal physicians. The Medical Faculty in Strasbourg also played an important role in the vaccination campaign, functioning both as vaccine committee and as health council and preparing annual reports on the progress of vaccination in the department. The early years of vaccination went well in the Bas-Rhin, owing to local initiative and the cooperation of the prefect, the Medical Faculty, and the health officers. Good results were being obtained there by 1810 without intervention from the national government and even before the establishment of the system of cantonal physicians. Strict measures were applied: no school or welfare for the unvaccinated and, from 1811, no work either. After 1810, the cantonal physicians played a major role in distributing vaccine in rural areas. Thirty-four salaried cantonal physicians were in charge of public health and medical care of the poor, with vaccination being one of their essential functions. All vaccinations were free, and doctors were required to keep exact records. Each generally announced vaccination session was preceded by a preparatory one to guarantee enough fresh vaccine for all. Mayors cooperated by submitting quarterly lists of newborns to physicians, with the birth date, the parents' names, and a column left blank to insert the date of vaccination, the name of the vaccinating physician, and if the vaccination had failed or had not been done and why. The names of those still unvaccinated were put at the top of the next quarterly list. A separate list was kept of smallpox cases. The result was that in many areas of the Bas-Rhin, even as early as 1811, the number of vaccinations almost equaled the number of births. The situation was so good that by 1819 there had been for that year only one case of smallpox in the whole department (imported by a foreigner), and the prefect proclaimed that the disease no longer existed in the Bas-Rhin.[42]

The Bas-Rhin was not typical of the country as a whole. Smallpox

41 A.N., F⁸113, Rapport sur la vaccination des nouveau-nés; Minister of the Interior to Prefect of the Loire-Inférieure, August 4, 1820; A.N., F⁸113, prefect of the Loire-Inférieure to Minister of the Interior, June 9, 1825.
42 Sussman, "Cantonal Physicians." All of this information on the Bas-Rhin in A.N., F⁸120, Reisseissen, "Rapport." A.N., F⁸120, prefect of the Bas-Rhin to Minister of the Interior, October 17, 1820.

epidemics continued to occur in many areas of France in spite of education, active campaigns, encouragement, and even notable success in some areas. For example, in the arrondissement of Savenay (Loire-Inférieure) in 1818 there were 1,698 cases of smallpox, almost equal to the number of vaccinations (1,786) and 336 deaths. In the department of the Loire-Inférieure for 1818 there were 3,353 cases of smallpox and 528 deaths. Smallpox was endemic in Lille from 1815 to 1824. During the Paris epidemic of 1822 there were 2,160 deaths, and an 1825 epidemic in that city took the lives of 2,193 people. In Marseilles, an 1818 epidemic resulted in 1,154 cases and 274 deaths; in 1823 there were 952 cases with 105 deaths; and in an 1828 epidemic, 1,488 people out of a population of about 120,000 died.[43]

After the 1820s, the early confidence in and euphoria about vaccination and the possibility of eradicating smallpox ended. Whereas in 1819 the prefect of the Bas-Rhin had been able to declare that the disease had been eliminated in his department, by 1839 the health council reported that there was smallpox in the Bas-Rhin every year. In addition, events of the early 1830s were harmful to the overall vaccination effort: Revolution (1830), working-class uprisings (1834), and cholera (1832–5) diverted the attention of national and local governments away from vaccination.[44] Furthermore, questions arose about the nature and efficacy of vaccine. The Paris epidemic of 1825 and the Marseilles epidemic of 1828 made some physicians doubt the preventive nature of vaccine, because in both epidemics there was a small but significant minority of vaccinated people who contracted the disease. Up to this time, two characteristics generally accepted about vaccine were its unalterability and its permanent protection against smallpox. By the 1830s there was a growing debate over the truth of these propositions, some physicians wondering if vaccination was only temporary and whether revaccination at stated intervals was necessary for continued prevention.[45]

43 A.N., F^{8}113, Tableau des vaccinations pratiquées dans le département de la Loire-Inférieure...Exercice 1818. A.N., F^{8}118, Tableaux des vaccinations...1815–1824. The worst year was 1818, with 2,854 reported cases and 588 deaths. For the 1822 epidemic, see A.N., F^{8}124, Tableau de vaccinations...Exercice 1822. For the 1825 epidemic, see G. Chabrol de Volvic, *Recherches statistiques sur la ville de Paris*, 5 vols. (Paris: Imprimerie municipale, 1821–44), 4 (1829); Moléon, *Rapports généraux*, 1825, pp. 335–6; A.N., F^{8}103, Tableau de vaccinations...Exercice 1818, Exercice 1823. On the 1828 epidemic, see *Rapport général, 1828–1829 et 1830*, pp. 8–41.

44 V. Stoeber, *Rapport du Conseil de salubrité publique du département du Bas-Rhin à M. le préfet sur les vaccinations opérées par les médecins cantonnaux du département* (Strasbourg: Silbermann, 1840), p. 6; see, for example, *Journal des Débats*, June 27, 1832, p. 2.

45 Moléon, *Rapports généraux*, 1825, pp. 335–6. One smallpox authority, Dr. Fiard, had been in communication with the Academy of Medicine since 1831 on this point. See Thomas M. L. Fiard, *Nécessité de la revaccination* (Paris: Locquin, 1838), p. 2. See also Charles Roesch, "Histoire d'une épidémie de variole: Revaccination

In 1836, a new strain of vaccine was discovered when cowpox was reported in Passy, Amiens, and Rambouillet. As a result, the debate on vaccine was enlarged to include a controversy over the comparative effectiveness of the new and old strains. In the late 1830s and early 1840s, the Royal Academy of Medicine, which had consistently argued for the efficacy of vaccination, was the scene of several major discussions on the nature of vaccine and the desirability of revaccination. In 1838, the Royal Academy of Sciences addressed the vaccination question by opening a contest for the best essay on vaccine dealing with its preventive qualities, duration of protection, and the question of revaccination. The commission judging the contest concluded (March 10, 1845) that vaccine was not 100 percent effective; that after ten to twelve years it sometimes lost its preventive qualities; that therefore revaccination was necessary in some cases; and that the old vaccine was as effective as the new.[46]

By the 1830s and 1840s, the government's goal of having the number of vaccinations equal the number of births was far from being attained for the nation in spite of considerable success in some places. For example, in 1836, the vaccine commission of the Royal Academy of Medicine reported that with all departments responding for 1835, there had been 518,734 vaccinations and 745,445 births. Out of 13,726 smallpox cases reported, 1,486 people had been left infirm or disfigured, and there had been 1,823 deaths. Statistics for 1840 showed 836,789 births and 525,509 vaccinations for all of France, with 14,470 cases of smallpox reported and 1,668 deaths. Yet progress had been made, as a comparison of figures from the 1830s with those from 1816 indicates. In 1816 the Central Vaccine Committee, compiling information from seventy-six departments, reported that out of 626,641 babies born, only 201,116 had been vaccinated.[47]

pratiquée à la suite: Nature de la varioloïde: Valeur de la revaccination," *Annales d'hygiène publique* 18 (1837): 73–164, in which he observed that vaccinated people were contracting smallpox; therefore he recommended revaccination every ten to twelve years, noting that those who had been revaccinated within seven to ten years rarely got the disease.

46 *Bull. de l'Acad. Roy. de Méd.* 1 (1836–7): 809–18; 3 (1838–9): 6–19, 45–60; 5 (1840): 36–63; 6 (1840–1): 671–82; 7 (1841–2): 699–706; 9(1843–4): 20–32, 90–109. The Royal Academy of Sciences was one of the four academies of the Institute that was reorganized by a royal ordinance of March 21, 1816. See *Mémoires de l'Académie Royale des Sciences de l'Institut de France* 1 (1816): V–X; *Comptes-rendus de l'Académie Royale des Sciences* 7 (1838): 358; For the report, see "Rapport fait à l'Académie royale des Sciences sur le prix de vaccine," reproduced in its entirety in *Annales d'hygiène publique* 33 (1845): 437–58. Members of the commission were Magendie, Breschet, Duméril, Roux, and Serres (chairman). The winner was Jean-Baptiste Bousquet for his essay, which was published as a book in 1848, *Nouveau traité de la vaccine et des éruptions varioleuses…*(Paris: Baillière, 1848). The first edition of this work, published in 1833, had been written under the auspices of the vaccine commission of the Royal Academy of Medicine.

47 *Bull. de l'Acad. Roy. de Méd.* 1 (1836): 808–22; 7 (1841–2): 705. For reports on earlier years, see Villermé's compilation of tables for the eighteen years preceding

The vaccination campaign was one of the most important national public health programs because effective prevention was possible. Physicians and administrators made great strides in the propagation of vaccination during the Restoration; yet smallpox epidemics continued to occur, and prevention was less effective than reformers had hoped. Two explanations account for the less than complete success of the program. First, popular opposition to vaccination remained substantial. Second, no national compulsory vaccination law was passed. Compulsory vaccination raised the basic public health question, then as now: the right of individual liberty versus the good of society. Those who favored compulsory vaccination, as one Bordelais doctor explained, thought that an individual should give up a portion of his liberty in order to enjoy the other portion in such a way that no harm was done to others; to transmit a contagious disease was to do harm, and therefore obligatory public health measures were justified and did not undermine the concept of individual liberty.[48] But Baron Capelle, speaking in 1821, better expressed the mood of individual liberty that prevailed under the Restoration and the July Monarchy with regard to obligatory public health measures: "The return to conservative ideas of order and liberty must then make us push away more and more from such measures...; we must seek to enlighten men on their real interests: but it is persuasion and not constraint which can dispel prejudices and assure the success of useful discoveries."[49]

CONCLUSION

From the 1770s to the 1820s, physician-hygienists and reforming administrators articulated and institutionalized the public health idea. During the Revolution the national government had accepted responsibility for the nation's health and both Napoleon and the Bourbons took up the charge, instituting a variety of public health policies and programs. By the 1820s several health programs were in place: the nationwide vaccination admin-

1829 in "Tableau relatif aux vaccinations pratiquées en France, et aux petites véroles," *Annales d'hygiène publique* 1 (1829): 400–4. The proportion of vaccinations to births varied widely from one department to another. In the Meurthe, for example, which had an active vaccine committee, in 1818 for 13,007 births there were 10,307 vaccinations. See Sébastien Serrières, *Notice historique sur les progrès de la vaccine dans le département de la Meurthe* (Nancy: Haener et Dard, 1829), reviewed in *Annales d'hygiène publique* 2 (1829): 497–8. The vaccine commission pointed out that the number of vaccinations could not be known, exactly, as many doctors did not send in figures, and in some departments, mothers and others who were not doctors vaccinated a certain number of children. See *Bull. de l'Acad. Roy. de Méd.* 7 (1841–2): 700; *Journal des Débats*, January 15, 1817.

48 A.N., F⁸110, Vaccine Committee to prefect, 1815, unsigned, undated.
49 A.N., F⁸124, Circular no. 38 to prefects from Baron Capelle, Secretary-General of the Ministry of the Interior, September 4, 1821.

istration; a two-tiered national health care program of epidemic physicians and health officers; a national administration of sanitary intendancies and, as its helm, a Superior Health Council. Public health institutions had been established at the national level: the Royal Academy of Medicine and the Superior Health Council; and at the local level, municipal and departmental health councils, the most important of which was the Paris council. The Royal Academy of Medicine, barely in place by the 1820s, exemplified the public health idea inherited from the Royal Society of Medicine.

Carrying out the mission:
Institutionalization, investigation, moralization, and practical reform

4

Institutionalization: The health councils

Although some public health concerns such as epidemics, vaccination, and child labor attracted the attention of the national government, public health administration was principally a municipal and departmental affair. The creation of advisory health councils (*conseils de salubrité*) at the municipal and departmental levels to assist prefects and mayors in regulating public health was characteristic of the period. The idea of a permanent advisory commission on public health dated from the Revolution, and the first French health council, the Paris health council, which became the model for all French councils, was founded in 1802 by the prefect of police of Paris, Dubois.[1] By the 1830s, when the French public health movement was at the height of its activity, the health council idea had spread to other cities and departments, and Nantes, Lyon, Marseilles, Lille, Strasbourg, Bordeaux, Rouen, Troyes, and Toulouse had their own advisory councils.

THE PARISIAN PUBLIC HEALTH ADMINISTRATION: THE PREFECTURE OF POLICE AND THE PARIS HEALTH COUNCIL

The Parisian public health administration consisted of the prefecture of police, the institution in charge of public health for the city, and the Paris

---

1 Dora B. Weiner, "Le Droit de l'homme à la santé – une belle idée devant l'Assemblée constituante: 1790–1791," *Clio Medica* 5 (1970): 209–23, but esp. pp. 216–17; Henry Ingrand, *Le Comité de salubrité de l'Assemblée nationale constituante (1790–91)* (Thesis, University of Paris, 1934), pp. 81–6. There had been boards of health in Italy as far back as the fifteenth century; see Carlo Cipolla, *Public Health and the Medical Profession in the Renaissance* (Cambridge: Cambridge University Press, 1976), pp. 11–66. There were boards of medicine (*Collegium medicum*) and sanitary boards (*Collegium sanitatis*) in Brandenburg-Prussia, but neither seems to have been equivalent to the French health councils. See Reinhold August Dorwart, *The Prussian Welfare State before 1740* (Cambridge, MA: Harvard University Press, 1971), pp. 240–54. The *Collegium medicum* appears to have been a common institution in other German states as well, but was more concerned with regulating the practice of medicine than other aspects of public health. For another example, see Mary Lindemann, "Quacks, Bread-Thieves, and Interlopers: The Economics of Medical Practice in Braunschweig-Wolfenbüttel, 1750–1820," paper presented at

health council, the advisory body to the prefect of police and the one institution devoted solely to the preservation of the public health in Paris.[2] Paris and the department of the Seine were governed by two magistrates, the prefect of the Seine and the prefect of police, each appointed by the Minister of the Interior.[3] The prefect of the Seine was in charge of major public health–related works such as water supply, sewer construction, and road building, and the prefect of police was specifically empowered to administer the pubic health, in addition to other administrative duties related to political police, public safety, and the preservation of law and order.

Public health was one of the major duties of the prefect of police but, depending on the situation, not always the most important. For example, Henri Gisquet, prefect of police from 1831 to 1836, was primarily occupied with the political police, crushing strikes, and consolidating the new regime, whereas Gabriel Delessert, prefect of police from 1836 to 1848, devoted more time to administrative police, including public health.[4]

the annual meeting of the American Association for the History of Medicine, Rochester, New York, May 2, 1986.

2 From 1802 to 1848 health council members prepared yearly 150 to 500 reports on various aspects of public health in Paris and the department of the Seine. Annually they prepared a report summarizing the year's work and analyzing the most important problems they had investigated. These annual reports were published at varying intervals, and provide a complete record of the activities of the council and a good picture of the state of public health in Paris. Individual manuscript reports for 1808–25 are available at the Archives of the Prefecture of Police in Paris. Some provincial councils also published annual reports, such as the Nord (Lille), Bouches-du-Rhône (Marseilles), and Loire-Inférieure (Nantes). On the Paris health council, see Dora B. Weiner, "Public Health Under Napoleon: The Conseil de salubrité de Paris, 1802–1815," *Clio Medica* 9 (1974): 271–84 and Ann Fowler La Berge, "The Paris Health Council, 1802–1848," *Bull. Hist. Med.* 49 (1975): 339–52.

3 Also included in the jurisdiction were the communes of St.-Cloud, Sèvres, and Meudon in the Department of Seine-et-Oise. The government of Paris and the Departments of the Seine differed from those of the rest of the departments and cities of France. At the head of every other department was a prefect, appointed by the Minister of the Interior, whose duties included public health. The departments were divided into arrondissements administered by a subprefect, who also had public health responsibilities. Each commune (town or city) had a mayor, elected by the municipal council but responsible to the prefect. Mayors were in charge of public health in their towns or cities.

4 Jean Tulard, *La préfecture de police sous la monarchie de juillet* (Paris: Imprimerie nationale, 1964), p. 111. For a list of the prefects of police from 1815 to 1849, see Appendix 4. See Henri Gisquet, *Mémoires d'un préfet de police écrits par lui-même*, 4 vols. (Paris: Marchant, 1840); in the Archives of the Prefecture of Police there are reconstituted dossiers of Anglès, Delaveau, Debelleyme, Vivien, Gisquet, and Delessert; they contain little new information, consisting primarily of newspaper clippings, copies of printed articles, and excerpts from biographical dictionaries; they contain no original manuscript material. There is also a dossier for Delessert in the National Archives, F 158[12], but it contains no information on him as prefect of police.

Specific public health duties of the prefect of police included control and surveillance of prostitution, inspection of markets and slaughterhouses, street and sewer cleaning, public lighting, surveillance and authorization of industrial establishments, supervision of animal diseases, destruction of stray animals, salubrity of public places, and control of charlatans. After the passage of the child labor law in 1841, the prefect of police became responsible for its administration.[5] The prefect of police issued and enforced public health ordinances. Health council reports reveal, however, that prefects often neglected their enforcement responsibilities.[6] As an advisory board, the health council had no real power, but its influence on public health policies was considerable. Technical personnel attached to the prefecture of police included inspectors of markets and slaughterhouses, wine tasters, architects concerned with public works (*la petite voirie*), engineers attached to the division in control of dangerous establishments (such as chemical match factories), physicians who examined prostitutes at the Dispensary, inspectors of wet-nursing establishments and nursing homes (*maisons de santé*), and prison personnel.[7]

The money for the prefecture of police came from the Paris municipal council, which allocated funds from the city budget. The municipal council exercised considerable control over the purse strings, and many programs suggested by the health council were never effected owing to the municipal council's refusal or inability to provide the necessary funds. The budgets of the prefecture of police ranged from 5,197,831 francs in 1819 to 7,111,77 francs in 1828 to 7,240,191 francs in 1836 to 10,720,072 francs in 1847.[8] The prefect of police's salary was fixed at 30,000 francs a year in 1818; the salaries of division heads at 9,000 to 10,000 francs a year; the salaries of heads of bureaus at 4,500 francs; and the salaries of assistant heads at 3,000 francs. Additionally, salaries were paid to the 5,000 other people who worked for the prefecture.[9] From a total budget of 10,720,072 francs in 1847, approximately 3,240,610 was spent for public health-related expenses, including both salaries and materials. The largest single

5 Alexandre Vivien, *Etudes administratives. Le préfet de police* (Paris: Fournier, 1842), pp. 34–40. For the organization of the office of the prefect of police, see Appendix 5.
6 *Rapports généraux du Conseil de salubrité de la ville de Paris, 1802–1848*, passim. See also Tulard, *La préfecture de police*, p. 77, and *Annales d'hygiène publique*, 1829–48.
7 Tulard, *La préfecture de police*, p. 64. According to Tulard (p. 39), during the July Monarchy, the Paris prefecture of police had an administration equalling that of certain ministries in importance. There were 200 employees at the prefecture of police and about 5,000 people attached in various ways to the service.
8 Tulard, *La préfecture de police*, pp. 39, 68–9. See also APP, Da 79, Ville de Paris, Budget des Dépenses de la Préfecture de police pour l'exercice 1847. Annexe au Budget de la Ville de Paris pour ledit Exercice.
9 APP, Da 69. Personnel. Budget de 1831; Budget de la Préfecture de Police 1832.

expenditure was for street lighting (1,622,220 francs), and the next largest was for street and sewer cleaning (1,086,750 francs).[10]

The Paris health council was established in 1802. As the story goes, Count Dubois, the first prefect of police, was in the habit of consulting specialists for public health advice; depending on the question, a physician, veterinarian, chemist, or pharmacist was consulted. When he needed the opinion of more than one specialist, Dubois convened a temporary commission. In 1802, one of the experts who had been consulted often, pharmacist Charles-Louis Cadet de Gassicourt, proposed that Dubois create a permanent health council. On July 6, 1802, the Paris health council, consisting of four members, was founded. During its first five years the council had only limited duties, including examination of adulterated drinks; investigation of epizootics, unhealthy factories, workshops, and prisons; and providing first aid to persons in danger of drowning or asphyxiation. In 1807, when the health council received its definitive organization, its duties were increased to include most aspects of public health. The council was henceforth to report on epidemics, markets, rivers, cemeteries, slaughterhouses and slaughteryards, dumps, dissection rooms, and public baths. The council also compiled medical statistics and mortality tables and conducted research on the sanitary reform of public places, industrial processes, and secret remedies. Also included among its duties were the elimination of quackery and determination of the best methods of heating and lighting.[11]

As Paris became more urbanized and industrialized, health council activity increased from 2,524 reports from 1811 to 1820, to 2,886 in the next decade, and then to 4,228 reports between 1831 and 1840.[12] This increase was not necessarily a sign of more widespread attention to all areas of public health, however, but corresponded to the growing industrialization of the Parisian area after 1830.[13] The investigation of requests for in-

10 APP, Da 79, Ville de Paris, Compte, du 17 mai 1848, des Dépenses de la Préfecture de police pour l'exercice 1847, suivi du compte des recettes dont le recouvrement est opéré ou suivi par ladite Préfecture. For a comparison of the budgets of the prefecture of police for 1831 and 1847 and money spent on various aspects of public health administration, see Appendix 6.

11 Victor de Moléon, *Rapports généraux sur les travaux du Conseil de salubrité de la ville de Paris et du département de la Seine exécutés depuis l'année 1802 jusqu'à l'année 1826 inclusivement* (Paris: au bureau du "Recueil industriel," 1828), 1817, pp. 99–103; hereafter referred to as Moléon, *R. G.*, followed by the year of the report. For a good account of the founding, early years, and administrative history of the pre-1850 Paris health council, see Adolphe Trébuchet, ed., *Rapport général sur les travaux du Conseil d'hygiène publique et de salubrité depuis 1849 jusqu'à 1858 inclusivement* (Paris: Boucquin, imprimerie de la Préfecture de police, 1861).

12 *Rapports généraux des travaux du Conseil de salubrité pendant les années 1840–1845 inclusivement* (Paris: Imprimerie municipale, 1847), 1842, p. 146; hereafter referred to as *R. G.*, followed by the year of the report.

13 In other areas health council duties were limited, due primarily to the emergence of other organizations whose duties included public health. For example, when the Royal Society for the Improvement of Prisons was founded in 1819, that body

dustrial authorization accounted for the great expansion in health council activity after 1830. This duty dated from an imperial decree of 1810 that provided for the classification of industries in three areas, depending on how dangerous, unhealthy, or obnoxious they were. According to the decree, persons wishing to establish a factory or workshop had to seek authorization from the prefect of police. Before authorization was granted, the health council would inspect and classify (in the case of a new industry) the establishment and prepare a report either recommending or denying authorization.[14] The inspection of industrial establishments became one of the most time-consuming duties of the health council, and by 1841 this task had become its habitual daily work. The reports pointed out that Paris and the department of the Seine were no longer a center of production destined only for food and the consumption of its inhabitants, but that Paris had become an industrial manufacturing area whose products were sold throughout France and in most foreign countries. An example of the relative importance of inspection of requests for industrial authorization as part of the whole spectrum of health council activities is furnished by figures from the 1842 report. Out of 590 reports prepared by the health council that year, 516 dealt with industrial establishments; of these, 54 were complaints and 462 were requests for authorizations.[15]

In 1807, membership in the health council increased from four to seven. Recruiting new members was the responsibility of the prefect of police, who chose one of three candidates nominated by the health council.[16]

took over most of the health council's duties related to prison inspection – at least until its demise in 1829. After the founding of the Royal Academy of Medicine in 1820, that institution took over former health council duties related to epidemics, research on secret remedies, and the elimination of quackery. Moléon, *R. G.*, 1819, pp. 154–5; 1820, p. 169; 1826, p. 372; *Mém. de l'Acad. Roy. de Méd.* 1 (1828): 2; in fact, the health council had been stripped of its duties with regard to epidemics as early as 1811, when the control of epidemics, which since 1800 had been one of the duties of the prefect of police, became one of the areas of responsibility of the prefect of the Seine; see Moléon, *R. G.*, 1811, p. 57; 1817, pp. 103–4, 111.

14   Moléon, *R. G.*, 1809, p. 39; 1810, p. 40; for the 1810 decree on dangerous trades, see *Recueil des textes officiels concernant la protection de la santé publique, 1790 à 1935*, 9 vols. (Paris: Ministère de la Santé Publique, 1957), 1: 165–7; for the royal ordinance of 1815 reinforcing the Napoleonic decree, see ibid., 1: 209, or *Moniteur universel*, February 16, 1815, pp. 187–8; see also Adolphe Trébuchet, *Code administratif des établissemens dangereux, insalubres ou incommodes* (Paris: Béchet jeune, 1832). Trébuchet's book is the definitive work on this subject. See the review by Pierre Girard, "Rapport sur un ouvrage intitulé: *Code administratif des établissemens dangereux, insalubres ou incommodes*, par M. Adolphe Trébuchet," *Annales d'hygiène publique* 10 (1833): 197–201.

15   For example, both the 1837 and 1838 reports emphasized the effect that increasing industrialization of the Parisian area was having on health council activities. See *Rapports généraux des travaux du Conseil de salubrité pendant les années 1829 à 1839 inclusivement* (Paris: Imprimerie municipale, 1840), 1837, pp. 145, 158; 1838, p. 95. *R. G.*, 1841, p. 95. *R. G.*, 1842, p. 147.

16   Moléon, *R.G.*, pp. 1–4; see also A. J. B. Parent-Duchâtelet, "Quelques considérations sur le Conseil de salubrité de Paris," *Hygiène publique*, 2 vols. (Paris: Baillière, 1836), 1: 8–10.

From 1802 to 1848 the members of the Paris health council were an illustrious group, well known in their particular specialties. In 1807, the members were Charles-Louis Cadet de Gassicourt, chemist and pharmacist; Nicolas Deyeux, who held the chair of chemistry at the Paris Faculty; Guillaume Dupuytren, second surgeon at the Hôtel-Dieu; Jean-Baptiste Huzard, inspector-general of the Veterinary School of France; Antoine-Augustin Parmentier, pharmacist and chemist, who introduced the potato to France;[17] Michel-Augustin Thouret, dean of the Faculty of Medicine and author of many works on hygiene; and Jean-Jacques Leroux, who succeeded Thouret in 1810 as dean of the Faculty of Medicine.[18]

By 1828 the number of council members had increased to twenty-two. Those appointed to the health council between 1807 and 1828 included Etienne Pariset, a physician who would become permanent secretary of the Royal Academy of Medicine (1808); Joseph d'Arcet, a chemist well known for his research on the improvement of industrial processes (1815); Charles C. H. Marc, a legal medicine specialist and personal physician of the Duc d'Orléans, later King Louis Philippe (1815); Pierre Girard, chief engineer in charge of bridges and highways for the department of the Seine (1819); Joseph Pelletier, pharmacist and chemist, discoverer (with Caventou) of quinine (1821); Antoine-Germain Labarraque, chemist and pharmacist, credited with the discovery of the disinfectant *eau de Javel* (1828); and, of course, Parent-Duchâtelet (1825).[19] From 1831 to 1836 Villermé was an adjunct member.[20]

After 1828 the health council included twelve titular members who were appointed for life and paid 1,200 francs a year, six adjunct members, and numerous honorary members.[21] The honorary members (from 1832) included the dean of the Paris Faculty of Medicine, the professors of public hygiene and legal medicine at the Paris Faculty, and (from 1838) persons who possessed special technical or administrative competence. This last category included the chief mining engineer of the department of the Seine, the engineer in charge of bridges and highways for the department of the Seine, the chief engineer in charge of the Paris water supply, the

---

17 Parmentier's essay *Examen chimique des pommes de terre* (Paris: Didot le jeune, 1773) won the prize offered by the Academy of Besançon for the best essay on the most appropriate vegetable to replace bread. See *La grande encyclopédie*, 31 vols. (Paris: Société anonyme de la Grande Encyclopédie, 1886–1902), 25: 1177–8. On Cadet de Gassicourt, see Alex Berman, "The Cadet Circle: An Era in French Pharmacy," *Bull. Hist. Med.* 40 (1966): 101–11.

18 Moléon, R. G., pp. xv–xxvi.

19 Parent-Duchâtelet was a member until his death in 1836. At the time of his death he was vice-president of the health council.

20 Moléon, R.G., pp. xv–xl. For a complete list of the members of the council, see Jean François and Fernand Prunet, *Le Conseil d'hygiène publique et de salubrité du département de la Seine. Sa création. Ses modifications. Sa composition de 1802 à 1935*. In APP, 2779–20, pp. 4–40, for the year 1815–48.

21 A titular member was a permanent, salaried member; an adjunct member was an unpaid associate member.

architect-commissioner of small public works, the head of the second division of the prefecture of police (the division in charge of public health and public works), and the head of the sanitary office at the prefecture of police.[22]

The official function of the Paris council remained the same throughout the first half of the century: Members investigated public health problems and requests for industrial authorizations and prepared between 150 and 600 reports a year. The council had considerable influence in three areas: (1) Upon the council's recommendation, the prefect of police issued police ordinances regulating the public health; (2) public health measures and programs were effected following health council recommendations; and (3) industries were authorized or denied authorization based on the health council's investigation. Public health in Paris was regulated by ordinances issued by the prefect of police that had the force of law.[23] New public health ordinances typically resulted from health council recommendations. Between 1829 and 1845 ordinances addressed problems associated with toxic coloring in food, use of copper utensils, adulteration of salt, first aid to the drowning and asphyxiated, deposits of mud and garbage in rural communes, cleaning of wells, adulteration and sale of explosives, classification of new industries, anatomy amphitheaters, butchershops, animals with contagious diseases, the transportation of unhealthy materials, and the manufacture and transportation of chemical matches, a new and dangerous industry. An example of how the process worked was the ordinance of July 1832 on the use of copper utensils. Research done by hygienists on copper and lead utensils revealed that these substances were hazardous to health. The ordinance regulated their use, providing for periodic inspection of public establishments that used them. Another ordinance forbade the use of mineral substances in food coloring and provided for annual inspections of candy factories. (It is interesting to note that annual visits were considered frequent enough to provide adequate enforcement.)[24]

Lack of law enforcement was one of the major frustrations of health

22 François and Prunet, *Le conseil*, pp. 4–5; A.N., F⁸171, Note pour M. le Ministre 185_. This note contains all the decrees regulating the organization of the Paris health council. François and Prunet, *Le conseil*, p. 8, say that the salary of titular members was 1,200 francs a year, dating from 1803. The note in the A.N. gives the date as 1832. For the new members added in 1838, see François and Prunet, *Le conseil*, p. 60.

23 A. Vivien, *Etudes administratives*, p. 13.

24 Adolphe Trébuchet, "Rapports généraux des travaux du Conseil de Salubrité, depuis 1829 jusqu'en 1839," *Annales d'hygiène publique*, 25 (1841): 98–9 (this and the following article by Trébuchet are summaries of the *Rapports généraux* for the given years). See "Ordonnance de police concernant la salubrité," *Annales d'hygiène publique*, 16 (1836): 463–6; [Adolphe Trébuchet], "Rapports généraux des travaux du Conseil de Salubrité depuis 1840 jusqu'à 1845 inclusivement," *Annales d'hygiène publique*, 38 (1847): 149. See, for example, "Ordonnance concernant les liqueurs, sucreries, dragées et pastillages coloriés," *Annales d'hygiène publique*, 29 (1843): 359–60.

council members.[25] Public health ordinances were not regularly enforced in the 1820s and early 1830s, perhaps because in these years the Paris police gave priority to rooting out subversives, ending strikes, and coping with working-class troubles and crime.[26] As far as the Parisian administration was concerned, except for the 1832 cholera epidemic, there were more immediate problems for the Paris police to tackle than the enforcement of public health ordinances. Gabriel Delessert, prefect of police from 1836 to 1848, extended the public health duties of that office by reissuing and attempting to enforce many ordinances that had been ignored and forgotten. Nevertheless, enforcement was still not as rigorous as the health council would have liked. Historian Jean Tulard explained the lack of regular enforcement during the July Monarchy as a reaction to the strict regulation of Parisian life under Napoleon and the first prefect of police, Dubois. Tulard suggested that the administrators of the July Monarchy were convinced liberals who were trying to break away from an earlier tradition of interventionism that they had inherited.[27]

Public health measures and programs were initiated upon the health council's recommendation. The first example of the health council's influence on public health policy was the 1810 imperial decree on dangerous industries, which was based on a health council report prepared in 1809.[28] Another example involved a sewer cleaning project undertaken in the 1820s by the Parisian administration. By the mid-1820s many Parisian sewers were in desperate need of a good cleaning. In 1826, when the administration decided to clean out one of the largest right bank sewers, the prefect of police named a commission, which included members of the health council, to determine hygienic precautions. Traditionally, one of the worst problems associated with sewer cleaning had been asphyxiation of sewer workers. The recommendations of the health council provided for adequate ventilation and disinfection with chloride of lime. The five-

25 See Tulard, *La préfecture de police*, p. 77. The health council reports furnish numerous examples of the lack of law enforcement. See Moléon, *R. G.*, 1815, p. 86; 1818, p. 132; 1820, p. 172; 1829, p. 26; 1837, p. 157; 1843, p. 225; *Rapports généraux des travaux du Conseil de salubrité pendant les années 1846, 1847 et 1848* (Paris: Imprimerie municipale, 1855), 1846, p. 36. See also Adolphe Trébuchet, ed., *Bulletin administratif et judiciaire de la préfecture de police et de la ville de Paris*, No. 1, January 1835, pp. 3–4. Apparently the bulletin ceased publication after No. 2 of February 1835.

26 See the inventory of the Bulletins of Paris, addressed daily from the prefect of police to the Minister of the Interior for the years 1830–48 in Tulard, *La préfecture de police*, pp. 118ff. These bulletins generally do not deal with public health, but rather with political activity and economic troubles. See also Tulard, *La préfecture de police*, pp. 77–111. See Vivien, *Etudes administratives*, pp. 14–39; John Phillip Stead, *The Police of Paris* (London: Staples Press, 1957), pp. 99–109.

27 Tulard, *La préfecture de police*, pp. 77–8, 97–111. See also, the health council reports, passim, where all these generalizations are supported.

28 See Moléon, *R. G.*, 1809, p. 39; 1818, p. 40.

month project was a success, since not only were lives spared and good health maintained, but the sewers were cleaned.[29]

Further evidence of the health council's influence is illustrated by its handling of the problems associated with *équarrissage*, the industry of the cutting up and flaying of horses and other animals. The success of the municipal slaughterhouses that had been built under Napoleon[30] had led city administrators to investigate the construction of a central slaughterhouse for *équarrissage*. According to the administrators' plan, not only could all the small industries that used animal debris be brought together, but at least a major portion of the city dump at Montfaucon could be suppressed, a reform proposal that antedated the revolution of 1789. The administration asked the health council to consider the advantages of a central slaughterhouse and to make recommendations for its construction. Members opposed the administration's plan to build a grandiose, monumental slaughterhouse, because they deemed it a waste of money and unnecessary, given the improvements that had occurred in the industry: Steam power and disinfectants had improved industrial processes so that the industry was no longer as offensive as it once had been. The health council suggested that the city simply purchase a tract of land and set up a central slaughteryard where individual proprietors could practice their trades. Having become convinced of the soundness of the health council's recommendations, the administration decided in 1838 to establish a slaughteryard in Aubervilliers, outside Paris. All precautions and hygienic measures recommended by the health council, such as adequate water supply and drainage and the application of modern processes involving the use of steam power and disinfectants, were used. The health council considered the establishment of the slaughteryard an important public health measure, since it made possible the final suppression of the city dump at Montfaucon in 1841.[31]

29 Moléon, *R. G.*, 1826, pp. 365–71; see also the report itself: A. J. B. Parent-Duchâtelet, chairman, "Rapport sur le curage des égouts Amelot, de la Roquette, St.-Martin et autres, ou exposé des moyens qui ont été mis en usage pour exécuter cette grande opération, sans compromettre la salubrité publique et la santé des ouvriers qui y ont été employés," *Hygiène publique*, 1: 308–437.

30 The health council had not been consulted on their construction. See Moléon, *R. G.*, 1819, p. 143. The fact that the council was consulted in the 1830s suggests increasing influence and authority.

31 Moléon, *R. G.*, 1824, p. 299; 1835, pp. 105–6; 1837, pp. 172–3; 1838, pp. 207–9; 1839, pp. 233–5; 1840, pp. 42–5; 1841, pp. 101–2; see Parent-Duchâtelet, "Projet d'un rapport demandé par M. le préfet de la Seine sur la construction d'un clos central d'équarrissage pour la ville de Paris," *Hygiène publique*, 2: 309–26. For the new processes that made the industry practically inoffensive, see Parent-Duchâtelet, chairman, "Rapport sur les nouveaux procédés de MM. Salmon, Payen et Compagnie, pour la dessication des chevaux morts et la désinfection instantanée des matières fécales; précédé de quelques considérations sur les voiries de la ville de Paris," *Hygiène publique*, 2: 285–308; this report was done by a health council commission.

The Paris cholera epidemic of 1832 offers another example of the health council's influence. In 1831, as cholera was moving westward across Europe, Parisian administrators and hygienists began making plans to keep the disease out of the city and to manage it if it did arrive. The prefect of police asked the health council to prepare a report outlining preventive measures. This report served as the basis of administrative measures taken against cholera, including specific ways to improve the city's sanitary state.[32] Although a major clean-up campaign was launched in Paris, cholera was not deterred. When the epidemic hit, health council recommendations had already been put into effect: first aid stations, ambulance service, temporary hospitals, maintenance of accurate statistical records, services to provide for sanitary burials, curtailment of public gatherings, and disinfection and continual cleaning on public and private levels.

On the other hand, the health council recommended some programs and measures that were not adopted. When the administration failed to accept the recommendations of the health council, the reason cited was usually money. A good example involved garbage and mud disposal. In the 1820s the health council proposed a plan providing for daily garbage and mud pickup, with their transportation on barges to locations outside the city, where they could ferment, eventually to be used as fertilizer. The plan was never adopted, ostensibly because it was too expensive, but resistance from ragpickers and garbage collectors played a role in the decision.[33] The health council deplored the mud and garbage deposits on land surrounding Paris, but the practice became less offensive and less of a health hazard in the 1830s after the application of a newly discovered disinfectant.[34]

Another example of the administration's failure to adopt a health council recommendation involved water drainage in the rural communes outside Paris, where sewer systems were primitive. Upon investigation, the health council recommended the construction of a complete drainage system including paving streets and constructing sewers, for as members pointed

32 R. G., 1830–4, pp. 75–80. These five annual reports were published as one report. On this, see also George Sussman, "From Yellow Fever to Cholera: A Study of French Government Policy, Medical Professionalism, and Popular Movements in the Epidemic Crises of the Restoration and the July Monarchy" (Ph.D. dissertation, Yale University, 1971), pp. 214–77. See also François Delaporte, *Disease and Civilization: The Cholera in Paris, 1832* (Cambridge, MA: MIT Press, 1986), and Patrice Bourdelais and Jean-Yves Raulot, *Une Peur bleue: Histoire du choléra en France, 1832–1854* (Paris: Payot, 1987).

33 On this, see Edwin Chadwick, ed. Michael W. Flinn, *Report on the Sanitary Condition of the Labouring Population of Great Britain, 1842* (Edinburgh: Edinburgh University Press, 1965), pp. 162–3; Sussman, "Yellow Fever to Cholera," pp. 290–303.

34 *Rapport général sur les travaux du Conseil de salubrité pendant l'année 1827* (Paris: Imprimerie municipale, 1828), pp. 35–8; "Rapport général des travaux du Conseil de salubrité de la ville de Paris pour l'année 1828, *Annales d'hygiène publique*, 2 (1829): 329–30; R. G., 1835, pp. 112–13; 1837, pp. 186–8; 1839, pp. 253–5.

out, an unhealthy situation in the communes could compromise the health of Paris. By the 1840s the suggested plan had not been effected. The health council reasoned that available funds were being spent for monuments instead of public health, and the problem of stagnant water in the rural communes went unsolved.[35]

The third major area in which the health council exerted its influence was industrial authorization and classification. When the proprietor of an industrial establishment sought authorization for his industry from the prefect of police, the health council conducted an investigation of the proposed establishment to determine the inconveniences to property owners and public health hazards. In the case of a new industry, the investigation would result in a recommended classification and approval or rejection of authorization. Posters were displayed in the locality of the industry, and inhabitants were asked to voice their complaints or approvals. In most cases, the health council recommended authorization with contingencies. For example, if smoke was the problem, the proprietor might be required to build a high chimney or use a smokeless fuel. In the case of a first-class, or obnoxious or dangerous industry, authorization could be granted only if the industry was located outside the city center. For this reason, by the 1840s much Parisian industry was growing in the communes surrounding the city. This improved public health in Paris but caused problems for the rapidly developing suburbs. Usually the prefect of police followed the recommendations of the health council with regard to classification, authorization, and the conditions to be imposed. Enforcement of required modifications often created problems, however, for the health council was powerless, being dependent upon the police to ensure that requirements were met. In many cases enforcement was lax, a situation the health council often lamented.[36]

The health council's influence on the Parisian public health administration varied, depending on who was prefect of police and the exigencies of the moment, but its influence and authority gradually increased. Publicity of council activities through its published reports and articles encouraged awareness within the Parisian and national administrations, highlighting the council's role as the leading public health authority in the nation. Especially after 1835, the council's influence grew as Prefect of the Seine Rambuteau and Prefect of Police Delessert gave more attention to urban health problems.[37]

---

35 *R. G.*, 1828, pp. 319–27; 1841, pp. 106–8; 1842, pp. 170–3; 1847, p. 105.
36 See, for example, *R. G.*, 1837, pp. 157–8. In fact, complaints against industrial establishments were evidence that the imposed conditions had not been adhered to. By 1844 the situation seemed to have improved. See *R. G.*, 1844, pp. 269–70.
37 Claude Rambuteau, *Mémoires du Comte de Rambuteau publiés par son petit-fils* (Paris: Lévy, 1905), pp. 267–93, 325–94; Tulard, *La préfecture de police*, pp. 102–11.

The general attitude of health council members was pragmatic. Their appointment to and continued service on the council being dependent on the approval of the prefect of police (and after 1832 of the Minister of Commerce also), they had to court his favor. Members realized that public health was only one of several important rights and interests of Parisian citizens, and not always the most important in the public opinion. They recognized that for many in the ruling classes the right of all to public health was secondary to the rights of a few to liberty and property. The council took as its charge the reconciliation of public health and the interests of liberty and property, a difficult task, for members shared a predominantly liberal outlook. Although in theory they adhered to the principle of government nonintervention in commerce and industry, in practice they often had to recommend intervention to protect public health and safety.

The Paris health council devoted much attention to the health problems created by urbanization and industrialization. As early as the 1820s, the council began to view the rapid growth of Paris as a public health menace. The influx of immigrants from the provinces between 1820 and 1848 made the need for housing critical. Council members noted that new construction came at the expense of public health by eliminating sunshine and air, and replacing trees, flowers, courtyards, and parks with new, often shoddily built edifices. They urged the administration to develop an urban planning program and to adopt a building code, so new construction would have to meet certain minimum health and safety standards. Until such a code was adopted, they pleaded with the administration to enforce existing ordinances regulating such matters as the height of buildings proportional to the width of streets. Health council recommendations were finally effected in 1848, when an ordinance regulating the salubrity of private dwellings was passed.[38]

The 1810 decree on dangerous trades had conferred special duties on the health council; therefore, the council devoted more attention to industrialization than urbanization. For health council members, industrialization meant the rapid increase in the number of small workshops, the application of steam power to industry – resulting in the growth of some large factories – and the development of home industry for the manufacture of capital goods. The industrial revolution (they used this term) that they saw taking place in Paris after 1830 was the mechanization of industry.[39] The council's

---

38 Moléon, R. G., 1824, pp. 308–11; 1825, pp. 357–62; 1827, p. 39; 1829, pp. 37–9; 1848, pp. 172–92. See Ann-Louise Shapiro, *Housing the Poor of Paris, 1850–1902* (Madison: University of Wisconsin Press, 1985).

39 Moléon, R. G., 1818, p. 121; 1820, p. 159; 1822, pp. 221–2; 1823, p. 260; 1824, pp. 281–4, 298–9; 1827, p. 7; 1837, p. 145; 1838, pp. 195, 200; 1841, p. 49; 1842, pp. 156–8.

outlook on industrialization was optimistic, for members considered it a sign of the progress of civilization. As long as industry did not infringe upon the rights of property holders or menace the public health, they encouraged industrial development, but reconciling their belief in laissez-faire with public health requirements caused consternation for some council members. Good liberals, they feared restrictions on the freedom of industry even for public health reasons, believing that wealth was essential to health. They believed public health had to be considered within a broader economic framework, for if the industrial system did not work, general poverty would result, adversely affecting the health of all. Villermé had already demonstrated the relationship between poverty and mortality, and most hygienists had accepted his hypothesis. Optimistic about the social and economic benefits of industrialization, hygienists believed it would result in a general increase in wealth that would filter down to the common worker. Increased wealth would result in greater consumption of goods, which would necessitate construction of more factories and work-shops, leading to more jobs and more wealth.[40]

Furthermore, although industrialization posed certain recognized public health hazards, it was in some cases beneficial. By the 1840s, mechaniza-tion and the improvement of industrial processes had eliminated many inconveniences associated with various industries in their infancy, such as *équarrissage*. Better processes, fuels, machines, and means of using and disposing of industrial wastes improved the healthfulness and safety of certain industries. Mechanization meant that some of the most hazardous and unhealthy jobs could be relegated to machines.[41] After 1830, when industrialization increased rapidly in Paris and the surrounding area, the health council began to favor increased government intervention to regu-late industry and enforce existing laws, since there was a tendency among industrialists to ignore health measures imposed by industrial authoriza-tions. By the 1840s, the health council advocated the preparation of a uniform industrial code regulating all industries and ensuring freedom to industrialists, as long as public health and the rights of property owners were not compromised. The council included such a code in its 1845 report, but no action was taken, the government promulgating no formal industrial code before 1850.[42]

The Paris health council considered itself to be and was considered by others to be the leading French public health authority, owing to its

---

40 Moléon, *R. G.*, 1821, p. 208; 1824, pp. 281–4; 1827, p. 15; 1829, p. 38; 1838, pp. 216–17, 195–6; 1842, p. 157; 1846, pp. 2–4.
41 *R. G.*, 1835, pp. 88–9, 104–6; 1845, pp. 296–8; 1846, pp. 2–4, 57; 1848, pp. 207–8.
42 Moléon, *R. G.*, 1822, pp. 221–2; 1837, pp. 157–8; 1842, p. 157; 1843, pp. 225, 229; 1844, pp. 269–70; 1845, pp. 282–5; 1846, p. 2.

distinguished membership and the breadth of its research. The unique situation of Paris and the publicity of health council activities contributed to the significance of the problems it tackled and the decisions it made. Many scientific discoveries and technological innovations occurred in Paris; hence many new industries got their start there. Paris was also the home of the learned academies, several of which debated public health questions. Finally, during this period Paris was the medical capital of the Western world. Thus, the Paris health council was in a position to consider new discoveries, inventions, and ideas before provincial groups, and also to be in close touch with important medical and hygienic debates occurring in academies, faculties, and hospitals. For these reasons the Paris health council set the example for the rest of the nation, and provincial administrators and health councils used its decisions as guidelines.[43]

Publicity of health council activities kept French and foreign hygienists and administrators in touch with council work. From 1815, newspapers and journals regularly reported the work of the council. The *Annales d'hygiène publique*, many of whose editors and contributors were health council members, published both annual and individual health council reports, as well as analyses of ordinances passed on council recommendation.[44] When the annual reports of the council were published (at varying intervals), they became administrative reference works. Copies were sent to other health councils, to prefects, and to the Minister of Commerce, and were available in libraries and in administrative offices that managed public health.[45] Copies were sent to Britain and the United States.[46] Given

---

43 R. G., 1829, p. 35; 1837, p. 145; 1842, p. 189; 1843, pp. 191–2; 1844, pp. 247–8; 1846, p. 1; see also Parent-Duchâtelet, "Quelques considérations sur le Conseil de salubrité," pp. 4–7.

44 Moléon, *R. G.*, pp. vii–viii; see, for example, Peuchet, "Administration. Conseil de salubrité," *Moniteur universel*, December 13, 1828, p. 1822, for a summary of work done by the health council in 1827. See the summary for 1825 by Peuchet in *Moniteur*, December 14, 1827, p. 1702. See also, for example, *Archives générales de médecine*, 1823–9, passim, and *Annales d'hygiène publique*, 1829–48, passim.

45 A.N., F⁸171, Circulaire no. 12. Ministère du Commerce. Bureau sanitaire. Salubrité. Paris, le 19 mai 1835. In this circular the minister tried to convince the prefects of the advantages to be obtained from a departmental health council; he recommended that each of the general councils allocate eight francs for the purchase of the printed collection of Paris health council reports; A.N., F⁸171, Circulaire du Ministre de l'Agriculture et du Commerce, le 26 oct. 1843 à M. le préfet au sujet de l'envoi du 2e volume des actes de ce conseil. In a form letter of that same year the Minister of Agriculture and Commerce stated that the prefects should have copies of Volume 1 of the health council reports and said he was sending a copy of Volume 2 (1827–39). Both the Paris council and its reports were most favorably spoken of by the Minister of Agriculture and Commerce in A.N., F⁸171, Ministère de l'Agriculture et du Commerce. Bureau sanitaire. A M. le Préfet de – au sujet de salubrité, Octobre 1843.

46 See, for example, Chadwick, *Report on the Sanitary Condition*, pp. 319, 397; Lemuel Shattuck et al., *Report of the Sanitary Commission of Massachusetts, 1850*, foreword by C.-E.-A. Winslow (Cambridge, MA: Harvard University Press, 1948), pp. 16–24;

the preeminence of the Paris council in public health matters by the 1830s, it is not surprising that provincial mayors and prefects used it as a model for establishing their own health councils. By the 1830s, health councils had been established in several cities and departments.

PROVINCIAL HEALTH COUNCILS

At the departmental level prefects were responsible for public health and welfare.[47] When questions arose, prefects and mayors often relied on the advice of local medical and scientific societies, which were commonplace in middle-sized and large cities and towns. Sometimes a mayor or prefect formed a special advisory commission of local experts drawn from those institutions – usually preeminent physicians and pharmacists. Responding to the need for specialized advice on public health matters, mayors and prefects created health councils based on the Paris model. During the Restoration, prefects established health councils in Nantes (1817), Lyon (1822), Marseilles (1825), Lille (1828), and Strasbourg (1829). In the 1830s the proliferation of health councils continued, primarily as a response to the 1832 cholera epidemic, councils being founded in Troyes (1830), Rouen and Bordeaux (1831), and Toulouse (1832).[48]

Although the organization, membership, and duties of the provincial councils closely resembled those of the Paris council, there were noticeable variations, since provincial councils were adapted to local needs and circumstances. Like the Paris council, provincial health councils were advisory only, and their organization was basically the same as that of the Paris council. Their membership included physicians and pharmacists – who dominated the councils – and often an engineer, a veterinarian, and an architect. Members were unsalaried, in contrast to the Paris council. Some councils gave out tokens worth a few francs to encourage attendance. Most councils had departmentwide organizations, but those that did not hoped to extend their influence throughout the department, since the plan was that councils in each arrondissement would communicate regularly with

Lemuel Shattuck, *Report on a General Plan for the Promotion of Public and Personal Health* (Boston: Dutton and Wentworth, 1850), p. 539. The two works by Shattuck are the same; the 1850 edition, however, contains an important appendix.

47 Alan B. Spitzer, "The Bureaucrat as Proconsul: The Restoration Prefect and the *police générale*," *Comparative Studies in Society and History* 7 (1964–5): 371–392; Nicholas Richardson, *The French Prefectoral Corps, 1814–1830* (Cambridge: Cambridge University Press, 1966); Brian Chapman, *The Prefects and Provincial France* (London: Allen and Unwin, 1955), pp. 11–43; and on prefectoral history, Guy Thuillier and Vincent Wright, "Notes sur les sources de l'histoire du corps préfectoral (1800–1880)," *Revue historique*, 253 (1975): 139–54.

48 Bourdelais and Raulot indicate the founding of a number of other health councils in response to cholera. See *Histoire du choléra*, pp. 179–86. Little is known about these councils.

the departmental council. Duties varied from one council to the next, but with the exception of the Bas-Rhin council, the most important function was the investigation and authorization of industrial establishments. The activity and utility of the councils varied, depending on the use the mayor and prefect made of them and the council's ability to solve local health problems. One of the most active was the Nantes council; others, such as the Rouen council, were little more than debating clubs, meeting rarely and conducting little business.

A common outlook prevailed among provincial health council members regarding their *mission civilisatrice* to rural folk. Like many French physicians from the late eighteenth century on, provincial health council members believed their mission was to practice medicine and spread enlightened ideas in rural areas. They complained incessantly about the insouciance of rural folk, their lack of concern for hygiene, aversion to novelty, and preference for charlatans. Provincial health council members agreed on major urban problems, their primary concern being the water supply – the lack of adequate running water and public baths. Debating the relative advantages of well water and river water, they concluded that river water was probably cleaner, because urban well water had been polluted by cesspool seepage. Members lamented the habitual filthiness of streets and squares, attributing it to insufficient water, bad habits, and lack of police enforcement. They voiced concern over inadequate sewage disposal, which was the accomplished by the traditional cesspool system with its accompanying *vidange*. As in Paris, health council members considered the horsebutchering industry and city dumps major public health hazards. Because so much of the work of the provincial councils concentrated on the investigation and authorization of industrial establishments, members supported regular industrial inspection and enforcement of health council recommendations. Several councils (Rouen, Nord-Lille) proposed the appointment of an inspector of dangerous and unhealthy establishments.

The first provincial health council was founded in Nantes in 1817 by Prefect de Brosses on the suggestion of the major of Nantes, Louis de St.-Aignan.[49] It was modeled on the Paris council, but its duties were more circumscribed. Whereas the Paris council's duties were broad, the Nantes health council was created as a permanent commission to give its opinion on unhealthy and incommodious establishments, in compliance with the 1810 decree. Within a few years of its creation, however, the duties of its

---

49 The prefect of the Haut-Rhin wanted to set up a health council in Colmar in 1804, but when a commission of the Paris Faculty of Medicine, which advised the national government on public health matters, voiced its opposition, the project was abandoned. A.N., F^{8}75, Rhin (Bas), Rhin (Haut), Rhône, Extrait des registres des délibérations de l'Ecole de Médecine de Paris, séance du 27 floréal, an XII, and several related letters in the same file, and Extrait des registres de la Préfecture du Département du Haut-Rhin du 11 jour de Ventôse an XII.

three members, a physician (Julien Fouré) and two pharmacists (Le Sant
and Hectot), were broadened to include areas of more general public health
interest. By 1824, when Alban de Villeneuve-Bargemont arrived in Nantes
as prefect, the health council had advised the mayor and prefect on
slaughterhouses, cemeteries, water supply, epizootics, prison construction,
swamp drainage, and rabies, in addition to industrial establishments. The
investigation of goods that came through customs became a major focus
of health council activities by 1828, distinguishing it from other councils.
Members checked to see if alterations of food and drink were hazardous to
health, and in case of spoilage or adulteration recommended destruction of
the goods.[50]

Jean-Paul Alban de Villeneuve-Bargement (1784–1850) is best known to
historians as a Christian economist and humanitarian.[51] Less well known
are the details of his twenty-six-year administrative career, particularly his
public health contributions while prefect of the Loire-Inférieure from 1824
to 1828 and of the Nord from 1828 to 1830. He expanded the Nantes
health council to create the first departmentwide public health board in
France (the model for the post-1848 health council organization) and established the same institution in the Nord. After serving in the French
administration for almost twenty years, Villeneuve-Bargemont was trans-
ferred in 1824 from the prefecture of the Meurthe at Nancy to the prefecture of the Loire-Inférieure at Nantes. During his tenure (1824–8)
the Nantes council was very active. Villeneuve-Bargemont consulted the
health council regularly on a wide range of public health matters: dangers
posed by heat and drought, altered water supplies, hemp retting, public
health hazards associated with the construction of the Brittany canal from
Nantes to Brest, charlatanism, rabies, prejudices against vaccination, adulteration of food and drink, public health dangers resulting from flooding of
the Loire valley, the sanitary state of the Nantes prison, and the salubrity
of a proposed insane asylum. He was prompt and conscientious in acting
on the health council's recommendations, issuing circulars, corresponding with subprefects and mayors, distributing copies of health council
instructions for posting, and enlisting the council's help in preparing his
annual reports on the state of the department. How much he valued the
institution is reflected in a letter he wrote to the council in 1826:

You have seen equally, sirs, by my correspondence, how much importance I have
attached to your propositions, which I have always either adopted or consulted in
my decisions. It is thus that I had publicized in the countryside your observations
on the methods of purifying water altered by the summer heat; that I did what was

50 *Rapport général sur les travaux du conseil de salubrité de Nantes (depuis le 4 mars 1817,
jusqu'au 31 décembre 1825* (Nantes: Mellinet-Malassis, 1826).
51 His best-known work is *Economie politique chrétienne, ou recherches sur la nature et les
causes du paupérisme en France et en Europe,* 3 vols. (Paris: Paulin, 1834).

in my domain to repress the illicit practice of medicine; that I welcomed your views on hydrophobia and stray dogs; it is thus especially that your opinions served to direct the administration in all the affairs concerning the formation of unhealthy establishments.[52]

The single most ambitious project undertaken by the health council during Villeneuve-Bargemont's administration was its investigation of the tallow melting industry. Hoping to discover a method to eliminate the pollution associated with the industry, the council sent out inquiries and received replies from well-known chemists throughout France and Europe – Faraday in London, Berzelius in Stockholm, Vogel in Munich, and d'Arcet in Paris. The members conducted experiments with various processes, and even though they found no pollution-free method, they developed an improved process of tallow melting, which proved useful to other health councils and administrators. By 1826, the Nantes health council was making important contributions to public health in Nantes, and its members and Villeneuve-Bargemont wanted it enlarged to a departmental institution. Therefore, in May 1826, Villeneuve-Bargemont increased the membership from three to seven, set up secondary councils at Paimboeuf and Ancenis, which were to correspond regularly with the central council in Nantes, and named correspondents of the Nantes council in major towns of the department. In creating the first departmental council, Villeneuve-Bargemont hoped that the new organization would establish communication between secondary councils and the central council in Nantes, benefitting public health by eliminating local causes of insalubrity and combatting prejudices and practices contrary to health.[53]

52 A.D., Loire-Atlantique, 1 M1373; 1 M6753, dossiers 4, 5, 6, lettres de la préfecture 1826, 1827, 1828, and the health council reports for these years: *Rapport général sur les travaux du conseil de salubrité de Nantes pendant l'année 1826* (Nantes: Mellinet-Malassis, 1827); *Rapport sur les travaux du conseil de salubrité de Nantes pendant l'année 1827* (Nantes: Mellinet-Malassis, 1828); *Rapport général sur les travaux du conseil de salubrité de Nantes, pendant l'année 1828* (Nantes: Mellinet-Malassis, 1829). These reports hereafter cited as *R. G., Nantes*, followed by the year and page number. A.D., Loire-Atlantique, 1 M1373, prefect to Nantes health council, June 23, 1827; prefect to Nantes health council, July 10, 1827. On Villeneuve-Bargemont and his public health contributions, see Ann F. La Berge, "A Restoration Prefect and Public Health: Alban de Villeneuve-Bargemont at Nantes and Lille, 1824–1830," *Proceedings of the Fifth Annual Meeting of the Western Society for French History, 1977*, 5 (1978): 128–37. Quotation is from A.D. Loire-Atlantique, 1M6753, prefect to Nantes health council, April 5, 1826.

53 A.D., Loire-Atlantique, 1M6753, dossier Abattoir, Pièces relatives à la fonte de suif en branches. This dossier contains the replies from the health council's inquiries. See also, *R. G.*, 1827, pp. 14–32. A.D., Loire-Atlantique, 1 M1373. Secrétariat général. Organisation du service de salubrité dans le département. Du 27 mai 1826. Préfet de la Loire-Inférieure. The four new members were the physicians A. Laennec, Marion de Procé, and Sallion, and the pharmacist Prével. See also *R. G., Nantes*, 1826. In December 1827 Villeneuve-Bargemont further increased the number of correspondents and set up a secondary health council at Savenay. See A.D., Loire-Atlantique, 1 M1373. Extrait des registres de la préfecture du département. Du déc. 1827.

In the early 1830s, the Nantes health council entered a period of decline, perhaps due to the death of two of its most active members or because, after Villeneuve-Bargemont's departure for the Nord in 1828, leadership was lacking.[54] The secondary health councils and correspondents ceased to function. Although the cholera epidemic acted as a stimulus to the creation of health councils in some cities, the epidemic decreased the authority of the Nantes council, for other institutions – the sanitary intendancy and health commissions – were empowered to deal with the emergency. As the Minister of Commerce explained, the health councils were consultative bodies, whereas the sanitary intendancies of Nantes and health commissions (*comités de salubrité*) were authorities that, in case the department were placed under the sanitary regime, had the power to make decisions and apply laws and regulations.[55] Basically, the Nantes health council was to act as a clearinghouse between the sanitary intendancy and the health commissions. In the 1840s, the Nantes council underwent a revival and functioned effectively for the city, but not as a departmentwide institution. Its scope of interest was much narrower than it had been in the 1820s; it returned to its original duties: the inspection of goods coming through customs, and the investigation and authorization of industrial establishments.[56]

The second provincial health council founded during the Restoration was the Rhône council, established in 1822 by Prefect Tournon to serve both him and the mayor of Lyon as a public health advisory commission. Members, like those of other health councils, came from a variety of backgrounds. For example, in 1829, the Rhône council had nine unsalaried members: six physicians, a chemist, an engineer, and a veterinarian. In 1846 the membership included five physicians, two chemists, and two engineers. In its first twenty years, the council prepared an average of 30 reports a year, compared with the Paris council's 300 to 500 reports. Monfalcon and Polinière, health council members and among the most

54 The 1829 report was not printed but is available in manuscript form in A.D., Loire-Atlantique, 1 M1373, Conseil de salubrité de la ville de Nantes. Rapport général. 1829. *Rapport général sur les travaux du Conseil central de salubrité pendant l'année 1835* (Nantes: Mellinet, 1836), p. 6; there were no annual reports, printed or manuscript, between 1830 and 1835. There were no annual reports, printed or manuscript, between 1835 and 1844, apparently; see *Rapport général sur les travaux du Conseil central de salubrité de Nantes et du département de la Loire-Inférieure* (Nantes: Mellinet, 1844), p. 5.

55 A.D., Loire-Atlantique, 1 M1373, letter from Minister of Commerce and Public Works to prefect of Loire-Inférieure, December 28, 1831; A.D., Loire-Atlantique, 1 M1373, Nantes health council to prefect October 27, 1831.

56 *R. G., Nantes, 1844; Rapport général sur les travaux du Conseil central de salubrité de Nantes et du département de la Loire-Inférieure pendant l'année 1845* (Nantes: Mellinet, 1846); *Rapport général sur les affaires traitées par le Conseil central de salubrité de Nantes et du département de la Loire-Inférieure, pendant l'année 1846* (Nantes: Mellinet, 1847); *Rapport général sur les travaux de Conseil central de salubrité de Nantes et du département de la Loire-Inférieure pendant les années 1847 et 1848* (Nantes: Mellinet, 1849).

active and influential of the Lyonnais physician-hygienists, explained the difference in workload between the Paris and Rhône councils by suggesting that in Paris many industries were submitted to preliminary investigation by the health council before any authorization, whereas in Lyon the opinion of the health council was sought only if there was opposition to the industry.[57]

An administrative problem weakened the authority of the Rhône health council, for public health duties were legally split between the prefect of the Rhône and the mayor of Lyon. The prefect was in charge of the epidemic service (*service des épidémies*), prisons, and dangerous and unhealthy establishments, whereas the mayor was responsible for inspection of prostitutes, the dispensary, first-aid boxes for the drowning and asphyxiated, and policing of food and drink. From 1822 to 1830 the Rhône health council served both the major and the prefect, but when Gabriel Prunelle became mayor of Lyon in 1830, he set up a separate municipal health council to advise him. Gabriel Prunelle, physician and former professor at the Medical Faculty at Montpellier, became mayor of Lyon after the July Revolution. He created his own health council, probably because of many disagreements between him and the prefect.[58] After 1830, there were two health councils in Lyon. The overlapping jurisdiction was a curious situation, since many of the hygienists sat on both councils. Health council members deplored the administrative duplication, urging the unification of the councils into one authoritative body serving both mayor and prefect, as in Lille, Nantes, and Bordeaux, but several attempts to merge the councils – the last in 1840 – were unsuccessful. Thus, neither council functioned as a competent public health authority on all matters, and no departmentwide organization was established in the Rhône. Health council correspondents were not appointed throughout the department, though members advocated such a move. Lack of cooperation between the prefect and the health council and between the prefect and the mayor lessened the influence of both health councils.[59]

57 Etienne Sainte-Marie, *Lectures relatives à la police médicale faites au Conseil de salubrité de Lyon et du département du Rhône pendant les années 1826, 1827, et 1828* (Paris: Baillière, 1829); Jean-Baptiste Monfalcon and A. P. Isidore de Polinière, *Hygiène de Lyon* (Paris: Baillière, 1846), pp. 517–18. Members in 1829 included the physicians Jean-Marie Viricel, Etienne Martin, Jean-Baptiste Monfalcon, Isidore Polinière, Louis-Vincent Cartier, and Etienne Sainte-Marie; the chemist Nicolas Tissier, the engineer Henry Tabareau; and the veterinarian Louis-Furcy Grognier. Members in 1846 included the physicians Jean-Marie Viricel, Etienne Martin, Jean-Baptiste Monfalcon, Isidore Polinière, and Fleury Imbert; the chemists Nicolas Tissier and Alphonse Dupasquier; and the engineers Henry Tabareau and Gabriel Pigeon. Monfalcon and Polinière, *Hygiène de Lyon*, pp. 522–3.
58 On this, see Jean-Baptiste Monfalcon, *Histoire monumentale de la ville de Lyon*, 9 vols. (Lyon: Bibliothèque de la ville de Lyon, 1866), 4: 105, and Robert Bezucha, *The Lyon Uprising of 1834* (Cambridge, MA: Harvard University Press, 1974), pp. 58–9.
59 Little might be known about the work of the Rhône and Lyon health councils had

Both health councils were copies of the Paris council, being advisory boards only, possessing no initiative or power of enforcement. Despite these limitations, they exerted considerable influence at the local level, concentrating on the investigation and authorization of industrial establishments. The Rhône health council, like many health councils, desired more work and authority than it had, but suffered from lack of cooperation with the prefect and mayor. At least half of its duties were neglected. Writing in 1834, the physician Bertrand Julia de Cazères suggested merging the two councils and paying members a salary in order to help improve public health in Lyon.[60]

The situation in Marseilles was different from that in Lyon. Marseilles had a long tradition of public health institutions, namely, the sanitary intendancy, which was in charge of preventing the importation of epidemics by sea. Public health in Marseilles had traditionally been a matter of epidemic prevention, or *la police du port*. During the Napoleonic era and the first years of the Restoration, when the administration needed advice on other public health problems, it turned to the local medical society (*Société de médecine*). For example, during the Restoration the Société académique de médecine de Marseilles was in charge of compiling the quarterly reports on the prevalent diseases, which were then sent to the

it not been for the work of a few prominent hygienists – Etienne Sainte-Marie, Jean-Baptiste Monfalcon, and A. P. Isidore de Polinière – and later Louis Rougier and Alexandre Glénard, who published independent works dealing primarily with the work of the health councils, for unlike the Paris health council and many of the provincial health councils, neither of the Lyonnais health councils published its annual reports. The only published annual report was the 1824 report. See *Rapport sur l'établissement et les premiers travaux du Conseil de salubrité de la ville de Lyon...* (Lyon: Ballanche, 1824) in Archives municipales de Lyon, I⁵2. In fact, this was the health council of the Rhône, established by the prefect. For the 1820s see Sainte-Marie, *Lectures relatives à la police médicale*. Sainte-Marie was a physician trained at Montpellier, a member of the Rhône health council, the Medical Society of Lyon, and consulting physician for the Société protestante de prévoyance et de secours mutuels. See also his *Précis élémentaire de police médicale* (Paris: Baillière, 1824), which contains information on the origins of public health in France and on public health terminology. Principal sources of information are Monfalcon and Polinière, *Hygiène de Lyon*, the second part of *Traité de la salubrité dans les grandes villes* (Paris: Baillière, 1846), and *Traité de la salubrité*. Both *Hygiène de Lyon* and *Traité de la salubrité* deal in large part with the work of the health councils and of the leading hygienists, most of whom served on one or both health councils. For the 1850s and for general background on public health in Lyon in the first half of the nineteenth century, see Louis-Auguste Rougier and Alexandre Glénard, *Hygiène de Lyon. Compte-rendu des travaux du Conseil d'hygiène et de salubrité du département du Rhône du 1er janv. 1851 au 31 déc. 1859* (Lyon: Vingtrinier, 1860). Rougier was vice-president of the health council and a former physician at the Hôtel-Dieu; Glénard was secretary of the health council and a professor of chemistry at the preparatory school of medicine in Lyon.

60 Bertrand Julia de Cazères, *Rapport sur l'ouvrage de MM. Monfalcon et de Polinière intitulé Hygiène de la ville de Lyon, ou Opinions et Rapports du Conseil de Salubrité de Lyon* (Lyon: Savy jeune, 1845), p. 12; Julia de Cazères, who reviewed the first edition of the work, was assistant physician at the military hospital of Lyon.

prefect, who forwarded them to the Minister of the Interior.[61] When the nine-member Marseilles health council was founded in 1825 by Prefect Christophe de Villeneuve-Bargemont (brother of Alban), it occupied a secondary position vis-à-vis the long-established sanitary intendancy (before the nineteenth century, called the *Bureau de Santé*). The prefect considered the health council a sister institution to the sanitary intendancy. The main purpose of the health council was to prevent disease *within* national boundaries, a counterpart to the sanitary intendancy, whose task was to prevent *imported* diseases. The principal concerns of the health council in the 1820s were marshy, swampy areas and stagnant water with its resultant intermittent fevers, the industrial development of Marseilles, and the construction of the Provence canal.

Commenting on public health in Marseilles in 1826–7, the council noted that the city was basically healthy, being endowed with a good water supply. Its two major public health problems were piles of garbage in the streets and the insanitary state of the port, due primarily to the increased number of industries that discharged polluted water. Other problems were stray, possibly rabid dogs, intermittent fevers, the misery of many inhabitants, and the adulteration of food.[62] By 1831, the membership of the council had increased from nine to fourteen, to include civil engineers from the department of bridges and highways and the engineer of mines. Correspondents had also been named in the principal cities of the department. Both changes were typical of the direction taken by other health councils: diversification of membership to include members other than physicians and pharmacists and expansion on a departmentwide scale.

Although a separate agency was in charge of vaccinations, the health council could not help but get involved in the 1828 smallpox epidemic, which killed 1,488 out of approximately 120,000 Marseillais. The health council attributed the extreme violence of the disease to the widespread indifference of the Marseillais to vaccination. In spite of physicians' efforts, free vaccinations, cooperation of the clergy, and the threat of denial of welfare (*secours*), many parents refused to have their children vaccinated because of their repugnance for the procedure. The 1828 smallpox epi-

---

61 A.N., F⁸37, La Société académique de médecine à Monsieur le Comte de Villeneuve, Préfet du Département des Bouches-du-Rhône, Rapports sur les Maladies qui ont regné à Marseille depuis le Mois de Novembre dernier, le 10 janvier 1816.

62 *Rapport général sur les travaux du Conseil de salubrité du département des Bouches-du-Rhône pendant les années 1826 et 1827* (Marseille: Richard, 1828). There was duplication of membership with the Société académique de médecine; for example, Lautard and Robert, health council members, had been active in the Société at least since the beginning of the Restoration. The health council members in 1828 were Robert, vice-president; Martin, Dugas, Ducros, Cauvière, Lautard, Laurens, Moulaud, and Robert, nephew, secretary and chairman.

demic offers a good example of the inefficiency of public health administration and lack of cooperation between "public health" institutions. The municipal authority asked the health council for advice on managing the epidemic. The health council wrote to the two local medical societies, but neither cooperated with the health council, sending their documents and observations instead to the municipal authority. These medical societies (*Société royale de médecine de Marseilles* and *Société académique de médecine*) were in the habit of giving public health advice and probably resented the intrusion of the recently created health council, or so the health council believed. The Marseilles health council was still functioning in 1840, but lack of documentation makes it impossible to know its activities after 1831. It is likely that the death of Villeneuve-Bargemont in 1829 deprived the council of the leadership needed to function effectively.[63]

Christophe de Villeneuve-Bargemont's brother, Alban, established the health council of the Nord in June 1828, shortly after his arrival in Lille to take up his prefectoral assignment. After his years in the Loire-Inférieure, Alban de Villeneuve-Bargement was convinced of the benefits of a departmentwide health council, and two months later he established secondary councils at Douai, Dunkirk, Cambrai, and Valenciennes, with cantonal correspondents throughout the department, copying the basic organization he had used in the Loire-Inférieure. He justified the importance of the health council in a letter to the 1828 session of the general council of the department:

Sirs, the maintenance of public health is one of the special duties of the municipal authority; it includes the salubrity of air, water, food, and drink, and medications....The superior administrative authority must therefore intervene in most of the health questions; the laws and regulations attribute to it the knowledge of works of health which are related to cities and communes, as well as the authorization or prohibition of setting up incommodious or unhealthy establishments. In a department where all types of industry and commerce are multiplying [industrial] establishments and population, how many various causes of insalubrity challenge the attention of the administration?...These motives have by no means escaped the administrators of the large cities of the kingdom. Councils composed of doctors and chemists are constantly being consulted on all questions of hygiene and health raised by the execution of the laws and police regulations. In order that this department and its principal cities may benefit from the same advantages, I have just formed a central health council at Lille and secondary councils at Dunkirk, Valenciennes, Douai, and Cambrai....This institution was lacking in such a highly populated department whose population is so industrious. It will doubtless gain

63 *Rapport général sur les travaux du Conseil de salubrité du département des Bouches-du-Rhône pendant les années 1828, 1829 et 1830* (Marseille: Achard, 1831), pp. 22–3. *Règlement du Conseil de salubrité du département des Bouches-du-Rhône* (Marseille: Achard, 1840).

your approval and I will ask you to vote from the funds used for unexpected expenses a sum of 1200 francs for the office expenses of the council.[64]

In its first two years the health council of the Nord (Lille) investigated sixty-seven industrial establishments, including the white lead and tallow melting industries, and focused its efforts on combatting venereal disease and prostitution and improving street conditions and bathing facilities. The council prepared major reports on an insane asylum for women, construction at the St.-Sauveur hospital, the adulteration of bread, and the safety of eating meat from tubercular cows.[65]

After Villeneuve-Bargemont resigned in August 1830, the Lille council continued to function actively throughout the 1840s, devoting most of its attention to the investigation and authorization of industrial establishments and occasionally undertaking major studies on problems such as the unhealthiness of working-class dwellings.[66] The fate of the secondary councils varied. The Douai council remained fairly active, but others barely functioned due to lack of time, interest, and motivation. The Avesnes council, for example, did not meet from 1833 to 1848; the Hazebrouck council functioned sporadically, its president consulting by himself with the subprefect if public health questions arose.[67]

The last health council established in the precholera era was the health council of the Bas-Rhin, established in Strasbourg in 1829 by Prefect Esmangart as an agency to centralize the correspondence of the department's agricultural committees (*comités agricoles*), cantonal physicians, and

64 A.D. Nord, M256/1, Extrait des registres des actes de la préfecture, du 25 juin 1828, pp. 1–2; A.D. Nord, M256/4, Extrait des registres des actes de la préfecture du août 1828. See also *Rapport du Conseil central de salubrité du département du Nord à M. le préfet du département* (Lille: Danel, 1830), pp. 1–2. Quotation from A.D. Nord. M257/8, prefect to the general council of the department of the Nord, 1828 session.

65 *Rapport du conseil central...du Nord (1830)*.

66 There were supposed to be printed reports for 1832 and 1833–7, but I found these neither at the Bibliothèque nationale nor in the departmental archives. But one can still get a general idea, especially as the 1848–9 report gives a summary of all the health council's work since 1828. See *Rapport sur les travaux du Conseil central de salubrité du département du Nord, pendant les années 1838, 1839, et 1840* (Lille: Ducrocq, 1842); *Rapport sur les travaux du Conseil central de salubrité du Nord pendant les années 1841 et 1842* (Lille: Ducrocq, 1843); *Rapport sur les travaux du Conseil central de salubrité du département du Nord pendant les années 1845 et 1846* (Lille: Ducrocq, 1847); *Rapport sur les travaux du Conseil central de salubrité du département du Nord pendant les années 1847, 1848, et 1849* (Lille: Ducrocq, 1849). See two major reports on the sanitary state of workers' dwellings: "Assainissement des habitations de la classe pauvre de la ville de Lille," *Rapport, Nord 1841–1842*, pp. 26–61; "Assainissement des maisons et des caves servant à l'habitation des indigents," *Rapport, Nord 1845–6*, pp. 60–80.

67 A.D. Nord, M257/8, subprefect of Avesnes to prefect of Nord, July 15, 1839; and Conseil général, 1848; A.D. Nord, M257/8, president of Hazebrouck health council to prefect, undated; president of health council to prefect, March 9, 1841.

veterinarians. Esmangart's stated goal in establishing a health council was to gain more accurate knowledge of the sanitary state of rural areas and to facilitate the diffusion of public health knowledge.[68] One of his specific aims was to have the health council examine existing sanitary regulations in order to prepare a uniform health code for local authorities.[69] The council was also to oversee the vaccination program, give advice on epidemics and epizootics, publish instructions in case of natural calamities that might lead to famine or disease, and examine all existing regulations regarding the *police sanitaire* in urban areas in order to abrogate useless ones and propose new regulations.[70] The Bas-Rhin council differed from other health councils in that its principal activity – official duties notwithstanding – was the examination of candidates for the position of cantonal physician. Another major difference was that the Bas-Rhin council was not involved with the investigation of industrial establishments, the principal activity, by the 1830s and 1840s, of most French health councils.[71]

By 1831, health council activity had dwindled. The proposed health code had not been completed, and the health council's only task seems to have been judging the prefect's candidates for the position of cantonal physician. The prefect was apparently too busy to attend meetings. Fodéré complained to him, emphasizing the importance of a health council to good prefectoral administration: "To put the health council of this department on a level with those of other large cities of the kingdom will be a great good...which will always honor your administration."[72] Probably in response to Fodéré's complaints, Esmangart added eight new members to the council, even though he himself by this time expressed no

68 A.D., Bas-Rhin, 5 M1, Circulaire à MM les maires, relative à la formation d'un conseil de salubrité publique, 20 October 1829.
69 A.D., Bas-Rhin, 5 M1, prefect to M. Goupil, member of health council, November 27, 1829; A.D., Bas-Rhin, 5 M1, Police médicale. Salubrité publique. Bordereau des pièces communiquées à M. Goupil, membre de la commission de salubrité publique; A.D., Bas-Rhin, 5 M1, Fodéré to prefect, November 24, 1829, Indication de quelques articles de police de salubrité, by F. E. Fodéré.
70 A.D., Bas-Rhin, 5 M1, prefect Esmangart to deans of Faculty of Medicine, Strasbourg, October 22, 1829.
71 A.D., Bas-Rhin, 5 M1, prefect Esmangart to deans of Faculty of Medicine, Strasbourg, October 22, 1829. Members of the Bas-Rhin health council included physicians François Fodéré and Coze, professors at the Faculty of Medicine in Strasbourg; Schweighauser, head physician at the civilian hospital in Strasbourg; Goupil, permanent secretary of the Société des Sciences, Arts et Agriculture; Fabulet, head pharmacist at the military hospital; and Thiéry, head of the Royal Depot of Stallions. Fodéré was one of the leading French public hygienists, well known for his contributions to epidemiology. François-Emmanuel Fodéré, *Leçons sur les épidémies et l'hygiène publique*, 4 vols. (Paris: Levrault, 1822–4); and *Traité de médecine légale et d'hygiéne publique ou de police de santé* (Paris: Mame, 1813).
72 A.D., Bas-Rhin, 5 M1, health council (signed Fodéré) to prefect, July 4, 1831. "Mettre le conseil de salubrité de ce département à l'instar de ceux des autres grandes villes du Royaume, sera un grand bien que vous opérér, et qui honnera à toujours votre administration."

great interest in public health.[73] By 1833, the council had taken on the added duty of acting as a departmental clearinghouse for public health information. That year the new prefect called on mayors and cantonal physicians to assist health councils by providing data on local epidemics and epizootics, sanitary measures, and illicit sales of secret remedies.[74] Later that same year, the prefect was still trying to drum up business for the health council, which had fewer and fewer meetings, because its members had nothing to discuss: None of the cantonal physicians responded to the prefect's request for public health information.[75] The prefect criticized them, noting how parochial they would become if they confined themselves to vaccinations and rounds during epidemics. He expressed disbelief that in the area of the canton confided to their care, they could not find any need for public health improvements.[76]

Lack of cooperation between the health council and cantonal physicians continued to be a problem, and by 1837 the health council had still not achieved its initial goals. Attendance at meetings was low. Usually only four or five out of sixteen members attended.[77] By 1837, twenty out of thirty-three cantonal physicians finally reported to the health council, although only two complete reports were submitted, both by physicians who were members of the council, and one of which was by Fodéré, clearly the leading hygienist in the Bas-Rhin. The council had by this time added to its duties the compilation of the annual vaccination reports to be submitted to the prefect. (Before this, these reports had been prepared by a commission from the Faculty of Medicine.) Preparing these reports and approving the candidacy of cantonal physicians constituted the regular work of the health council.[78] During the 1840s the Bas-Rhin council entered a period of inactivity, with only a few isolated health issues, such

73 Caillot, dean of the Faculty of Medicine; Ehrmann, professor of anatomy; Lobstein, professor of pathological anatomy; Duvernoy, professor of natural history; Boechtel, a cantonal physician; Spielmann and Zecht, pharmacists; and Vries, the veterinarian for the arrondissement of Strasbourg, in A.D., Bas-Rhin, 5 M1, prefect to Fodéré, July 5, 1831 and July 30, 1831. Two more members were added in August, raising the total membership of the health council to 16. A.D., Bas-Rhin, 5 M1, arrêté, 29 août 1831.

74 A.D., Bas-Rhin, 5 M1, Circulaire à MM les maires et à MM les médecins cantonnaux, relative au Conseil de salubrité publique crée par arrêté de 20 oct. 1829 in *Actes administratives: Recueil des actes de la préfecture*, 1 juillet 1832.

75 These letters in A.D., Bas-Rhin, 5 M1. See, for example, Stoeber, health council member, to prefect, September 22, 1832.

76 A.D., Bas-Rhin, 5 M1, préfet à MM les médecins cantonnaux, circulaire: renseignemens à fournir au Conseil de salubrité publique, 14 Novembre 1833.

77 A.D., Bas-Rhin, 5 M1, Conseil de salubrité, séance du 12 Octobre 1837.

78 A.D., Bas-Rhin, 5 M1, Rapport général sur les rapports adressés au Conseil de salubrité par MM les médecins cantonnaux du département, 1834, 1835, 1836. V. Stoeber, *Rapport du Conseil de salubrité publique de département du Bas-Rhin à M. le préfet sur les vaccinations opérées en 1839 par les médecins cantonnaux du département* (Strasbourg: Silbermann, 1840).

as accidental poisoning from the administration of sleeping potions to children, occupying the attention of its members.[79]

In May 1848, a prefectoral order replaced the Bas-Rhin health council with a medical council (*conseil médical*) of twenty members who were put in charge of public health and medical police. Its specific duties were broad, including surveillance of public establishments, approval of construction of public buildings, investigation and authorization of dangerous and unhealthy establishments, compilation of a medical and statistical topography of the department, selection of juries that named cantonal physicians, reorganization of the system of cantonal physicians, maintenance and propagation of vaccine, verification of deaths, and publication of annual lists of medical personnel. It was a large order, which the medical council could not handle. It was subsequently superseded in 1849 by departmental and arrondissement health councils (*conseils de salubrité et d'hygiène publique*) established in accordance with the 1848 national law on health councils.[80]

Four more provincial health councils were established in the early 1830s in response to cholera. The first of these was in Rouen. There had been some interest in creating a health council in Rouen during the 1820s: The prefect of the Seine-Inférieure corresponded with Villeneuve-Bargemont in 1827, asking for information on health councils and indicating his intention to establish a council.[81] He did not carry out his plans, however, and there is no indication of further interest until the summer of 1831, when the prefect again sent out requests for information, probably because of cholera.[82] Replies were quickly forthcoming, and in August 1831 the Rouen health council was established to serve both the mayor and the prefect. The first president was Achille Flaubert, father of the novelist, chief surgeon at the Hôtel-Dieu of Rouen, and director of the Preparatory School of Medicine in Rouen. Secondary councils were also established in Le Havre, Neufchâtel, Yvetot, and Dieppe. Cholera was the first order of business, and a committee was named that November to map out a clean-up program for the city. As in other cities, the local sanitary intendancy was in charge of specific measures against the disease, with the council

79 A.D., Bas-Rhin, 5 M1, Conseil de salubrité, séance du 23 décembre 1847.
80 A.D., Bas-Rhin, 5 M1, arrêté, 31 mai 1848, printed in *Actes administratives*, V: 46; A.D., Bas-Rhin, 5 M1, Arrêté, 23 juillet 1849. Organisation des conseils d'hygiène publique et de salubrité. Actes du département, vol. L, no. 45; Conseil de salubrité et d'hygiène publique, séance du 18 août 1849.
81 A.D., Loire-Atlantique, 1 M 1373, prefect of Loire-Inférieure to prefect of Seine-Inférieure, February 18, 1827; prefect of Loire-Inférieure to prefect of Seine-Inférieure, March 18, 1827; prefect of Seine-Inférieure to prefect of Loire-Inférieure, July 2, 1827.
82 A.D., Nord, M261/4, prefect of Seine-Inférieure to prefect of Nord, June 8, 1831; A.D., Loire-Atlantique, 1 M 1373, prefect of Seine-Inférieure to prefect of Seine-Inférieure, June 16, 1831.

being responsible for *assainissement*, or sanitary reform. Several health council members also served on the sanitary intendancy.

Whether the measures taken by the health council and the sanitary intendancy were effective or not, Rouen escaped cholera, and the council almost ceased to function. Between 1831 and 1848, only 1838 saw any activity by the health council. That year its main business was industrial investigations and authorizations, with reports also being published on horse flaying and chemical matches. Like other councils, such as that of the Nord, the Rouen health council also urged the appointment of a permanent inspector of dangerous and unhealthy establishments.[83] After 1844 the Rouen council barely functioned, meeting only twice a year. Since its main task had become industrial investigation and authorization, lack of activity may have been due to the commercial and industrial slump affecting France during those years. The Rouen council was less active than other health councils, publishing between 1831 and 1847 an average of only ten to twelve reports a year.[84]

Cholera was also the stimulus for the creation of the health council of the Haute-Garonne at Toulouse, founded April 1, 1832, by Prefect Barennes, who also established secondary councils throughout the department. The council recommended a citywide clean-up campaign, and one member later asserted that Toulouse escaped cholera because of sanitary improvements ordered by the health council.[85] Once fear of cholera abated, the council ceased to function, publishing no reports between 1832 and 1838. The rapid industrialization of Toulouse in the 1830s, however, convinced the mayor that a health council was necessary, and he established the health council of Toulouse in June 1838.[86] Until then, as in other cities, the municipal administration had relied upon local academies of

83 A.D., Seine-Maritime, 5 MP 2237, Rapports, ms. of Conseil de Salubrité, November 17, 1838; June 8, 1839; March 30, 1844; *Rapport, Nord, 1841 et 1842*, pp. 112–15.

84 All information on the Rouen health council is contained in A.D., Seine-Maritime, 5 MP 2236, the annual reports, mss, of the health council, and 5 MP 2237, the minutes and individual reports. No reports were printed, and it was noted (5 MP 2237, February 26, 1832) that the funds of the health council were insufficient to publish its reports; A.D., Seine-Maritime, 5 MP 2236. In 1832 there were only two reports; in 1838, eighteen.

85 Ducasse, *Rapport général sur les travaux du Conseil de salubrité du département de la Haute-Garonne séant à Toulouse pendant l'année 1832* (Toulouse: Jean-Matthieu Douladonne, 1832), pp. 1, 8–25.

86 A. Dassier, *Travaux du Conseil de salubrité de la ville de Toulouse du 21 juin 1838 au 31 déc. 1847* (Toulouse: Chauvin, 1847); the members were Barnard, professor at the Veterinary School; Boisgiraud, professor of chemistry at the Faculty of Sciences; Costes, a lawyer; Dr. A. Dassier, member of the Société de Médecine; Delaye, prof. suppléant at the Ecole de Médecine; Fourtaniès, king's attorney at the civil tribunal; Magnes-Lahens, a pharmacist; and Mather, a manufacturer. At the time, Arnoux was mayor of Toulouse and O. de Bréville was prefect of the Haute-Garonne.

science and medicine for public health advice. Even after the health council's creation, the mayor still turned over some public health problems
to commissions outside the health council. This was common practice in
Lyon and Paris as well, although such commissions usually included health
council members. The Toulouse health council, like others, dealt primarily
with industrial authorizations and investigations, following the example of
the Paris council.[87]

The health council of the Gironde (Bordeaux) was founded in 1831 with
twenty-one members, including the epidemic physician for the department
(Léon Marchant), physicians and surgeons from the hospitals, the Ecole de
Médecine, the local medical society, and chemists and pharmacists. Health
council correspondents were named throughout the department, one for
each canton. Although there is no indication that the Gironde council was
established specifically because of cholera, the date of its founding –
August 9, 1831 – suggests that this was the case. As in other cities, before
the founding of the Gironde health council, the local medical society
(*Société royale de médecine*) and the scientific academy (*Académie des Sciences*)
advised authorities on public health issues. The council corresponded with
the local sanitary intendancy, and together they worked on disease prevention, sanitary reform, aid to the sick, and plans for burial of cholera
victims. Cholera took a few lives in Bordeaux in the late summer of 1832,
but by October the danger had passed.[88]

Draining of marshes and urban water supply were the major preoccupa-
tions of the Gironde health council. Between one-third and two-thirds of
the department was covered with marshes, most of which were privately
owned. The owners neither appreciated the advantages of drainage nor
cared to go to the expense. Physicians considered swamps a foyer for intermittent fever, urging drainage by canalization and cleaning river beds so
that water would flow more rapidly.[89] The health council of the Gironde
also devoted much attention to the Bordeaux water supply, which, as
in most French cities, was insufficient. The water service of Bordeaux
had no hydraulic system, and wells were used for drinking water and

87 All this in Dassier, *Travaux*. Toulouse in fact may not have had many of the typical
    urban health problems, for the city was atypical in that it had a good system of
    water distribution. See *J. des Débats*, September 27, 1838, "Lettres du Midi," pp.
    3–4. The most interesting and significant report done by the Toulouse health
    council was an 1845 report on "Assainissement des établissements publics."
88 Léon Marchant, *Rapport général des travaux du conseil central de salubrité du département
    de la Gironde depuis son organisation jusqu'à 1er janvier de l'année courante* (Bordeaux:
    Teycheney, 1833); Léon Marchant, *Rapport général des travaux du Conseil central de
    salubrité du département de la Gironde pour les années 1833 et 1834* (Bordeaux:
    Teycheney, 1835).
89 Léon Marchant, *Rapport général des travaux du Conseil central de salubrité du
    département de la Gironde* (Bordeaux: Teycheney, 1837).

irrigation. The health council spent much time searching for new water sources.[90]

A major question investigated by the Gironde health council was a disease called *pellagra des Landes*. One health council correspondent, Dr. Hameau of La Teste, claimed the disease, discovered in the Landes in 1818, was the same as *mal de la rosa*, found in Lombardy-Venetia. The health council, along with its correspondents and the epidemic physicians – many of whom were health council correspondents – looked into the question. The health council held a contest in 1838 to award two 100-franc medals to the authors of the best essays on pellagra and its preventive and curative measures. Six manuscripts were submitted, and Dr. Hameau, who had been working on the disease since 1829, and Dr. Lalesque won. The question continued to occupy the attention of health council members, and in 1840 Léon Marchant, secretary of the health council and epidemic physician for the department, published a major report on the disease.[91]

One major project of canalization and drainage in the Gironde involved a private company that was interested in the exploitation and colonization of the Landes, an unhealthy marshy area plagued with intermittent fevers, of which only one-fourth was cultivated. The administrators of the enterprise formed a health council that included well-known Parisian physicians and scientists: Matthew Orfila, Alexandre Parent-Duchâtelet, Joseph Pelletier, and Joseph d'Arcet. Paul Jolly, a physician, conducted an on-the-spot investigation to determine the nature of the unhealthy conditions, reforms needed, and sanitary measures that would be required by canalization. Jolly's report provides good insights into rural hygiene problems, canalization, and swamp drainage.[92]

The Aube (Troyes) health council was also founded in response to the cholera epidemic. Although the council was established in 1830, its actual organization dated from 1833 when a departmentwide organization was instituted, probably as a result of the cholera epidemic. Activity was restricted to the central council in Troyes in the first few years after its

90 Marchant, *R. G. Gironde, 1833 et 1834*; Léon Marchant, *Rapport général des travaux du conseil central de salubrité pour les années 1839 et 1840* (Bordeaux: Ramadié, 1841). The Gironde health council set the ordinary needs of inhabitants of a large city at twenty liters a day (five gallons), but if water for fires, cleaning the city, and industry were added, then that amount was increased to forty liters a day. See Léon Marchant, *Collection des rapports du Conseil central de salubrité du département de la Gironde pour les années 1845 et 1846* (Bordeaux: Durand, 1847).

91 Marchant, *R. G. Gironde, 1839 et 1840*; Léon Marchant, *Etude de la pellagre des Landes...rapport au Conseil central de salubrité du département de la Gironde* (Bordeaux: P. Faye, 1840).

92 Paul Jolly, *Rapport fait au Conseil de salubrité institué près la compagnie d'exploitation et de colonisation des Landes de Bordeaux sur l'état sanitaire et les moyens de l'assainissement de cette partie de la France* (Paris: Pillet, 1834).

foundation.[93] Members of the Troyes council included Dr. Pigeotte, a physician; Lhoste, an engineer; Gréau, a merchant and former artillery officer; two other physicians; and a pharmacist. The council undertook few investigations and published few reports: Dr. Pigeotte published a short report in 1834; two reports were published in 1835, and then in 1836 the council published instructions on first aid to the drowning.[94] Some indication of the low level of activity of the Aube council is that between 1832 and 1867 the council prepared only eighty reports, or an average of just over two reports a year, most of which concerned industrial establishments.[95]

The usual precautions against cholera were taken in the Aube. Arrondissement health councils were created with authority to maintain cleanliness in cities, and to eliminate foyers of infection and adulteration of food and drink. A network of cantonal correspondents was established to act as cantonal physicians, or physicians or the poor (*médecins des pauvres*). Cantonal correspondents were put in charge of vaccine, first-aid boxes for the drowning and asphyxiated, equipment for performing autopsies and dispensing medications, and foundlings and their wet nurses. They were also expected to give free care to poor families with chronic diseases, such as skin ailments and syphilis. According to the proposed plan, health councils would be consulted on dangerous and unhealthy establishments, on the construction of public works such as prisons, hospitals, barracks, and schools, and on general public health concerns. Cantonal correspondents would communicate with health councils on measures to be taken in case of epidemics or epizootics and would notify the authority of abuses in the sale of food, drink, and medicines.[96] One distinguishing feature of the Aube council was that the position of physician or surgeon of hospitals and prisons was accorded by preference to health council members. Also, since there were no epidemic physicians in the Aube before 1852, health council

93 The history of the Troyes health council is found in A. Vauthier, *Rapport général sur les travaux du Conseil d'hygiène de Troyes et sur les communications qui lui ont été adressés depuis sa fondation en 1830 jusqu'à 1867 exclusivement* (Troyes: Dufour-Bouquot, 1867), in A.D. Aube, M1615.

94 Pigeotte, *Précis des travaux du Conseil de salubrité de la ville de Troyes* (Troyes: d'Anner-André, 1834), in A.D. Aube, M1615; *Recueil des principaux travaux du Conseil de salubrité du département de l'Aube* (Troyes: Cardon, February 1835, and Bouquot, September 1835). Contained in the September reports are two very interesting reports on hygienic conditions in two rural communes: "Recherches hygiéniques sur la commune de Rouilly-Saint-Loup (pp. 22–42) and "Recherches hygiéniques sur la commune de Villemaur (pp. 42–64). The September 1835 report on these communes was mainly the work of Patin, Desguerrois, Clément-Mullet, and Charles des Etangs.

95 The procès-verbaux are in Vauthier, *R. G. Troyes*; most reports concerned industrial establishments.

96 "Organisation et composition des conseils," in *Recueil des travaux*, February 1835.

members fulfilled these functions as well. Basically, after a short burst of activity in 1834 and 1835, the Aube health council barely functioned.

Although provincial health councils proliferated in the 1820s and 1830s, there was no central organization of health councils, nor did the health councils become a nationwide institution until 1848. According to Patrice Bourdelais and Jean-Yves Raulot, other councils besides those just discussed were founded, but leading hygienists were unaware of them. Nor were their activities reported in the *Annales d'hygiène publique*.[97]

THE HEALTH COUNCIL AS A NATIONWIDE PROGRAM

As early as 1815 the members of the Paris health council suggested that institution coordinate a nationwide system of health councils, serving as a central point of correspondence with provincial prefectures. However, the prefect of police was not receptive to the idea, and nothing came of it. But by the 1830s, the reputation of the Paris council was well secured, with its activities and those of some provincial health councils receiving enough publicity that the national administration began to view a nationwide system of health councils with more favor.[98]

The interest of the national government in the health councils dated from the 1830s and was directly related to the failure of the Restoration government's sanitary policy. Once cholera invaded France in the spring of 1832, the sanitary policy was abandoned. Actually, the government had been scaling down the expenditures for the sanitary administration since the late 1820s, but the sanitary program was revived in the fall of 1831 to combat cholera.[99] In the summer and fall of 1831 sanitary intendancies and newly created health commissions were empowered to deal with the epidemic, but in the spring of 1832, when, in spite of all precautions, cholera invaded France, the program was disbanded and health councils,

---

97 Ibid.; Vauthier, *R. G. Troyes*, p. 61. Three members of the Aube health council published an article in the *Annales d'hygiène publique* in 1834: Pigeotte, Lhoste, and Gréau, "Rapport fait au conseil de salubrité de Troyes, sur les accidens auxquels sont exposés les ouvriers employés dans les filatures de laine et de coton," *Annales d'hygiène publique* 12 (1834): 5–30. See Charles C. H. Marc, chairman, "Rapport d'une commission de l'Académie royale de Médecine, à M. le Ministre du Commerce et des Travaux Publics sur l'établissement de Conseils de salubrité départementaux," *Annales d'hygiène publique* 18 (1837): 5–36. Bourdelais and Raulot, *Histoire du choléra*, pp. 179–86.

98 Moléon, *R. G.*, 1815, p. 88. This was not a new idea, having been debated by the Health Committee of the National Constituent Assembly in 1790–1. See Ingrand, *Le comité de salubrité*, pp. 32–84, and Weiner, "Le droit de l'homme à la santé," pp. 216–17.

99 *Documents statistiques sur la France publiés par le Ministre de Commerce*, 1 (1835): 148–9. This is the first part of the complete collection, *Statistique générale de la France*, 34 vols. (Paris: Imprimerie royale, 1835–73).

where they existed, were merged with intendancies.[100] Cities and towns that were spared, such as Lyon and Rouen, attributed their good fortune to local programs of sanitary reform, and since health councils and health commissions had been in charge of such programs, national officials began to view them with more favor.

In the mid-1830s, Minister of Commerce Tanneguy Duchâtel, who had jurisdiction over public health, became interested in a nationwide network of health councils. At his request a commission of the Royal Academy of Medicine prepared a report on the health councils and proposed that councils be established throughout the nation at departmental and arrondissement levels. The Academy suggested that the Paris health council serve as a model, but also advocated local variations as necessary. The Royal Academy of Medicine put itself – and not the Paris health council – at the head of the proposed nationwide health council organization in much the same way that it coordinated the national vaccination program. Each health council would submit its general reports to the Academy, which would issue an annual report on the activities of all the health councils.[101]

The proposed plan did not materialize under the government of the July Monarchy. From the mid-1830s, the interest of the national government in the health councils waned until after the revolution of 1848, when a national law instituted health councils throughout the nation at the departmental and arrondissement levels.[102] The 1848 law left the organization of the existing health councils basically unchanged, and it did not remedy the fundamental problem of the health councils, which was their lack of legal authority and coercive power.[103] The results of the nationwide program were not so gratifying as many hygienists had hoped. By the late 1850s, many of the recently established health councils were do-nothing

100 *Recueil des textes officiels*, 2: 30–6, for ordinances regulating the importation of goods, quarantine, and the formation of sanitary intendancies and commissions to combat the importation of cholera. See also, 2: 41. Such was the case in Nantes and Lille, for example.

101 A.N., F⁸171, Circulaire No. 12. Ministère du Commerce. Bureau sanitaire. Salubrité. Paris le 19 mai 1835. Marc, "Rapport sur l'établissement de conseils de salubrité départementaux"; other members of the commission were Orfila, Pariset, Villermé, Adelon, Villeneuve, and Dupuy.

102 A.N., F⁸171. Ministère de l'Agriculture et du Commerce. Bureau sanitaire. A M. le Préfet de _____ au sujet de salubrité. October 1843; A.N. F⁸171, Ministère de l'Agriculture et du Commerce. Comité consultatif d'hygiène publique. République française...; for the 1848 law see *Recueil des textes officiels*, 2: 231–2. Even in 1848 the original plan of the Health Committee of the National Constituent Assembly was not realized, for the health councils remained strictly advisory boards, not being invested with independent power, as the Health Committee had envisaged.

103 A.N., F⁸171, decree of 15 déc. 1851 regarding the organization of the Paris health council; A.N., F⁸171, Prefect of police to Minister of Commerce and Agriculture, November 20, 1849.

organizations either because of lack of interest or lack of funds. Writing in 1861, Maxime Vernois, industrial hygienist and member of the Paris health council, reluctantly concluded that practical and administrative hygiene in France were still in their early stages of development.[104] Thus, throughout the Second Empire, the health councils continued to function in an advisory capacity only, much as they had during the Restoration and the July Monarchy.

THE HEALTH COUNCIL MODEL

The health councils had the potential for much utility as advisory bodies only, and indeed, some prefects and mayors used the institution to good advantage. Unless a prefect or mayor consulted the health council regularly and acted on its advice, however, the health council, possessing no initiative of its own and powerless, could and often did degenerate into a debating club. Unlike the boards of health in fifteenth- and sixteenth-century Italy, or the boards of health that were established in England and in the United States in the second half of the nineteenth century, the French health councils could not make and enforce policy.[105] Councils were further hampered by the fact that, with the exception of the Paris council, members were unsalaried. This was undoubtedly the chief reason that many of the councils functioned only sporadically, and why, in some places, subprefects had great difficulty even getting physicians and pharmacists to serve on arrondissement councils.

The health councils are central to an understanding of the French public health movement, in spite of their weaknesses and the unevenness of their accomplishments. A study of health council reports tells us a lot about the public health problems faced by cities and industrial towns in the early nineteenth century. The institution of the health councils demonstrates how some prefects and mayors attempted to solve local public health problems by establishing their own advisory boards. In addition, the organization and activities of the health councils typify the concept of public health that prevailed in the early nineteenth century, when public health as a discipline was in the process of definition. Before the nineteenth century in France, public health was synonymous with epidemic prevention, with boards of health temporarily set up to deal with emergency situations. Once the danger ended, restrictions were lifted and the boards were disbanded. Public hygienists of the late eighteenth and early nine-

104 Maxime Vernois, "Des rapports généraux des Conseils d'hygiène de l'Empire," *Annales d'hygiène publique* 2 série 15 (1861): 453–69.
105 Cipolla, *Public Health*, pp. 11–66. As one historian has suggested, had the French health councils been invested with power of their own, as had been envisaged by the Health Committee of the Constituent Assembly, the history of public health in France would have been different; see Ingrand, *Le comité de salubrité*, p. 84.

teenth centuries broadened the traditional concept of public health to include anything that was in any way related to health. The breadth of health council activities demonstrates the all-encompassing view of public health held by the hygienists. Because its scope was so broad, public hygienists came to consider public health a permanent goal. For that reason, the Paris health council and some of the provincial councils functioned as permanent advisory boards. Public health measures were no longer to be merely restrictions imposed in time of emergency, but regulations to be obeyed at all times.

The Paris health council should be singled out, because it was the principal institution through which the public health movement developed. By the 1830s it had become the preeminent public health authority in France, with an international reputation. Its distinguished membership, the breadth of its research, and its methods of investigation all contributed to its stature at home and abroad. It researched and reported on most of the urban health problems of the era, and its opinions and conclusions were held in high esteem in France and elsewhere.

The model typified by the Paris council was one of the most important contributions of the early-nineteenth-century French public health movement. The health council model included, first of all, a permanent institution that investigated day-to-day public health problems. Second, it consisted of a board of technical experts – public hygienists instead of citizen volunteers or appointed officials – to advise local authorities on public health. Third, the health council was the embodiment, the institutionalization of *hygiène publique*, the scientific discipline of public hygiene. The Paris health council model was copied throughout France in the provincial health councils, and outside France as well. In the 1830s, Belgium modeled its health councils on the French institution; in 1847, the Kingdom of Sardinia established a central health council and branch councils on the Paris model. And in 1866, the Council of Hygiene of New York City used the French model as a basis for the establishment of the New York City Board of Health.[106]

The health councils illustrate the success of the hygienists in achieving two of their goals: the institutionalization of the public health idea and their investigative mission. The function of the councils was investigative and advisory. Investigation was the principal means hygienists used to address occupational hygiene and the perceived socioeconomic dislocation of industrialization. Investigation was the first step toward another goal, moralization, the means by which the working class was to be incorporated into French society.

---

106 Ambroise Tardieu, "Introduction" to the second edition of *Dictionnaire d'hygiène publique et de salubrité*, 4 vols. (Paris: Baillière, 1862), 1: viii–x.

5

Investigation and moralization: Occupational hygiene and industrialization

Before 1850, most French workers were employed in traditional artisanal industries located in small workshops and workers' cottages, but some areas of northern France, namely, the Nord, Loire, Seine-Inférieure, Alsace, and greater Paris industrialized rapidly. Both handcraft and domestic industries and new mechanized, factory-based industries attracted the attention of sociomedical investigators.[1] Industrialization generated a new interest among public hygienists and social reformers in the health of the working classes, because it seemed to threaten the health of factory workers.[2] Statistics gathered in England and France showed that mortality

1 On French industrialization, see the older but still useful works by Arthur Dunham, *The Industrial Revolution in France, 1815–1914* (New York: Exposition Press, 1955), and J. H. Clapham, *The Economic Development of France and Germany, 1815–1914*, 4th ed. (Cambridge: Cambridge University Press, 1968). Recent works to be consulted include William Reddy, *The Rise of Market Culture: The Textile Trade and French Society, 1750–1900* (New York: Cambridge University Press, 1984); William Sewell, *Work and Revolution in France: The Language of Labor from the Old Regime to 1848* (New York: Cambridge University Press, 1980); and Peter Stearns, *Paths to Authority: The Middle Class and the Industrial Labor Force in France, 1820–1848* (Chicago: University of Illinois Press, 1978). The two best contemporary sources, which deal mainly with the textile industry, are Louis-René Villermé, *Tableau de l'état physique et moral des ouvriers employés dans les manufactures de coton, de laine et de soie*, 2 vols. (Paris: Renouard, 1840), and Jean-Pierre Thouvenin, "De l'influence que l'industrie exerce sur la santé des populations dans les grands centres manufacturiers," *Annales d'hygiène publique* 36 (1846): 16–46, 277–96, and 37 (1847): 83–111. For more information on the extent of industrialization and the working-class population, see Appendix 1.
2 In this study the terms *working class* and *working classes* refer to workers of several types: handcraft workers (artisans), those employed in the domestic (putting-out) system, and factory workers, some of whom were handcraft workers. The French working class in the nineteenth century included proletarians (factory, industrial workers), the laboring classes (a term usually used to denote preindustrial workers) and the poor, who were often employed as day laborers. The authors of working-class inquiries used the terms *ouvriers* (Villermé and Blanqui), *des classes laborieuses* (Buret), and *des classes dangereuses* (Frégier); Thouvenin referred to "la population dans les grands centres manufacturiers." Louis Chevalier has analyzed *des classes laborieuses et dangereuses* in *Classes laborieuses et dangereuses à Paris pendant la première moitié du XIXe siècle* (Paris: Plon, 1958). See Jurgen Kuczynski, *The Rise of the Working Class*, trans. C. T. A. Ray (New York: McGraw-Hill, 1967), pp. 188–96.

was much higher in industrial than agricultural areas and that army rejections were greater among the working classes than among the comfortable classes.[3] Hygienists and reformers investigated the condition of the working class to determine how industry and industrialization affected workers' health. At stake, hygienists believed, was the military and productive strength of the nation.

Hygienists identified two principal ways in which industry could affect workers' health: Industrial and occupational processes and working conditions in factories and workshops could cause health problems; and workers' living conditions could affect their health directly or indirectly. Although the hygienists' role was primarily investigative, they advocated socioeconomic reform and legislative measures to improve workers' health. Underlying their recommendations was the strong need for moral reform, or the moralization of workers. This was especially true in the case of Villermé. Sociomedical investigations led to increased awareness of industrial health problems, but they did not lead to effective national legislation. The hygienists' failure to effect legislative reform can be explained primarily in terms of the predominant liberal ideology, which favored nonintervention.

OCCUPATIONAL HYGIENE

Hygienists sought to determine if certain processes were injurious to health and if there was a relationship between occupations and mortality rates.[4] They also wanted to find out if mechanization of industry was a health and safety hazard. Although mechanization could eliminate dangerous and unhealthy processes, sometimes it caused industrial accidents.[5] Hygienists also wanted to know if industrialization posed public health problems resulting from pollution, noise, and fire. Alexandre Parent-Duchâtelet, Louis-René Villermé, Alphonse Chevallier, Joseph d'Arcet, and others investigated these concerns to discover if industry and industrial processes were a cause of workers' disease and mortality. The interest of hygienists in occupational hygiene is demonstrated by the numerous articles that appeared in the *Annales d'hygiène publique*. The Paris health council also

3 L. R. Villermé, "Sur la population de la Grande-Bretagne considérée principalement et comparativement dans les districts agricoles, dans les districts manufacturiers et dans les grandes villes," *Annales d'hygiène publique* 12 (1834): 247–71; Villermé, *Tableau,* 1:280–317.

4 See Chapter 2 for further discussion of the relationship between occupations and mortality rates. A comprehensive history of occupational medicine is Michel Valentin, *Travail des hommes et savants oubliés: Histoire de la médecine de travail, de la sécurité et de l'ergonomie* (Paris: Editions Docis, 1978). See especially chs. 8–10.

5 See, for example, Pigeotte, Lhoste, and Gréau, "Rapport fait au conseil de salubrité de Troyes, sur les accidens auxquels sont exposés les ouvriers employés dans les filatures de laine et de coton," *Annales d'hygiène publique* 12 (1834): 5–30.

devoted much of its attention to occupational hygiene, the authorization of industrial establishments being one of its primary duties.[6]

Hygienists investigated reputedly dangerous and unhealthy industries such as the white lead, explosives, and phosphorus match industries, all of which they found to be injurious to the health of workers and the public. The white lead industry, recognized by all as dangerous and unhealthy, received more attention from hygienists than any other industry. Hygienists also examined lead-related occupations, such as painting, for the relationship between working with lead and the consequent development of lead poisoning and lead colic was recognized. Pharmacist-chemist Alphonse Chevallier and industrial chemist Joseph d'Arcet, acting under the auspices of the Paris health council, conducted an extensive study into the health dangers associated with the white lead industry,[7] and Louis Tanquerel des Planches examined diseases that afflicted workers in lead-related industries.[8] These investigators found that hygienic precautions were usually not taken in factories and workshops where lead was worked; consequently, lead colic sooner or later afflicted almost all workers. Chevallier observed that even in factories where precautions were taken, it was difficult to get workers to cooperate. Many workers simply did not practice basic rules of personal hygiene, such as washing hands before eating. Hygienists suggested that part of the solution to lead disease was hygienic and recommended personal cleanliness to avoid ingestion of lead particles. Factory owners, they stated, should also provide adequate ventilation to prevent workers from absorbing dust particles. Reflecting the predominant liberal ideology, hygienists urged workers and factory owners to take responsibility for these measures so that no government regulation, surveillance, or intervention would be necessary.[9]

6 See Chapter 4 for a discussion of this duty. On occupational hygiene in the *Annales d'hygiène publique*, see Bernard Lécuyer, "Les maladies professionnelles dans les 'Annales d'hygiène publique et de médecine légale' ou une première approche de l'usure du travail," *Mouvement social* 124 (1983): 45–69.

7 Alphonse Chevallier, "Sur l'hygiène des ouvriers en général, et sur celle des cérusiers en particulier," *Annales d'hygiène publique* 48 (1852): 331–8, for a résumé of the health council's investigation of the industry.

8 *Traité des maladies de plomb*, 2 vols. (Paris: Ferra, 1839). The work was abridged and translated into English by Samuel L. Dana, published as *Lead Diseases* (Boston: D. Bixby and Co., 1848).

9 Alphonse Chevallier, "Recherches sur les causes de la maladie dite colique de plomb, chez les ouvriers qui préparent la céruse," *Annales d'hygiène publique* 15 (1836): 5–67. See also by Chevallier, "Notes statistiques sur les ouvriers atteints de la colique de plomb traités dans les hôpitaux de Paris en 1840," *Annales d'hygiène publique* 26 (1841): 451–3, in which Chevallier pointed out that the incidence of lead colic was on the increase. For an article on a lead-related industry, see Alphonse Dalmenesche, "Observations sur les causes de la colique de plomb chez les tisserands à la Jacquart; moyens d'y remédier," *Annales d'hygiène publique* 27

The chemical (phosphorus) match industry, whose development began in France in the 1830s as a result of mechanization, was another industry that hygienists found to be unhealthy to workers and dangerous to public safety, due to the inflammable nature of its product. Before that date, match production had been a slow process and had employed about 100 workers in Paris. But after mechanization, by 1846, there were about 4,000 match workers in Paris, and one worker could produce 1,200,000 to 1,800,000 matches daily. Dipping matches in phosphorus revolutionized the industry but also created health and safety hazards for workers. In his definitive study of the match industry, physician-hygienist Théophile Roussel noted that workers were commonly afflicted with coughs and sore throats, sometimes developing a serious disease, maxillary necrosis (necrosis of the jawbone, or "phossy jaw"), caused by phosphorus emanations. Furthermore, many accidents had been associated with the industry. Fires and explosions had occurred within factories and in the transport, sale, and use of matches. The only administrative measure regulating the match industry was an 1838 ordinance that made the transport of chemical matches subject to the same regulations as explosives. However, the ordinance was poorly enforced, so accidents continued. Roussel contended that the main problem was that the industry had remained outside administrative regulations, since it had never been classified as dangerous and unhealthy. Because of this, the government had given industrialists no directions for the internal plan of the factories. Roussel argued that industrial legislation had kept pace neither with developments in old industries nor with the creation of new ones. He noted that in spite of the 1810 law on dangerous trades – the basis of the public health regulations concerning industry – many industries established since 1810 developed and survived outside existing regulations. In spite of more efficient and complete regulations after 1830, some industries were still not being covered by the law. Roussel's solution to the health problems related to the chemical match industry was twofold: administrative measures to regulate the industry for the health and safety of workers and the public, and hygienic measures to be applied in factories by owners and workers. Roussel went even further, advocating uniform regulations to protect workers' health in all dangerous and unhealthy industries. Other industries, especially those that produced chemical products, posed public health problems, owing to

(1842): 205–11. An interesting article giving a history of the white lead factory of Clichy, in the Paris suburbs, is Bréchot, fils, "Mémoire sur les accidens résultant de la fabrication de la céruse," *Annales d'hygiène publique* 12 (1834): 72–80. Bréchot's father owned the factory. On liberal ideology and public hygiene, see William Coleman, *Death Is a Social Disease: Public Health and Political Economy in Early Industrial France* (Madison: University of Wisconsin Press, 1982).

inadequate means of industrial waste disposal, resulting in pollution of air and water. Solutions were hard to find until new and better processes were invented, and often the only measure available was isolation of such industries from populated areas.[10]

Hygienists proposed three ways to manage public health problems caused by dangerous and unhealthy industries: (1) administrative measures – government intervention to regulate industry;[11] (2) hygienic precautions taken by both employers and employees;[12] and (3) the invention and application of new processes either by mechanization or by scientific and technological innovations.[13] All three were tried. Government intervention and regulation dated from the 1810 law on dangerous and unhealthy trades, reissued by Louis XVIII in 1815. According to this law, industries were to be classified into one of three areas, depending on how dangerous, unhealthy, or obnoxious they were. Unhealthy or dangerous industries were classified first class and had to be located away from populated areas; second-class industries were considered obnoxious and offensive, but not dangerous or unhealthy, and could be tolerated within the city. In the third class were industries that could be safely established in populated areas without any inconvenience to inhabitants. All persons wishing to establish an industry or workshop had to seek authorization. If the industry was first class, the approval of the *Conseil d'état* was necessary. For second- and third-class industries the approval of the prefect of police (in Paris) or the departmental prefect was required for authorization. Before the prefect granted authorization, the health council – if there was one – would

10 Théophile Roussel, *Recherches sur les maladies des ouvriers employés à la fabrication des allumettes chimiques, sur les accidents qui résultent du transport et de l'usage de ces allumettes et sur les mesures hygiéniques et administratives nécessaires pour assainir cette industrie* (Paris: Labé, 1846), pp. 1–17, 22–60, 66–9. This is the same Roussel after whom the Roussel Law for the Protection of Infants and Children (1874) was named. Damage to the environment was not an issue examined by the public hygienists. On the dangers and inconveniences of chemical industries, see, for example, Braconnet and Simonin, "Note sur des émanations des fabriques de produits chimiques," *Annales d'hygiène publique* 40 (1848): 128–36; Alexandre Parent-Duchâtelet, "Des inconvéniens que peuvent avoir, dans quelques circonstances, les huiles pyrogénées et le goudron provenant de la distillation de la houille," *Hygiène publique*, 2 vols. (Paris: Baillière, 1836), 2:426–39.

11 See, for example, Pigeotte, Lhoste, and Gréau, "Accidens auxquels sont exposés les ouvriers," pp. 26–30; Edouard Duchesne, *Essai sur la colique de plomb* (Paris, M.D. thesis, 1827), pp. 29–30; Roussel, *Recherches*, pp. 70–6.

12 Tanquerel des Planches, *Lead Diseases*, pp. 330–63; Chevallier, "Recherches sur la colique de plomb," pp. 26–55, Dalmenesche, "Observations sur la colique de plomb," pp. 205–11; Bréchot, "Fabrication de la céruse," pp. 79–80; Alphonse Guérard, "Note sur la ventilation des filatures," *Annales d'hygiène publique* 30 (1843): 115–16.

13 See, for example, Joseph d'Arcet, Henri Gaultier de Claubry, and Alexandre Parent-Duchâtelet, "Mémoire sur un moyen mécanique nouvellement proposé pour respirer impunément les gaz délétères et pénétrer avec facilité dans les lieux qui en sont remplis," *Hygiène publique*, 1:67–97.

inspect, classify, and report on the industry, recommending whether authorization should be given or not, and in some cases requiring that certain conditions be imposed on the industry before final authorization.[14]

It is debatable to what extent the 1810 law was a public health law and how effective it was. First, since industries already in existence in 1810 were not covered, many industries were excluded, contributing to the law's ineffectiveness.[15] Second, although the law was purported to reconcile the interests of industry, property (the rights of property owners living in the vicinity of the industry), and public health, in practice it addressed primarily industrial and propertied interests. Although public hygienists considered the 1810 law an important public health law, they argued that too often it was interpreted to protect the rights of property owners and industrialists, to the neglect of public health concerns.

Resolving this tension between statism and liberalism occupied the attention of hygienists. A timeless question with which reformers and governments have had to wrestle is: How far does the role of the state as guardian of the public health extend? Chevallier phrased it another way: If an occupation or industry was found to be harmful to public health, did the administration have the right to prohibit its existence or regulate it in the interest of all citizens? Although most hygienists advocated regulation, their liberalism conflicted with a statist, regulatory approach. When public health and the rights of factory owners came into conflict, they typically decided in favor of free enterprise.[16] Nevertheless, the existence of the law indicates governmental awareness of industrial health problems and the need to regulate and impose restrictions on new industry.

Other royal and local police ordinances regulated dangerous and unhealthy industries, such as the traditional nuisance trades: tanning of leather, slaughtering of animals, and dyeing and degreasing of hides. Enforcement

14 The basis of the 1810 decree was a report done by the Paris health council in 1810. See V. de Moléon, *Rapports généraux sur les travaux du Conseil de salubrité de la ville de Paris et du département de la Seine exécutés depuis l'année 1802 jusqu'à l'année 1826 inclusivement* (Paris: Imprimerie municipale, 1828); 1809, p. 39; 1810, p. 40. For the 1810 decree on dangerous trades, see *Recueil des textes officiels concernant la protection de la santé publique, 1790 à 1935*, 9 vols. (Paris: Ministère de la Santé Publique, 1957), 1:165–7; for the royal ordinance of 1815 see *Recueil des textes*, 1:209, or *Moniteur universel*, February 16, 1815, pp. 187–8. The definitive work on the subject is Adolphe Trébuchet, *Code administratif des établissemens dangereux, insalubres, ou incommodes...* (Paris: Béchet jeune, 1832). See also the article by Pierre Girard about the work, "Rapport sur un ouvrage intitulé: *Code administratif des établissemens dangereux, insalubres et incommodes* par M. Adolphe Trébuchet," *Annales d'hygiène publique* 10 (1833): 197–201.

15 Adolphe Trébuchet, ed., *Bulletin administratif et judiciaire de la préfecture de police et de la ville de Paris* 1 (January 1835), p. 33.

16 Alphonse Chevallier, "Essai sur les maladies qui atteignent les ouvriers qui préparent le vert arsénical et les ouvriers en papiers peints qui emploient dans la préparation de ces papiers le vert schweinfurt; moyens de les prévenir," *Annales d'hygiène publique* 38 (1847): 56–7, note 1.

varied, but judging from local health council reports, it was often lax. Hygientists reported that in some factories employers and employees practiced preventive hygienic measures. But many factories and small workshops were poorly ventilated, hot, and dirty, and workers' personal hygiene was nonexistent. In certain industries, improvement of industrial processes solved some health problems but created others. Mechanization, for example, made some textile processes less hazardous, but, in turn, technological innovations could create new problems, such as machinery accidents and disposal of chemical wastes.

Although hygienists identified a few industries that presented definite occupational health hazards, the prevailing opinion of leading hygienists – Villermé, Chevallier, and Parent-Duchâtelet – was that it was not occupations per se that caused workers' health problems, but living conditions resulting from poverty. In the 1820s and 1830s there was a debunking attitude among hygienists that lent strength to this point of view. The traditional interpretation of occupational diseases presented in the early eighteenth century by Bernardino Ramazzini and translated into French by Antoine Fourcroy in 1777 was the object of repeated attacks by French hygienists.[17] According to Ramazzini and his followers, most occupations were hazardous to workers' health because of (1) dust vapors breathed in by workers; (2) conditions of constant humidity in workshops and factories; and (3) excess or lack of exercise – the occupation being either too physically demanding or sedentary. Hygienists debunked what they regarded as myths about the dangers of various occupations.[18] None of them denied that there were industrial processes injurious to health, but they argued that many processes that had been assumed to be dangerous and unhealthy had never been tested and proved dangerous; that in many cases – probably most – workers' bad health was due to causes other than occupational hazards. In some instances, mechanization made a dangerous procedure safer; in others, new preventive measures had been applied or new industrial processes invented. Hygienists argued that in most cases, the real cause of workers' diseases was not found in their occupations.

17 *De Morbis Artificum Diatriba* (Mutinae: A. Capponi, 1700). On Ramazzini, see Valentin, *Histoire de la médecine de travail*, ch. 4. Antoine Fourcroy, trans., *Essai sur les maladies des artisans* (Paris: Moutard, 1777); on Fourcroy and occupational diseases in eighteenth-century France, see Arlette Farge, "Les artisans malades de leur travail," *Annales: E.S.C.* 32 (1977): 993–1006.

18 Philibert Patissier, *Traité des maladies des artisans et de celles qui résultent de diverses professions d'après Ramazzini* (Paris: Baillière, 1822). See A. L. Gosse, *Propositions générales sur les maladies causées par l'exercice des professions* (Paris: M.D. thesis, 1816), p. 9, in which he states that most authors who have published works on occupational diseases since Ramazzini have copied him. See also Parent-Duchâtelet, "Mémoire sur les débardeurs de la ville de Paris," *Hygiène publique*, 2: 614–21, and Bernard Lécuyer, "Démographie statistique et hygiène publique sous la monarchie censitaire," *Annales de démographie historique* (1977): 241–5.

In 1829, Parent-Duchâtelet and d'Arcet embarked on a systematic study of Parisian trades and industries, their goal being to test scientifically all that had been said about occupational health hazards. The articles that resulted from this project, the work of Parent-Duchâtelet, d'Arcet, and Chevallier, constituted the first major break with the traditional interpretation of occupational medicine and hygiene.[19] Parent-Duchâtelet intended to apply scientific methodology to the study of the professions and their influence on health. Such a study was needed, he contended, because of the failure of the traditional authorities and their modern commentators to examine occupations scientifically. As he explained:

This manner of proceeding [empirical investigation] has demonstrated that the works about which we speak, far from being the fruit of long observation, have been composed in the silence of the study, by men who have only caught a glimpse of artisans and factories; and who, generalizing some facts that have been haphazardly presented to them, have singularly exaggerated the inconveniences of several professions and attributed to others influences that they are far from having.[20]

Parent-Duchâtelet and d'Arcet first expressed the debunking idea in an article on the tobacco industry. Rather than repeating what other authors had said, they suggested that each occupation should be scientifically investigated. Hygienists should consult historical documents and official regulations, gather statistical data, interview workers and foremen, and conduct on-site factory investigations. Using this methodology, Parent-Duchâtelet began an ambitious project that would have ultimately resulted in the investigation of all Parisian trades and industries. Although he died in 1836 before completing the project, he left detailed reports on the horsebutchering industry, the dock workers (stevedores) of Paris, sewer workers, tobacco workers, and the hemp-retting industry. Because he conducted his studies before the period of major French industrialization, his works on occupational hygiene deal with traditional industries and occupations.[21]

19 Parent-Duchâtelet and J. P. Joseph d'Arcet, "Mémoire sur les véritables influences que le tabac peut avoir sur la santé des ouvriers," *Hygiène publique*, 2:559; Parent-Duchâtelet, "Mémoire sur les débardeurs de la ville de Paris," *Hygiène publique*, 2: 614–15.

20 Parent-Duchâtelet and d'Arcet, "Mémoire sur les véritables influences que le tabac peut avoir," p. 559.

21 "Mémoire sur les véritables influences que le tabac peut avoir," *Hygiène publique*, 2: 559–606, and *Annales d'hygiène publique* 1 (1829): 9–227. On Parent-Duchâtelet, see Ann Fowler La Berge, "A. J. B. Parent-Duchâtelet: Hygienist of Paris, 1821–1836," *Clio Medica* 12 (1977): 279–301; "Les chantiers d'équarrissage de la ville de Paris envisagés sous le rapport de l'hygiène publique," *Hygiène publique*, 2: 123–256; "Mémoire sur les débardeurs de la ville de Paris," *Hygiène publique*, 2: 607–43; "Essai sur les cloaques ou égouts de la ville de Paris," *Hygiène publique*, 1: 156–307; "Le rouissage du chanvre considéré sous le rapport de l'hygiène publique," *Hygiène publique*, 2: 479–558.

Parent-Duchâtelet and d'Arcet investigated the tobacco industry, because authorities had asserted the dangerous influence of tobacco emanations on workers' health. They questioned foremen and physicians employed by the Paris factory, which had over 1,000 workers. They also sent out questionnaires to each of the other ten tobacco factories in the nation, employing a total of over 4,500 workers. After analyzing the data they collected, they flatly disagreed with what other authorities had said, contending that many diseases attributed to tobacco workers were pure fantasy, and that most workers were discharged because of old age, not bad health. Furthermore, during the sixteen years the Paris factory had been in operation, local authorities had received no complaints from neighboring establishments. Physicians practicing in the vicinity of the factory had found no harmful influence of tobacco emanations on health; nor had mortality rates been affected.[22]

Parent-Duchâtelet, who had been frequenting sewers, dumps, and workshops, both for his personal research and as a health council member, noticed that there was a great discrepancy between the health of the workers he observed and what the traditional authorities and their modern commentators asserted. One such group of workers was the stevedores of Paris. His investigation of the stevedores, published in 1830, was one of the most important occupational studies undertaken as part of his major project. The traditional authorities – Ramazzini, Fourcroy, and, most recently, Philibert Patissier – had maintained that people who worked with their lower extremities in water were subject to a variety of afflictions, especially leg ulcers. There was a consensus among both physicians and humanitarians that the occupation of stevedore was harmful to health. Parent-Duchâtelet wondered if this was really the case, if anyone had ever closely studied the stevedores. He thus conducted a detailed sociohygienic investigation into the occupation of stevedore, which included the study of over 600 workers in the Paris area. He reached conclusions quite opposite to the traditional and prevailing opinions, suggesting that "most of the diseases attributed to stevedores were pure suppositions, and that if their occupation was one of the most arduous, one could rank it in the class of the least unhealthy."[23]

But why, then, should there have been such a discrepancy between his findings and the pronouncements of the traditional authorities? Parent-Duchâtelet offered this explanation: "It is certainly due to that tendency of most men to generalize and to construct theories in the calm and silence of the study, and above all to the laziness of readers who prefer to believe without examination rather than to go to the trouble of research and verification."[24]

22 "Mémoire sur les véritables influences que le tabac peut avoir."
23 "Mémoire sur les débardeurs," p. 639.
24 Ibid., p. 640.

The traditional authorities had argued reasonably and by analogy, but had not based their arguments on firsthand observation, the proper method of procedure for the public hygienist. Parent-Duchâtelet wondered why no one had challenged the assertions of the authorities. He concluded:

...we have acquired the sad conviction that opinions are often transmitted from generation to generation and become the doctrine of a school by the sole reason that a dreamer in his study has recorded them in an agreeably written book, or that they have been uttered by a man with a great reputation.[25]

Criticizing physicians and their methods of studying occupational hygiene, Parent-Duchâtelet commented:

Among the numerous physicians at present and those becoming physicians every day, how is it that one finds so few who in ceasing to believe the works of the masters dare to doubt for one instant and try to verify the exactitude of that which is taught to them? If one of them had taken the trouble to go down to one of the ports of Paris and to question several workers, he would well have recognized like us that the diseases attributed to the stevedores did not exist, and that these workers had diseases or indispositions about which no one had ever spoken;[26]

Parent-Duchâtelet's 1824 work on the sewers of Paris exemplified his use of firsthand observation and the interview method in order to investigate sewers and sewer workers. This study, like his later report on the stevedores of Paris, clearly shows him to have been a scientific hygienist and a forerunner of empirical sociology. Here is Parent-Duchâtelet's description of how he proceeded:

I was not content to read what had been written on the matter and to question superficially workers and employers; *I walked over all the places that I describe* [his italics], I had frequent conversations with all those who are occupied or who have been occupied in the sewers, from the most distinguished academician to the lowliest worker; I attended more than once the work of the latter; I asked [the workers] for information both in the sewers and in their dwellings; I questioned them in a group and individually, to have if possible, contradictory reports, which have often served to put me on the track of new questions and to correct some errors.[27]

Other investigators expressed opinions similar to those of Parent-Duchâtelet and d'Arcet. After examining the relation of phthisis to occupation and finding little correlation, statistician-hygienist Benoiston de Châteauneuf suggested that a higher correlation might be found by studying the relation of affluence and poverty to phthisis.[28] Physician-hygienist Alphonse Guérard voiced similar opinions. He opposed those who

25 Ibid., p. 641.
26 Ibid.
27 Parent-Duchâtelet, "Mémoires sur les cloaques ou égouts," pp. 159–60.
28 L. F. Benoiston de Châteauneuf, "De l'influence de certaines professions sur le développement de la phthisie pulmonaire," *Annales d'hygiène publique* 6 (1831): 45.

thought each profession had its special disease and showed that occupational diseases did not differ from those produced under other similar etiological influences. Guérard argued that workers' bad habits rather than the unhealthiness of occupations were the cause of many occupational diseases, and that the frequency of morbidity among workers was related more to low wages than to occupational hazards.[29] Genevan statistician H. C. Lombard related the influence of professions to longevity and found that the main determining factor was the affluence or poverty associated with the profession.[30] In England, Charles Turner Thackrah disputed the findings first of Ramazzini, then of Patissier. He found many of Patissier's contentions unsupportable; in fact, his findings often flatly contradicted those of Patissier. Familiar with the work of d'Arcet and Parent-Duchâtelet on tobacco workers, Thackrah noted that the results of their investigations agreed with his. As Thackrah said in a statement that could just as well have been made by d'Arcet or Parent-Duchâtelet: "The want of close personal and fair examination we have often occasion to regret, as well in the interesting work of Ramazzini, as in that of his French commentator [Patissier]."[31] In 1835 Chevallier issued a debunking manifesto of his own, urging sociomedical investigators to abandon their libraries and go into the workshops to determine if diseases that had traditionally been considered dangerous and unhealthy really were. Chevallier showed, for example, that most printers' diseases were not occupation related. After Parent-Duchâtelet's death, Chevallier continued the project that Parent-Duchâtelet had started.[32]

Although Parent-Duchâtelet may have initiated what Isidore Bricheteau of the Royal Academy of Medicine called a "salutary reaction," later work by other investigators in the 1840s and 1850s suggested that in their zeal to debunk unproved theories, Parent-Duchâtelet and his colleagues may have exaggerated the safety of many industries. Investigating the tobacco industry in the 1840s, physician-hygienist François Mélier praised Parent-Duchâtelet for his contributions to occupational hygiene but argued that he had overestimated the innocuousness of some trades. Mélier pointed out

29 T. Gaillard, "M. Alphonse Guérard," *Annales d'hygiène publique*, 2e série 62 (1874): 458–78.
30 H. C. Lombard, "De l'influence des professions sur la durée de la vie," *Annales d'hygiène publique* 14 (1835): 5–45.
31 Charles Turner Thackrah, *The Effects of Arts, Trades, and Professions, and of Civil States and Habits of Living, on Health and Longevity*, 2nd ed., enlarged (London: Longman, Rees, 1832), pp. 8–63, 192–233; the quotation is from p. 60.
32 Alphonse Chevallier, "De la nécessité de faire de nouvelles recherches sur les maladies qui affligent les ouvriers et observations sur celles qui se font remarquer chez les imprimeurs," *Annales d'hygiène publique* 13 (1835): 304–44. On Chevallier and this manifesto, see Alex Berman, "J. B. A. Chevallier, Pharmacist-Chemist: A Major Figure in 19th Century French Public Health," *Bull. Hist. Med.* 52 (1978): 200–13.

shortcomings of Parent-Duchâtelet's approach, contending that because he had been afraid to attribute to an industry inconveniences that did not exist, he had ignored some that did. Mélier concurred with Parent-Duchâtelet, however, in concluding that in the case of tobacco workers, salary was the major consideration: Most tobacco workers were in good health because they had a comparatively high salary.[33] Mélier and other critics were justified in their criticism of Parent-Duchâtelet. The debunkers were indeed too lenient, failing to consider long-range effects of industrial processes and pollution on workers' health. In an 1852 article Chevallier recognized this very problem, noting that in certain cases it could take as long as thirty years for effects to become noticeable. He contended that although occupational diseases were not – with few exceptions – as serious as had been claimed, many diseases peculiar to industrial workers had up to then escaped the investigation of public hygienists.[34]

The central idea of the debunkers was that workers' health – with few exceptions – was not directly related to their occupations, but rather to their standard of living. The debunkers suggested that, first of all, factors other than occupation-related causes had to be examined; and second, that the variable with the highest correlation to workers' health was salary. The implication was that although the reform of industrial processes and the application of hygienic measures were beneficial, if the health of workers was to be improved, then poverty and its concomitant unhealthy living conditions had to be addressed: those factors that were the real causes of workers' diseases – poor-quality and insufficient food, inadequate clothing and shelter, and fatigue. This attitude led hygienists and reformers interested in the influence of industry on workers' health to investigate the condition of the working classes.

INDUSTRIALIZATION AND THE CONDITION OF THE WORKING CLASSES

Hygienists and reformers were interested in the condition of the working classes for socioeconomic and public health reasons. France industrialized later than Britain, and by the 1820s and 1830s, reformers, politicians, and hygienists were already acquainted with some of the social consequences of British industrialization. By the 1830s, continental observers exhibited much interest in British industrialization. Villermé and social reformer

---

33   François Mélier, *De la santé des ouvriers employés dans les manufactures de tabac* (Paris: Baillière, 1845). For Bricheteau's comment, see p. 56. On Mélier, see William Coleman, "Medicine Against Malthus: François Mélier on the Relation between Subsistence and Mortality (1843)," *Bull. Hist. Med.* 54 (1980): 23–42, and William Coleman, "Epidemiological Method in the 1860s: Yellow Fever at Saint-Nazaire," *Bull. Hist. Med.* 58 (1984): 145–63.
34   "Sur l'hygiène des ouvriers," pp. 331–8.

Eugène Buret investigated working-class conditions in Britain in order better to understand what was happening in France and in the hope of avoiding what they saw as the disastrous consequences of British industrialization.[35] The question hygienists debated was: Is industrialization beneficial to workers or not, that is, will it improve their health, or is it hazardous to health? Liberals were optimistic that in the long run industrialization would improve the standard of living and health of all, including workers. Thus, they opposed interfering with economic laws in any way that would be harmful to business expansion and industrial growth. Some hygienists, such as Villermé, adopted the liberal position but conceded that intervention might in some cases be justified if workers' health was in danger. It is wrong, however, to see Villermé's liberal views as representative of the larger public health movement. Other hygienists, such as Parent-Duchâtelet, were strong advocates of government regulation and intervention to improve public health.[36]

Conservatives and socialists criticized industrialization and unregulated capitalism. For different reasons, they both favored government regulation to eliminate the worst aspects of the industrial system. Adopting this viewpoint were the interventionists of the 1820s and 1830s, who took the pessimistic view of industrialization. This gloomy side of industrialization was strikingly portrayed by J. C. L. Simonde de Sismondi, François Fodéré, Pierre Bigot de Morogues, Alban de Villeneuve-Bargement, and Eugène Buret, who argued that industrialization was destroying the fabric of society and portrayed factory workers as being worse off materially and spiritually than before industrialization. They urged a return to home industry, so that workers could remain close to the soil and to their families, and advocated government intervention to alleviate the terrible conditions in which they believed industrial workers were living and working.[37] The father of economic interventionism was J. C. L. Simonde de Sismondi, whose influential book, *Nouveaux principes d'économie politique*, was published in 1819. Essentially, Sismondi's work was a cry of alarm against the laissez-faire philosophy.[38] Other writers who wrote of

---

35 L. R. Villermé, "Sur la population de la Grande-Bretagne"; Eugène Buret, *De la misère des classes laborieuses en Angleterre et en France*, 2 vols. (Paris: Paulin, 1840).

36 Coleman, *Dealth Is a Social Disease*. Others, such as Ted Porter and Bruno Latour, have cited Coleman as their source for this interpretation. See Theodore Porter, *The Rise of Statistical Thinking, 1820–1900* (Princeton, NJ: Princeton University Press, 1986); and Bruno Latour, *The Pasteurization of France* (Cambridge, MA: Harvard University Press, 1987).

37 For a historiographical treatment of this aspect of the industrial revolution-pessimistic versus optimistic interpretations –, see George Rudé, *Debate on Europe, 1815–1850* (New York: Harper and Row, 1972), pp. 60–2, which deals with the standard of living controversy. See also Reddy, *Rise of Market Culture*.

38 Second ed., 2 vols. (Paris: Delaunay, 1827). The first edition was published in 1819. See G. Sotiroff, "Préface à la troisième édition," *Nouveaux principes d'économie politique*, 2 vols. (Geneva: Jeheber, 1951), 1:67.

the dangers of unregulated capitalism and the havoc being wrought on the manufacturing classes, such as Buret, Villeneuve-Bargemont, and Bigot de Morogues, were all influenced by Sismondi.

François-Emmanuel Fodéré, public hygienist and professor of legal medicine at the medical faculty at Strasbourg, wrote *Essai historique et moral sur la pauvreté des nations* (1825) as a rebuttal to Adam Smith's *Wealth of Nations*. Discussing the evils of unregulated capitalism and industry, Fodéré asserted that industrialization and civilization were increasing poverty and creating beggars. Mechanization was bad, he argued, because machines took jobs away from workers. Additionally, Fodéré contended, industrialization was dehumanizing, for when workers were treated like machines, as Fodéré thought was happening, a germ of social discord was planted. Fodéré portrayed capitalist entrepreneurs as a new aristocracy, more vicious than that of birth.[39]

Baron Pierre-Marie-Sébastien Bigot de Morogues set out to investigate the effects of free enterprise on laborers. He visited a factory and gathered data on wages and cost of living to try to determine what a subsistence wage actually was. Bigot de Morogues opposed the factory system and free competition in industry, because he believed it was harmful to workers. Instead, like other conservatives, he urged a return to a rural economy, emphasizing the advantages of the small farm. Like others, he opposed industrialization, because it was impoverishing workers and he feared the result would be the degradation of the working class.[40]

Using terms similar to those of Fodéré, Alban de Villeneuve-Bargemont, former prefect of the Loire-Inférieure (1824–8) and the Nord (1828–30), called capitalist entrepreneurs a new feudal class, more rapacious than the old, and described the capitalist-industrial system as the exploitation of one group of people by another. Villeneuve-Bargemont gathered evidence for his view of industrialization in the manufacturing city of Lille, where, as prefect of the Nord, he found one-sixth of the population living on public charity. This fact made him realize that the much publicized distress of English workers was common to French workers as well. In his major work, *Economie politique chrétienne*, Villeneuve-Bargemont advanced the idea that capitalization and industrialization of agriculture were the best way to achieve the well-being of the lower classes, pointing out that, by

39 François Fodéré, *Essai historique et moral sur la pauvreté des nations* (Paris: Huzard, 1825), pp. 23, 55–61, 243–89, 308–23, 280.

40 Pierre Bigot de Morogues, *Recherches des causes de la richesse et de la misère des peuples civilisés* (Paris: Delarue, n.d.). See the report on this work by Villermé, "Rapport verbal fait à l'Académie des Sciences Morales et Politiques de l'Institut de France," published in an undated pamphlet. The report was an extract from the *Revue mensuelle d'économie politique* 2 (1834). See also Villermé, "Rapport verbal," on Bigot de Morogue's book. For a discussion of Bigot de Morogues's work, see Reddy, *Rise of Market Culture*, pp. 147–9. My comments are based on Reddy.

contrast, the manufacturing system increased the wealth of the few at the expense of the many.[41]

By the mid-1830s the pessimistic view of industrialization had been publicized by interventionists such as Sismondi, as well as by socialists and social reformers. In response to this viewpoint, the Academy of Political and Moral Sciences, which had been reestablished under Guizot in 1832, initiated a major inquiry to determine the true condition of the French working classes.[42] Villermé's sociomedical investigation, *Tableau de l'état physique et moral des ouvriers*, was done at the request of the Academy in 1835 and 1836 and published in two volumes in 1840.[43] Other inquiries dealt with the same question. Eugène Buret's *De la misère des classes laborieuses* was also undertaken in response to a contest sponsored by the Academy of Political and Moral Sciences and was published in 1840. Honoré Frégier, an employee at the Prefecture of the Seine, examined the condition of the working and dangerous classes in Paris, with his 1840 work receiving favorable recognition from the Academy of Political and Moral Sciences.[44] In 1840 and 1841 the working-class newspaper *l'Atelier* published several inquiries into the condition of the working classes, and in 1846 an independent inquiry on working-class conditions by Jean-Pierre Thouvenin, a Lille physician, was published as a lengthy three-part article in the *Annales d'hygiène publique*.[45] Finally, in 1848 the Academy of Political and Moral Sciences sponsored another inquiry into working-class con-

41 *Economie politique chrétienne*, 3 vols. (Paris: Paulin, 1834), 1: 15–18, 386–98.

42 The Academy of Political and Moral Sciences was part of the Institute, founded in 1795. It was suppressed under Napoleon in 1803 and reestablished under Guizot in 1832. According to Hilde Rigaudias-Weiss, it became a conservative institution that defended the state against the attempts of the workers to vindicate the economic and social position in which they found themselves. See *Les enquêtes ouvrières en France entre 1830 et 1848* (Paris: Félix Alcan, 1936), pp. 25–6.

43 For a review of the work, see Ulysse Trélat, "Bibliographie," *Annales d'hygiène publique* 24 (1840): 454–78. Parts of the report were first published as articles in the *Annales d'hygiène publique* in 1839 and in the *Mémoires de l'Académie des Sciences Morales et Politiques* in 1839. See *Annales d'hygiène publique* 21 (1839): 339–420; 22 (1839): 98–109, and *Mém. de l'Acad. des Sci. Mor. et Pol.* 2 (1839): 329–94.

44 Honoré A. Frégier, *Des classes dangereuses de la population dans les grandes villes et des moyens de les rendre meilleures*, 2 vols. (Paris: Baillière, 1840). See *Mém. de l'Acad. des Sci. Mor. et Pol.* 2 (1839): 125–52, in which a report on the work is given by Charles Dunoyer.

45 See, for example, one of these inquiries, "Réforme industrielle. Enquête. De la condition misérable des hommes, femmes, et enfans dans les manufactures; des causes ce cette misère et des moyens d'y remédier," *l'Atelier*, January 1841, pp. 35–7. See also, for the inquiry of *Atelier*, Hilde Rigaudias-Weiss, *Les enquêtes ouvrières*, pp. 158–9. See Armand Cuvillier, *Un Journal d'ouvriers: l'Atelier (1840–50)* (Paris: Félix Alcan, 1914), pp. 131–2. Other working-class newspapers also conducted inquiries: *l'Artisan* in 1830 and *Le Populaire* in 1841. See Robert-Goetz-Girey, *Croissance et progrès à l'origine des sociétés industrielles* (Paris: Editions Montchrestien, 1966), p. 278; Jean-Pierre Thouvenin, "De l'influence que l'industrie exerce sur la santé des populations dans les grands centres manufacturiers."

ditions.[46] For the history of public health, the inquiries of Villermé and Thouvenin were the most important.

Villermé's reputation as one of the leading French public hygienists was well established when he was chosen by his colleagues in the Academy of Political and Moral Sciences to conduct an investigation into the condition of the French working classes. In 1834, when the Academy asked Villermé and Benoiston de Châteauneuf to investigate the condition of the French working classes, both men had already published several articles on the relation of poverty to mortality.[47] Villermé's two studies on varying mortality rates, which he published in the 1820s, had secured him an international reputation. He had also conducted investigations on the influence of industrialization on the health and longevity of British workers, an article appearing in the *Annales d'hygiène publique* that same year (1834). Examining Britain's population statistics, Villermé found mortality rates to be much higher in manufacturing than in agricultural areas. For example, whereas the average length of life for the whole country was thirty-three years, in Lancaster, the most highly industrialized county, it was only twenty-five; yet, in the agricultural county of York, it was forty.

---

46   Adolphe-Jérome Blanqui, "Rapport sur la situation des classes ouvrières en 1848," *Séances et trav. de l'Acad. des Sci. Mor. et Pol.* 13 (1848): 317–6; the full work is *Des classes ouvrières en France pendant l'année 1848* (Paris: Pagnerre, 1849). Secondary sources on the work of Fodéré, Sismondi, Villeneuve-Bargement, and Bigot de Morogues, as well as on the various inquiries into the condition of the working classes, include Rigaudias-Weiss, *Les enquêtes ouvrières*; Maurice Deslandres and Alfred Michelin, *Il y a cent ans: Etat physique et moral des ouvriers du temps du libéralisme – Témoignage de Villermé* (Paris: Spes, 1938); Louis Chevalier, *Classes laborieuses et classes dangereuses à Paris pendant la première moitié du XIXe siècle,* esp. pp. 149–62; Goetz-Girey, *Croissance et progrès,* esp. pp. 243–309; Michelle Perrot, *Enquêtes sur la condition ouvrière au XIXe siècle* (Paris: Microéditions Hachette, 1972). On Villermé, see Coleman, *Death Is a Social Disease*; Reddy, *Rise of Market Culture*; and Sewell, *Work and Revolution*.

47   Villermé does not give the date when he and Benoiston de Châteauneuf were commissioned to do the work. Goetz-Girey gives the date as 1834 in *Croissance et progrès*, p. 277. The Academy of Political and Moral Sciences originated with the creation of the Institute of France in 1795. It was one of the three main classes into which the Institute was divided, the other two being physical sciences and mathematics, and literature and fine arts. In 1803 Napoleon severely modified the Institute and in so doing completely eliminated the class that dealt with political and moral sciences. In 1816 the designation *class* was changed to *academy*, but still the section of political and moral sciences did not reappear. It was not until after the July Revolution of 1830 that the old class of the Institute was resuscitated as the Academy of Political and Moral Sciences (October 26, 1832). The Academy was divided into five sections: Section IV, Political Economy and Statistics, counted among its members Count Sieyès, Prince Talleyrand, Count de Laborde, Baron Dupin, F. Charles Comte, and Villermé. Benoiston de Châteauneuf was an "académicien libre"; foreign associates included Thomas Malthus of London and Simonde de Sismondi of Geneva. Among the corresponding members in the section of political economy and statistics were Adolphe Quetelet of Brussels and James Mill of London. This information in *Mém. de l'Acad. des Sci. Mor. et Pol.* 1 (1837): v–vii, I–VIII, XX–XXII.

Villermé concluded that average life expectancy was lowest in manufacturing districts and large cities and greatest in less populated and agricultural areas. He did not blame industrialization per se for high death rates
but postulated that the probable cause of excessive mortality in British
manufacturing districts was the low salaries of the workers, reaffirming his
well-known hypothesis on the relationship of poverty to mortality rates.[48]

The Academy of Political and Moral Sciences asked Villermé and
Benoiston de Châteauneuf to determine if industrialization was harmful
or beneficial to workers, in response to conservatives and socialists who
attacked industrialization and deplored the demoralization of French
workers. The hygienists' task was to answer the following questions posed
by the Academy: What was the actual physical and moral condition of the
French working classes? Was the condition of the working classes as bad
as critics claimed, and were reformers' protests over the abuses resulting
from mechanization exaggerated? Was industrialization harmful or beneficial to workers? The investigation was divided between the two men,
with Benoiston de Châteauneuf taking the central region of France and
the Atlantic coast and Villermé visiting departments with the highest
concentration of workers employed in the cotton, wool, and silk industries. As it turned out, only Villermé's portion of the work received widespread publicity. Motivated by the pessimistic view of industrialization
advanced by Fodéré, Bigot de Morogues, Villeneuve-Bargemont, and
other conservative and socialist writers, the Academy and Villermé may
also have been influenced by a similar work, although more limited in
scope, done by the British physician James Phillips Kay-Shuttleworth on
the condition of the textile workers in Manchester. Above all, the Academy hoped to be able to show that workers' claims and reformers' protests
over the physical and moral abuses resulting from rapid mechanization of
industry were exaggerated.[49]

The *Tableau* is divided into two parts. In part one are Villermé's
observations of textile workers, identified with date and locality. Villermé
went into factories and workers' homes, joined workers in their leisure
hours, and talked with both factory owners and workers. The reporting is
descriptive.[50] Part two is Villermé's discussion, interpretation, and analysis
of the condition of the working classes accompanied by suggestions for
reform. The latter, which Villermé considered the most important part of
the work, was published in its entirety in the *Mémoires* of the Academy of

48   "Sur la population de la Grande-Bretagne."
49   Rigaudias-Weiss, *Les enquêtes ouvrières*, pp. ix–x, 21–6, 30. Goetz-Girey, *Croissance
     et progrès*, p. 277; *The Moral and Physical Condition of the Working Class Employed in
     the Cotton Manufacture in Manchester* (Manchester: J. Ridgway, 1832). Deslandres et
     Michelin, *Il y a cent ans*, p. 155, note 1.
50   Villermé, *Tableau*, 1: vi.

Political and Moral Sciences, and two articles from it appeared in the
Annales d'hygiène publique.[51] The general tone of the *Tableau* was optimistic. From his observations in the French textile centers (1835–7), Villermé
concluded that the material condition of the working classes – with a few
exceptions – had improved by comparison with conditions in the seventeenth and eighteenth centuries, as reported by Arthur Young, Moheau
(Montyon), and Vauban. Villermé disagreed with the common assertion
that wealth and its advantages were the exclusive privilege of one class.
Instead, he shared the belief held by many French hygienists that as
civilization progressed, a people became wealthier, and that this wealth
became more widely distributed as it filtered down through the various
levels of society. Villermé accused writers of manipulating workers'
perceptions of reality. He maintained that so much publicity had been
given to the view that the working classes were worse off than they had
been in earlier times that workers themselves had become convinced that
their condition was deteriorating – even though in reality it was improving. Although Villermé observed overall improvement in the material
conditions of the working classes, certain groups of workers were exempt.
Common weavers and spinners – especially in the cotton industry – had
not shared in this improvement, being the poorest of all the workers he
observed.[52]

Villermé reported that many textile workers were living in insanitary
conditions, and his descriptions of workers' quarters in Lille, Rouen, and
Lyon are well known for their portrayal of horrible living conditions.
Describing the cotton workers in Lille, one of the most industrialized cities
in France, Villermé called them the most miserable of all French workers,
with a high incidence of scrofula and tuberculosis prevalent among them.
The Rouennais cotton workers were only slightly better off. Of all the
workers Villermé observed, the handloom weavers (*tisserands à bras*) fared
the worst. Villermé vividly described their bad health, attributing it to
harmful working conditions, long working hours, and inadequate nutri-
tion. Yet he also saw signs of improvement. For example, he found that
the condition of the Lyonnais silk workers, who were traditionally as
poverty-stricken as the Lille cotton workers, had improved. Villermé
described how silk workers lived and worked, their poor health and their
filthiness, but he pointed out that although their living conditions were
still bad, in the last twelve years their physical, moral, and intellectual

51 *Tableau*, 1: vii–viii, for Villermé's comments on this; articles that appeared in the
   Annales d'hygiène publique were "De la santé des ouvriers employés dans les
   fabriques de soie, de coton, de laine," *Annales d'hygiène publique* 21 (1839): 339–
   420, and "De l'ivrognerie principalement chez les ouvriers des manufactures,"
   Annales d'hygiène publique 22 (1839): 98–108.
52 *Tableau*, 2: 1–7, 25.

conditions had improved, so that by 1836 they compared favorably with workers in other large manufacturing areas. He found the Lyonnais silk weavers noticeably better off than the cotton weavers in Lille and in the Haut-Rhin, and commented favorably on their sobriety and intelligence.[53]

For Villermé, material conditions were closely related to moral conditions, for he believed that poor material conditions predisposed people to bad morals. He observed that the more miserable were the material conditions of workers, the more they tried to escape by drinking. Drunkenness was the scourge of the working class, but the blame could not be laid completely on workers. Villermé was quick to admonish factory owners for having little concern for workers' physical or moral condition and accused them of regarding workers as *machines à produire*: "many factory owners...only regard them [workers] as simple production machines."[54] Villermé maintained no false hopes for the humanitarianism of factory owners, asserting that they would improve workers' conditions only out of self-interest or by coercion. Comparing French factory owners with American, Villermé suggested that American factory owners were solicitous of workers, not because they were more paternalistic and humanitarian than their French counterparts but because it was in their self-interest. The difference was what historian Frederick Jackson Turner later referred to as the "safety-valve theory." If factory conditions deteriorated, Villermé maintained, American workers went west. To keep workers, American factory owners had to make concessions. By contrast, French workers, who did not have this outlet, were at the mercy of factory owners.[55]

Although his research on British manufacturing areas suggested that industrialization was detrimental to health, Villermé contended in the *Tableau* that – except for certain groups of workers like the common weavers – industrialization was improving workers' standard of living. Thus, Villermé believed that in the long run industrialization was beneficial to workers, since better health was concomitant with a higher standard of living. Villermé answered critics of industrialization who contended that industrialization was harmful, because mechanization deprived workers of their jobs, asserting that such dislocation was only temporary. Villermé also suggested that mechanization could promote health and safety by eliminating dangerous processes and making certain

53   Ibid., 1: 75–103, 135–60, 341–400, 445; 2: 238–41. On the Lyonnais silk workers during this period, see Robert Bezucha, *The Lyon Uprising of 1834* (Cambridge, MA: Harvard University Press, 1974), pp. 4–59. For a discussion of the historiography of the handloom weavers, see Reddy, *Rise of Market Culture*, pp. 4–7.
54   *Tableau*, 2: 34–37; "...beaucoup de maîtres de manufactures...ne les regardent que comme de simples machines à produire." Quote, p. 55.
55   *Tableau*, 2: 76–82.

tasks easier to perform.[56] But if industrialization was improving the material condition of workers and was ultimately beneficial to health, as Villermé asserted, then what were the causes of workers' morbidity and premature mortality? A question of continuing debate in hygienic circles in the 1830s and 1840s was whether industrial processes and working conditions were hazardous to workers' health or whether the real cause was their living conditions. Hygienists such as Parent-Duchâtelet and Chevallier had taken exception to the older view that most industrial processes were dangerous to health, and as a result, a continuing debate over the so-called condition of the working classes had emerged. Hygienists wanted to know the causes of the physical and moral deterioration of the working classes at a time when public health in general was improving. If better health was concomitant with the progress of civilization – as most hygienists optimistically maintained – why was this large segment of the French population exempt? As a result of his investigations, Villermé shared the views of Chevallier, Parent-Duchâtelet, and the debunkers that in most cases neither industrial processes nor the mechanization of industry was the main cause of the high morbidity and mortality of the working classes. Villermé observed that conditions in large factories were generally better than those in small shops or in working-class dwellings, and that many processes suspected of being unhealthy were not. Many supposedly unhealthy situations in workshops did not even exist. Although Villermé found health hazards associated with spinning mills and irritating dust in cotton factories to be a real problem, often resulting in a disease known as *cotton phthisis* or *cotton pneumonia*, he concluded that most critics had been misled in attributing workers' diseases to unhealthy factory conditions and industrial processes. The real causes of workers' diseases were too much work, too long working hours, inadequate sleep, lack of personal hygiene, insufficient and bad food, habits like drunkenness and debauchery, and salaries too low to satisfy basic needs. The principal cause of workers' bad health was poverty and its resulting living conditions, not industrialization or factory conditions.[57]

Citing statistics from the industrial town of Mulhouse, Villermé showed that mortality rates were closely related to occupation, based on the amount of affluence provided by the salary. Workers receiving high wages were healthier and had a lower mortality rate than workers paid low wages. The high infant mortality rates of poor workers illustrated the

56   This contradiction is noticeable in the works themselves but is also pointed out in Deslandres and Michelin, *Il y a cent ans*, p. 155. See the discussion of the question of optimism and pessimism vis-à-vis industrialization in Goetz-Girey, *Croissance et progrès*, pp. 8–40; *Tableau*, 2: 295–9.

57   *Tableau*, 2: 203–22.

point. For example, in Mulhouse, whereas half of the children born to manufacturers, bankers, and factory owners reached the age of twenty-nine, half of the children of common weavers and spinners died before the age of two. This led Villermé to conclude, "it is not the work of certain occupations which is harmful, but the profound misery of the poorest workers."[58] In summary, Villermé contended that occupations acted on the health and mortality of workers in an indirect manner: "It is in an indirect, mediate manner, either by conditions of food, clothing, lodging, fatigue, length of workday, habits, in which the workers find themselves, that occupations most often act for good or bad on their health and on that of their family. This rule out to be regarded as general."[59] Villermé maintained that "if, for a large number of them, the workday was shorter, the work better paid, if it did not expose them to the influence of dusts, it would exert no real influence on their health."[60] But the statistically proven fact was that industrialization appeared to have a deleterious effect on workers' health. Speaking of infant mortality among workers, traditionally one barometer of health of a group, class, or nation, Villermé argued that whether the causes of morbidity and mortality associated with industrialization were direct or indirect, they still had to be reckoned with:

But it matters little...whether they die...by the crowding together of families in dwellings which are too confined, or whether they are concentrated in the immediate neighborhood of factories, or from any other circumstance dependent upon the direct influence of these factories. If the crowded conditions in which they live and if the other circumstances are caused by the factories or by the conditions in which the workers are living, it comes to the same thing.[61]

According to Villermé, the solution to workers' health problems was better salaries, better factory conditions, and shorter working hours. Villermé was especially concerned about the long working hours in most

58 Ibid., 2: 243–57, "...ce n'est pas le travail de certaines professions qui est nuisible, mais la profonde misère des plus pauvres ouvriers." p. 247.
59 Ibid., 2: 258. "C'est d'une manière indirecte, médiate, ou par les conditions de nourriture, de vêtement, de logement, de fatigue, de durée du travail, de moeurs, etc., dans lesquelles se trouvent les ouvriers, que les professions agissent le plus souvent en bien ou en mal sur leur santé ou sur celle de leur famille. Cette règle doit être regardée comme générale."
60 Ibid., 2: 260–1. "Si pour un grand nombre d'entre eux, le travail était moins long, mieux retribué, s'il ne les exposait pas à l'influence des poussières, il n'exercerait vraisemblablement aucune influence sur leur santé."
61 Ibid., 2: 275. "Mais, peu importe,...qu'ils meurent...par l'entassement des familles dans les habitations trop étroites, ou elles se concentrent dans le voisinage immédiat des manufactures, ou par toute autre circonstance dépendante de l'influence directe de ces manufactures. Si l'encombrement des habitations et si les autres circonstances sont amenées par les fabriques ou par les conditions dans lesquelles vivent les ouvriers, cela revient au même."

factories. The ordinary working day for cotton and wool workers was fifteen and a half hours, which, considering breaks, came to thirteen hours of effective work. Children often worked the same long hours as adults. Villermé argued that the long working hours of children were not work but torture: "It is no longer work, a chore, it is torture."[62] Villermé championed the cause of child labor and the evils associated with it, arguing for a national law to regulate child labor. Since the main advantage of such a law would be the better health of children, the law would also be a public health law. Villermé recognized the problems associated with a child labor law but maintained that the benefits of preserving the health of working-class children would outweigh the inconveniences. He noted that such laws had already been passed in Great Britain, Austria, and Prussia, and that many French manufacturers wanted a child labor law. Villermé's liberalism did not allow him to advocate a general law to limit the working hours of adults, however, for he believed such a law would infringe on the economic freedom of industrialists and violate the liberal notion of "free contract."[63]

Villermé also blamed workers themselves for their misery, suggesting that at least part of their poverty was attributable to drunkenness and debauchery. Thus he proposed good conduct, or moralization, as a way for workers to attain a higher standard of living. Furthermore, workers should be educated to their true position and should be informed that they were economically better off than before, even if social critics denied it. Villermé also called on entrepreneurs to improve workers' conditions by treating workers as people, not machines. Hoping that a sense of community and personalization could be restored in relations between factory owner and worker, Villermé argued that the aid of industrialists was necessary if the moral and physical conditions of workers were to be improved.[64]

In the final analysis, Villermé's optimism with regard to industrialization was guarded. Although industrialization had raised the standard of living of many textile workers and mechanization had made some processes less onerous and unhealthy, Villermé believed that it also had the social effect of depersonalization, of destroying the sense of community that had existed between masters and workers. For Villermé, this was an unfortunate development, for when workers were dehumanized, the bonds

---

62 Ibid., 2: 83–91; "Ce n'est plus là un travail, une tâche, c'est une torture," p. 91. For further work by Villermé on the dangers to the health of working children, see "Rapport touchant l'Enquête faite en Angleterre, sur le travail et la condition des enfants et adolescents employés dans les mines," *Séances et trav. de l'Acad. des Sci. Mor. et Pol.* 3 (1843): 45–58.
63 Ibid., 2: 91–108, 355–67.
64 Ibid., 2: 342–8, 368–73.

between them and factory owners were severed, depriving workers of good examples and moral direction.[65]

Additionally, industrialization created new problems for workers, such as industrial crises and the dissolution of family life. Villermé concluded that of all the workers he observed, the best off materially and morally were those engaged in both industry and agriculture, who still participated in the putting-out system. These workers, Villermé contended, were less victimized by industrial crises than factory workers and still had a family life.[66] Thus, although he was an apologist for industrialization, Villermé ended on a contradictory note by recognizing the advantages of the old system, preferred by writers such as Villeneuve-Bargemont and Sismondi, whom he had initially set out to disprove.

Finally, Villermé considered whether the improvement of the condition of the working class would continue as industrialization became more widespread. He did not answer affirmatively. Industrial centers seemed to be harmful to workers, and it was becoming increasingly difficult for them to have the social mobility to become masters because of the large capital outlay required to set up a factory. The conversion to the factory system was also systematically destroying those workers who were at the time the best off materially – those engaged in domestic industry. Villermé concluded that industrialization had so far been beneficial and progressive, but he was uncertain about the future. Describing the mechanization of industry – the application of steam power to industry – Villermé spoke of an industrial revolution that was taking place in the Western world whose outcome was unknown: "A revolution has resulted, but it is not finished; it is ongoing, without our knowing where it will stop and what the outcome will be."[67]

Villermé's *Tableau* is important both as a working-class inquiry and as a public health treatise. The *Tableau* reflected a spirit of nineteenth-century liberal optimism and constituted a rebuttal to the contentions of socialist and conservative writers who portrayed industrialization as destroying the fabric of society and as threatening the material and moral conditions of the working classes. Certainly Villermé's optimism was in the end tempered by uncertainty. Although he contended that industrialization was more beneficial than detrimental to workers' health, Villermé recognized

---

65 Ibid., 2: 313–20.
66 Ibid., 1: 443–6.
67 Ibid., 2: 354, 325–6. "Une révolution en est résultée, mais elle n'est pas accomplie; elle marche encore, sans que nous sachions ou elle s'arrêtera et quelles en seront toutes les suites." Quotation, p. 326. On the origin and use of the term *industrial revolution*, see I. Bernard Cohen, *Revolutions in Science* (Cambridge, MA: Harvard University Press, 1985), pp. 264–5. Cohen says the term was first used in 1788 by Arthur Young and was in fairly common use in France by the time Villermé was writing.

its pernicious influence and viewed it as a complicated socioeconomic development fraught with problems. Villermé had faith that ultimately the mechanization of industry would benefit society in general and the working classes in particular, but he did not ignore its immediate pernicious effects, primarily socioeconomic dislocation and health problems.

The *Tableau* exemplifies the general debunking tendency among occupational hygienists. Like Chevallier, Parent-Duchâtelet, and d'Arcet, Villermé concluded that it was not primarily industrial processes and working conditions that caused the bad health and high mortality of French workers, but their unhealthy living conditions resulting from salaries too low to provide basic needs and working hours that were too long. According to Villermé, the solution was neither industrial hygiene nor improvement of industrial processes and factory conditions, but limited working hours and higher salaries. Since the working hours of children seemed the greatest threat to the health of future generations and the abuse most likely to generate immediate reform, Villermé came forward as a leading advocate of a French child labor law.

Villermé's conclusions reinforced his earlier hypothesis on the relation of poverty and mortality: that poverty and its resultant bad living conditions were the primary cause of disease and death. Thus the *Tableau*, like the rest of Villermé's hygienic work, exemplifies the social theory of epidemiology. Villermé and the proponents of the social theory of disease causation saw the root of disease in social conditions – mainly poverty and its ramifications – and advocated socioeconomic and individual moral reform to improve public health.

Villermé's *Tableau* and other French and English working-class inquiries drew attention to the public health problems associated with industrialization. Many critics agreed that one of the main evils of industrialization was child labor, which weakened children's health and decreased the chances that they would grow up to be useful citizen/soldiers. The motivating factors behind a child labor law were humanitarian and nationalistic. Alsatian industrialists, represented by the Société industrielle de Mulhouse, were among the first to advocate a law limiting working hours for children, and sent petitions to the Chambers asking that such a law be passed.[68] In 1840 and 1841 the law was discussed in the Chamber of Peers and the Chamber of Deputies.[69] Charles Dupin, an advocate of the legislation, pointed out that limiting the working hours of children in Britain had not harmed British industry, and he and other proponents claimed that justice and humanity required such a law. Skeptics pointed out that government intervention to regulate industrial matters would set a dangerous

---

68   *Moniteur universel*, January 12, 1840, p. 64, Ch. Peers, séance du 11 janv; February 23, 1840, Ch. Peers, séance du 22 fév., p. 351.

69   See *Moniteur universel*, January–March 1840; December 1840, January–March 1841.

precedent, and that, furthermore, the government would be interfering in families, challenging the father's authority. Some deputies argued that since England, Prussia, and Austria already had such laws, France should keep up with the times, and interventionists warned that unregulated industrialization could destroy the social fabric of the country. The law finally passed by a large majority in both chambers in 1841. But in its final form it had one major weakness: It did not provide for salaried inspectors to enforce the law. Another problem was that it only applied to factories employing more than twenty people or factories with steam engines. Since most French industry was still the handcraft type carried out in small workshops, the bulk of industry was exempt from the law.[70] Charles Dupin pointed out these weaknesses in a speech in the Chamber of Peers in 1847, when the law again came up for consideration. That same year, an amended law instituting salaried inspectors and extending the law to all factories and workshops employing at least ten people or five children was presented to the Chamber of Peers. The amended draft law was not adopted by both Chambers before 1848, however; thus the only major piece of early-nineteenth-century social legislation remained unenforceable and inapplicable to much of French industry.[71]

Other physicians and social reformers also investigated the condition of the working classes and the influence of industrialization on workers' health. Honoré Frégier, head of an office at the Prefecture of the Seine, prepared his study in response to a contest sponsored by the Academy of Political and Moral Sciences. The topic of the essay was:

Research according to positive observations what are the elements of which is composed in Paris, or in any other large city, that part of the population which forms a dangerous class because of its vices, its ignorance and its misery; indicate the means by which the administration, rich and affluent men, intellectual and hardworking workers might improve this dangerous and depraved class.[72]

The work was not, strictly speaking, a working-class inquiry at all. Instead, it was an attempt to analyze the poor and dangerous classes of

---

70 *Moniteur universel*, February 24, 1841, séance du 23 fév., p. 456. In the Chamber of Peers, out of 106 voting, 104 were in favor of the law and 2 were opposed; 12 mars 1841, séance du 11 mars, Ch. Dep., p. 626; out of 235 voting, 218 were in favor of the law and 17 were against it. For the final law, see *Moniteur universel*, March 24, 1841, p. 721. Loi relative au travail des enfants employés dans les manufactures, usines ou ateliers.

71 *Moniteur universel*, July 2, 1847, pp. 1839–47. Ch. Peers, addition à la séance de mardi, le 29 juin. On the child labor law, see two recent works: Katherine Lynch, *Family, Class, and Ideology in Early Industrial France: Social Policy and the Working-Class Family, 1825–1848* (Madison: University of Wisconsin Press, 1988); and Lee Shai Weissbach, *Child Labor Reform in Nineteenth-Century France: Assuring the Future Harvest* (Baton Rouge: LSU Press, 1989). See also Colin Heywood, *Childhood in Nineteenth-Century France: Work, Health and Education Among the "Classes Populaires"* (Cambridge: Cambridge University Press, 1988), which devotes much attention to working children and the 1841 law.

72 Frégier, *Des classes dangereuses de la population dans les grandes villes*. See 1: V.

Paris, dangerous from a criminal, insurrectionary, and public health point of view. In a sense, though, Frégier's work *was* a working-class inquiry, since it focused on the poorest element of the preindustrial Parisian laboring classes, who were materially worse off than the industrial classes. The main public health problem created by the poor, dangerous classes was that their filthy dwellings were considered foyers of infection. Frégier concluded that to ameliorate the condition of the dangerous classes, the government must intervene to regulate child labor and to improve the unhealthy dwellings in which they lived. Better material conditions would result in better moral conditions, Frégier believed.[73] The Academy had reservations about Frégier's work. In his report to the Academy, Charles Dunoyer criticized some of Frégier's ideas as inexact and potentially too dangerous for the Academy to sanction. For example, in comparing the salaries of workers and capitalists, Frégier implied that the great difference in remuneration was unjust. Furthermore, he advocated workers' coalitions and unions as a way for workers to improve their salaries. Because of these radical ideas, the section of the Academy that examined the work hesitated to award the prize to Frégier. Rather, they decided simply to give him a consolation prize of 2,000 francs and to ask him to modify certain passages that they found unacceptable.[74]

Another contest sponsored by the Academy of Political and Moral Sciences resulted in a major inquiry into the condition of the working classes in England and France by Eugène Buret. The topic chosen by the Academy in 1837 and again in 1840 (because none of the 1837 essays was judged good enough for the prize) was: "Determine what misery consists of and by what signs it manifests itself in various countries. Research the causes that produce it."[75] Buret, a disciple of Sismondi, located the source of working-class misery in the organization of work, which he called *industrial feudalism*, blaming the unregulated capitalist and industrial system. Buret, who was critical of the developing capitalist system – especially in England – advocated state regulation of capitalism. Buret was less

73 Ibid., 2: 23–5, 125–51.
74 *Mém. de l'Acad. des Sci. Mor. et Pol.* 2 (1839): 125–52.
75 See *Séances et trav. de l'Acad. des Sci. Mor. et Pol.* Comptes-rendus publiés dans le *Moniteur universel* par Ch. Vergé et Loiseau, 1840–1, pp. 1–7; see Villermé's oral report on Buret's work, pp. 289ff.; see the report by Adolphe Blanqui, ibid., pp. 299–303. The money for the prize given to the winner of the contest came from M. le Baron Félix de Beaujour, who set up a prize of 5,000 francs to be given every five years for the best essay on questions whose solution would indicate the means of preventing or alleviating misery in various countries, but especially in France. In 1837 five essays were submitted, but none was considered worthy of the prize. The contest was reopened in 1840, and at that time twenty-two essays were submitted. Villermé was chairman of the committee to decide on the prizes. Three essays were judged worthy of the prize, but the one by Buret received 2,500 francs as the best essay on misery. The rest of the money was split between the author of the second and third best essays. Buret's essay was published in 1840 as *De la misère des classes laborieuses en Angleterre et en France*.

optimistic than Villermé about the general improvement of the condition of the working class. Although he believed in the advance of civilization, Buret contended that the urban laboring classes had not shared in the progress. Army recruitment figures showed the degree to which misery had caused a deterioration in workers' health. Buret treated workers' poor health as an aspect of their misery, which had socioeconomic roots in the capitalistic, industrial system. Like Sismondi and other conservatives and socialists, Buret showed keen insight into the problems of displacement and lack of hierarchy in the new industrial structure, maintaining that the industrial order was a source of working-class misery and had destroyed the bonds that existed between worker and master. Thus, Buret advocated government intervention to regulate industry, suggesting that such intervention might restore community by forming a social hierarchy that would offer every member a sense of order and security.[76]

Three other working-class inquiries of note appeared: The inquiries of the artisan-run newspaper *Atelier* were published in 1840 and 1841 – contemporaneous with the works of Villermé, Frégier, and Buret – the inquiry of Jean-Pierre Thouvenin in 1846 and that of Adolphe Blanqui, prepared in 1848 at the request of the Academy of Political and Moral Sciences. The inquiries of *Atelier* consisted of short reports published in the issues of the newspaper, which examined working-class occupations, workers' budgets and salaries, the length of the working day, the administration of factories and workshops, and occupational health hazards. Authors of the articles asserted that industrialization was the cause of working-class misery and that child labor was leading to the wasting away of the working class. They contended that the physical degradation of the working class, illustrated by army recruitment figures, was a menacing symptom of national decadence, and argued that only government intervention and effective regulation could curb the worst abuses of the developing industrial system.[77]

The inquiry of Jean-Pierre Thouvenin, published in the *Annales d'hygiène publique* in 1846, ranks in importance with Villermé's for public health history. Thouvenin, a Lillois physician and factory inspector for the enforcement of the 1841 child labor law, entitled his work "De l'influence que l'industrie exerce sur la santé des populations dans les grands centres manufacturiers."[78] Thouvenin discussed major industries and their influ-

---

76   Rigaudias-Weiss, *Les enquêtes ouvrières*, pp. X, 32, 241; Buret, *De la misère*, 1: 357–9, 340–65, for his treatment of health and sanitary matters; 2: 30–4, 92ff., 340.

77   *L'Atelier*, 1840, 1841, passim; Armand Cuvillier, *Un journal d'ouvriers*, pp. 131–2. For an example of one of these inquiries, see "Réforme industrielle. Enquête."

78   *Annales d'hygiène publique* 36 (1846): 16–46, 277–96; 37 (1847): 83–111. Thouvenin, a member of the health council of the Nord, wrote two other hygienic works: *Hygiène populaire aux gens du monde pour se garantir du choléra* (Lille: Conseil, 1849) and *Rapport présenté au conseil de vaccine pour 1851* (Lille, 1852).

ence on health. He found little directly dangerous to workers' health stem-
ming from their occupations and industrial processes but argued that the
physical waning of the working class was a statistically established fact.
The real causes of the degradation of the working class had yet to be
found, according to Thouvenin. His analysis was reminiscent of Villermé's.
Thouvenin first stated that rural workers lived better than urban workers
and hence enjoyed better health. He argued that living conditions – food,
clothing, fatigue, and morals – not factory work, were the direct causes of
the physical deterioration of the working class. Opposing Villermé's belief
in the rise of the standard of living of the working classes since the Revolution, Thouvenin asserted that there had been no appreciable improvement
in the condition of Lille workers – the most degraded in France – in the last
ten or twenty years. Thouvenin examined faults and vices that contributed – even more than industrialization – to the degradation of working-
class health. He concluded that industry did not directly exert a harmful
influence on workers' health; the main causes of their unhealthiness were
their dirty, unsanitary dwellings, inherited diseases, lengthy working
hours, insufficient and poor-quality food, and immorality, especially
drunkenness. To improve the condition of the working class, Thouvenin,
like Villermé, called for industrial paternalism, claiming that factory
owners must take responsibility for workers, treating them like people,
not machines, and providing a role model for moral behavior.[79]

Adolphe Blanqui's inquiry of 1848 – like that of Villermé – was done in
response to accusations of socialists and other reformers that industrialization was increasing the misery of the working class. Blanqui's official aim
in traveling throughout France was to give a true picture of working-class
conditions in order to rectify the supposedly false ideas being spread by
critics. Thus, Blanqui's report was written with a particular agenda in
mind, and he seems to have known his conclusions even before gathering
his data. Blanqui found – as had Villermé and Buret – that working-class
conditions varied greatly from place to place; that in Lille and Rouen there
was severe misery, and workers' morbidity was high. Generally, workers
in northern cities, where the factory system was more developed, lived in
worse conditions than workers in the south, where the domestic system
was still the predominant form of production. Blanqui concluded by
suggesting that the material improvement of some workers coincided with
the increasing misery of others, owing to several factors: (1) crowded
living conditions, (2) unemployment, (3) variation in salaries, and (4)
abusive employment of children. These four conditions, Blanqui found,

79 "L'influence de l'industrie," 36 (1846): 16–46, 277–96, 37 (1847): 110–11, 91–2.
    On Lille and its working class, see Pierre Pierrard, *La vie ouvrière à Lille sous le
    Second Empire* (Paris: Bloud and Gay, 1965), pp. 43–78, 115–94, and p. 29 of the
    bibliography.

greatly contributed to increasing the misery and disease of the working classes.[80]

The condition of the working classes was a major public health question, because at stake was the health of an important segment of French society. Reformers and hygienists agreed that the causes of poor health were socioeconomic and moral, and advocated a number of solutions to alleviate and improve the situation. The solutions of Villermé, Thouvenin, Buret, Frégier, and *Atelier* were three: First, they advocated government intervention to regulate capitalism and industry in order to end such abuses as child labor and to improve working-class conditions. Although all favored some government intervention, Villermé and Thouvenin recommended more extensive intervention and regulation than the others. Villermé, Thouvenin, and Buret also called on enlightened factory owners to improve the condition of workers, citing the Société industrielle de Mulhouse as an example. Villermé argued that ultimately industrialization would improve working-class conditions and that its harmful nature was only a temporary phenomenon. The worst abuses, such as child labor, had to be regulated, however. Second, Buret advocated state intervention to regulate industry and restore a sense of community, which, he contended, had been destroyed with the abolition of guilds and corporations, only to be replaced by unregulated capitalism. Third, Villermé contended that workers also had to take responsibility for improving their own living conditions and health by temperance, clean living, hard work, and planning for the future. Moral reform, or the adoption of bourgeois values, would make it possible for workers to better their situation.

Calls by hygienists and reformers for government intervention and regulation fell on deaf ears. Other than the child labor law, no other major factory legislation was passed in France before 1848. French liberalism, Orleanism, was a more intransigent creed than its British counterpart. Whereas British liberals, as well as conservatives, were capable of major political reform, and of factory legislation and reform, the French government remained firm in its nonintervention. Considering the prevailing opinion of French liberals before 1848, it is surprising that even an ineffective child labor law was passed.[81] Just as Britons feared tampering with the constitution in order to pass the Catholic Emancipation Act and the Reform Bill of 1832, so French legislators and some members of the Academy of Political and Moral Sciences saw the passage of any factory legislation as an ominous portent, a dangerous precedent for the future.

---

80 Blanqui, "Rapport sur la situation des classes ouvrières en 1848," *Séances et trav. de l'Acad. des Sci. Mor. et Pol.* 13 (1848): 317–36. The complete work, published in 1849, was entitled *Des classes ouvrières en France pendant l'année 1848* (Paris: Firmin Didot, 1849).

81 On this point, see Jean Lhomme, *La grande bourgeoisie au pouvoir (1830–1880)* (Paris: Presses universitaires de France, 1960), p. 85.

Examining the influence of industrialization and industrial processes on workers' health, French hygienists found that such influences were indirect. Although some industries were definitely unhealthy and industrialization seemed to exert an unfavorable influence on health and mortality, the root of the problem, they concluded, was the socioeconomic situation of workers. Workers were not paid enough to have a standard of living adequate for maintaining health. In addition, they often had to work such long hours that they were constantly fatigued. This was especially true of children. Such problems, hygienists argued, could be managed by socioeconomic reform to ensure better wages and more humane working conditions. But the hygienists failed to achieve any real results in the area of legislation. Even the child labor law was ineffective, for it was unenforceable.

The practical failure of the hygienists in this area of public health was due to the prevailing opinions of the legislators concerning the government's role in regulating the economy, society, and public health. The prevailing belief of legislators was classical liberalism, which they could not reconcile with the government intervention hygienists said was necessary to solve some of the problems associated with industrialization. In Britain a compromise was effected, and from the 1830s, British liberals began to acknowledge the necessity of intervention, at least where health questions were concerned. French liberalism did not go through this transition before 1848. Thus, although the publication and work of the hygienists increased awareness of the public health problems associated with industrialization and industrial processes, the only legislative achievement of the hygienists was the child labor law. The involvement of the national government remained – with few exceptions – limited to certain traditional, well-defined areas.[82]

PUBLIC HYGIENISTS AND THE INVESTIGATIVE TRADITION

Investigation was at the core of the public health movement. Bill Coleman discussed the meliorist attitude of the hygienists, the belief that once a problem had been adequately investigated, it would be solved. Reform

---

82 For an interesting discussion on the child labor law and government intervention, see "Discussion entre MM. Blanqui, Passy, Dunoyer, de Beaumont, Franck et Mignet sur ce qu'il faut entendre par l'organisation du travail et sur les effets de la loi qui règle le travail des enfants dans les manufactures," *Séances et trav. de l'Acad. des Sci. Mor. et Pol.* 8 (1845): 189–202. Deslandres and Michelin say: "All things considered it is not excessive to argue that Villermé and his 'Tableau' are at the origin of our social legislation." *Il y a cent ans*, p. 256, note 1. On Villermé and this area of historical inquiry, see Lécuyer, "Démographie, statistique et hygiène publique sous la monarchie censitaire," and Coleman, *Death Is a Social Disease*.

would be forthcoming, hygienists believed, once those in authority were aware of the problem and understood it. Coleman suggested that socio-medical investigation was a precondition for reform. William Reddy has argued, however, that investigation was more than a precondition, that it in itself constituted social action: "Observers, in the act of observation, are engaging in social action; their desire is to change as much as to see." Sociomedical investigators had an agenda; a particular notion of reform informed their work. They never intended their work to be *merely* descriptive, but descriptive, interpretive, and prescriptive. This is an important point, one that is obvious when you recall, for example, why the *Tableau* was undertaken in the first place. The aim was to provide an alternative account to the gloomy portrayals of industrialization being presented by socialists and conservatives. A more evenhanded, optimistic picture was called for. This project was never intended or expected to be impartial, unbiased research (if indeed such a thing is possible).[83]

Coleman offered a sympathetic account of Villermé and the *Tableau*, but William Reddy and William Sewell both presented critiques of the same work. Reddy is very harsh on Villermé, charging him with arranging his evidence to advance his own views. He may well be guilty as charged, but would we expect him to do otherwise? What reasonable person would arrange evidence to advance a view he or she did not share? The accusation seems to be: Villermé had preconceived notions. He was not objective. A comparison between Villermé's *Tableau* and Chadwick's *Sanitary Report* shows them both to have had preconceived ideas and to have used both descriptive and statistical evidence to support their ideas. Statistical evidence was central to Villermé's work, not just in the *Tableau* but in most of his studies. Reddy took Villermé to task for his misuse of statistics in his section analyzing annual and subsistence wages. All Villermé's statistical studies can, and have been, justly criticized for faulty methodology, but the point is that Villermé like Parent-Duchâtelet and others, was trying to make public hygiene a scientific discipline, and the use of statistics was one way to do this. Still, we must recognize Villermé's use of statistics as rhetoric. Like Chadwick, he understood that numbers carried weight in influencing readers and that because numbers were regarded as objective and scientific, their use made any argument more convincing in a society becoming increasingly scientized.[84]

83 Coleman, *Death Is a Social Disease*, pp. 205–38; Reddy, *Rise of Market Culture*, pp. 138–84. Quote, p. 140.
84 Reddy, *Rise of Market Culture*, pp. 140–51; Sewell, *Work and Revolution*; Edwin Chadwick, *Report on the Sanitary Condition of the Labouring Population of Great Britain, 1842*, ed. M. W. Flinn (Edinburgh: Edinburgh University Press, 1965). On Chadwick's rhetorical use of statistics, see Michael Cullen, *The Statistical Movement in Early Victorian Britain: The Foundations of Empirical Social Research* (New York: Harvester, 1975), pp. 56–60.

Reddy's critique does not stop there. He accuses Villermé of playing on readers' emotions, of pointing out deplorable situations, described in rich descriptive language, for their shock value. The charge seems to be that Villermé was a skilled rhetorician, that he knew what to do to convince his readers and provoke them to action. It is hard to see what is wrong with this approach. Reddy rejects the possibility that Villermé could have actually been shocked or moved by the scenes of misery he saw, arguing that neither poverty nor slum neighborhoods were new. What he fails to consider is that until consciousness is raised, one can look at scenes of poverty and degradation for years and never really see them. The change need not be in the situation observed; it can be in the mind of the observer. Reddy portrays Villermé as a manipulator of readers' emotions but denies the possibility that Villermé might himself have had emotions, that it is indeed possible that he was shocked by what he saw, that his moral outrage was real, not just feigned for stylistic effect. In fact, if one reads the correspondence between Villermé and Quetelet, it is clear that Villermé was an emotional person with a keen sensitivity. Without denying his skillful use of rhetoric, we can at least allow for the possibility that Villermé experienced some shock as he traveled about observing working-class conditions, and, as a skilled writer, succeeded in conveying his feelings to his readers.[85]

Reddy accuses Villermé of writing from his own experience, of seeing the world through the eyes of middle-class liberalism, of judging workers according to bourgeois standards. Reddy would like for Villermé to have been an anthropologist, to have understood workers on their own terms, to have appreciated their culture without being judgmental. He criticizes Villermé for wanting to make workers into bourgeois. If Reddy could have viewed Villermé within the context of the public health movement, he would have understood that *embourgeoisement* was the mission of hygienists and liberal reformers. It was one of the main points of their reform program: Through education and example they hoped to inculcate in workers bourgeois values and habits. In short, I think Reddy does the same thing to Villermé and his liberal bourgeois culture that he criticizes Villermé for doing to working-class culture. Reddy seems to lack appreciation for the liberal reform tradition of which Villermé was an eloquent spokesman. Indeed, he wants Villermé and other sociohygienic investigators to use an anthropological approach in order to understand working-class culture. But Reddy does not take his own advice, failing adequately

---

85 Reddy, *Rise of Market Culture*, pp. 174–80; Villermé–Quetelet correspondence. Brussels. Bibliothèque royale. Académie royale des Sciences, des Lettres et des Beaux Arts de Belgique. Centre national d'histoire de Sciences. Correspondence Villermé-Quetelet. Cat. 2560 (1826–35) and 2561 (1839–63).

to understand the culture of which Villermé and other reforming physicians were a part.[86]

Finally, Reddy accuses Villermé of constructing working-class conditions to suit his own purposes. Reddy, like other historians, wants to provide a corrective to the traditional interpretation of a degraded, deteriorating, diseased working class portrayed by investigators and reformers. He thinks they exaggerated their claims for shock value generalized from a few experiences, and interpreted what they saw in a very gloomy fashion. But this would have been a peculiar tactic for Villermé, since, after all, he was a defender of industrialization. He sought only to regulate what he considered the worst abuse of the system, child labor, not to reform or abolish the whole industrial system, which he believed in the long run would be beneficial to workers and society in general.[87]

Thus, Reddy's analysis, although provocative, must be in part rejected. He seems to have misunderstood the main purpose of sociomedical investigation. These inquiries were intended to be rhetorical, to be exposés, to show social pathologies, to arouse concern, to provoke readers to action. They were not – nor were they intended to be – objective, scientific accounts. They were based on what hygienists considered to be scientific methods: firsthand observation, interviews, and use of statistical data. But the scientific data were interpreted in light of the world view and goals of the authors. There was always a particular agenda in mind. Some of the answers were already known; the outcome, predictable. Indeed, Villermé's *Tableau* was less predictable than most, because it contained contradictory interpretations and ended on a note of uncertainty. In spite of his rhetoric and his agenda, Villermé concluded his investigation less sure of his position than when he started. Unlike Chadwick's *Sanitary Report*, which had specific conclusions and recommendations for reform, the *Tableau* ended by raising as many questions as it answered.

INVESTIGATION AND MORALIZATION

The goal of much sociohygienic investigation was – Reddy has got it right – *embourgeoisement*, the liberal reformers' answer to dealing with the problems of the working class. Through education and moral example, they would be taught to emulate the middle class, and as their material condition improved, they could even become middle class. Sewell argues that Villermé provided a primarily moral interpretation of poverty. According to Sewell, "The crucial problem for him [Villermé] was not that workers received inadequate material remuneration but that they had

---

86 Reddy, *Rise of Market Culture*, pp. 182–3.
87 Ibid., pp. 180–4.

an inadequate moral constitution." Sewell is partly right, but his interpretation is as contradictory as Villermé's. He points out that on the one hand, Villermé saw moral degradation as the cause of material deprivation, but on the other hand, his theory of moralization was environmentalist: that immorality was the product of a bad environment. According to Sewell, Villermé's principal concept in discussions of moral standards was "demoralization," or the failure of workers to adopt middle-class values, practices, and habits. Sewell is correct in emphasizing that Villermé thought moral reform was up to individual workers as well as factory owners. Each had to do his or her part. The factory owner should take responsibility for setting an example of right behavior and provide the correct environment in the factory. Sewell provides a Foucaultian analysis of Villermé's prescription for moral reform: "If the moral degradation of workers is to be overcome, factories must be made into reformatories, into beneficial industrial prisons where the design of the work process, the paternal presence of the manufacturer, and the untiring eye of the overlooker banish disorder and immorality from from the worker's long day."[88]

Sewell has recognized a key feature of the hygienists' moralizing mission: Workers have to take responsibility for their own actions, but those in positions of authority must also create an environment that will enable workers to practice middle-class morality. Environmental reform had to occur at all levels if moral and material standards were to be raised. This is why hygienists could argue it both ways: Immorality was at the root of poverty and disease, but immorality could also result from poverty and disease.

According to Reddy and Sewell, the principal motivation for socio-hygienic investigation was moral reform, or moralization. Physicians like Villermé were also motivated out of a sense of humanitarianism. To ignore their humanitarian motivations would give a distorted view of the public health movement. It has become fashionable to see motivations only in terms of self-interest, what Katherine Lynch has referred to as the "hermeneutics of suspicion." But as she points out, self-interest and humanitarianism were not mutually exclusive. Humanitarianism always included self-interest, the goal of reforming hygienists being ultimately the healthy, well-ordered society. Nationalistic motivations also figured prominently. A perceived deterioration of the working class threatened the productive and military capacity of the nation, and a disorderly working

---

88 Sewell, *Work and Revolution*, pp. 223–6. Quotes, pp. 225, 229. See also Michel Foucault, *Discipline and Punish: The Birth of the Prison*, trans. Alan Sheridan (New York: Random House, 1979). Sewell reminds us that Villermé started out as a prison reformer, publishing in 1820 *Les prisons telles qu'elles sont et telles qu'elles devraient être* (Paris: Méquignon-Marvis, 1820).

class threatened the social order. The nineteenth-century "social problem," or what to do with the working class, how to integrate them into society and diffuse them as a threat, figured prominently in some of these writings. Sewell senses that Villermé too was motivated by the fear of the working classes, and understood that a class morally and materially degraded could become dangerous. The fear was, not only for Villermé but also for conservative social reformers, social disorder, a society out of control. This was Frégier's (and later Chevalier's) vision.[89]

The hygienists' program of moralization and *embourgeoisement* was in sharp contrast to the conservative point of view of most industrialists. In his analysis of early-nineteenth-century middle-class industrialists, Peter Stearns shows how, because they were neither liberals not intellectuals, these men did not share the common assumptions about reform, nor did they have the same attitudes toward workers. They did not address workers in the abstract – as a force – but associated with them on a daily basis as real people. Although this does not necessarily mean that they penetrated working-class culture, as Sewell and Reddy would have liked, industrialists, Stearns points out, were already actively involved in just the kinds of moralization programs Villermé was advocating, but with different attitudes and somewhat different goals. In fact, Villermé cited the example of some of the forward-looking industrialists, such as the Société industrielle de Mulhouse. Industrialists were motivated by self-interest and paternalism, and thought more along the lines of eighteenth-century corporatism than of liberalism. They neither feared their workers nor considered them a race apart. Stearns suggests that such an attitude toward workers may have been true in Paris and Lyon but was not true for most industrialists. In fact, it was not regularly employed industrial workers that urbanites feared, but nomads, day laborers, that marginal group that formed, at least in Paris, Frégier's dangerous classes. Industrialists wanted to keep their workers, and so provided benefits ranging from schooling to housing to medical care. Such fringe benefits allowed factory owners more control than high wages, which workers could spend indiscriminately. But the sharp difference between the liberal, reform point of view represented by Villermé and the paternalistic viewpoint of the industrialists was that the industrialists did not seek to make workers into bourgeois. They simply wanted to make them better workers who would keep their place in the social hierarchy. They did not expect them to be socially mobile or to adopt middle-class values and habits. The paternalistic approach was to keep them content, provide for them, and create a situation good enough so that they would be productive and not quit. If Stearns's account is

89 Frégier, *Des classes dangereuses*; Chevalier, *Classes laborieuses et classes dangereuses*; Sewell, *Work and Revolution*, pp. 226–31; Lynch, *Family, Class and Ideology*, pp. 26–7.

correct, we find a wide disparity between the liberalism of many of the hygienists and the government of the July Monarchy, and the conservative paternalism of the industrialists.[90]

In their investigation of industrialization and working-class conditions, Villermé and Thouvenin proposed moralization as one of the solutions to industrialization-induced public health problems. In addition to government intervention – the child labor law only – moralization was the key to improving the material and moral condition of workers. Both factory owners and workers would have to take responsibility for moral reform, which, like legislative reform, would lead to better health conditions among the working classes. For many of the sociohygienic investigators, investigation was the first step in moralization. Investigation was also a precondition for practical public health reform, another key goal of the overall mission of the hygienists. In attempting to solve urban health problems, investigation always preceded reform.

90 Stearns, *Paths to Authority*, pp. 160–6; see also Coleman, *Death Is a Social Disease*, pp. 211–14.

6

Investigation and practical reform: Public health in Paris

Investigation was central to the practice of public hygiene in Paris. Acting individually, as health council members, or as appointed members on a municipal commission, hygienists investigated problems referred to them by the municipal government or undertook such studies on their own initiative. Investigations varied in depth and scope, ranging from routine investigations of industrial establishments to studies of national problems such as working-class conditions. Several research methods predominated. Many hygienists employed historical research in archives and official collections, as well as interviews, questionnaires, on-site observations, and statistical data. Some public health problems required experimentation as well. Once the data were gathered, the investigation completed, a report prepared, and a conclusion reached, the investigator(s) proposed one or more solutions, which were sent to the official in charge – usually the prefect of police – who then determined what action to take.

Considering themselves scientific investigators, Parisian hygienists used the city as their laboratory, since it was "well equipped" with many problems and useful tools for investigation. For historical research there were the records of the prefecture of police and the municipal council to be surveyed. Manuscript records of the Paris health council dating from 1802 were available at the Prefecture of Police, and hospitals and the Prefecture of Police both collected statistical data that hygienists routinely used. The most important statistical resource was, however, the *Recherches statistiques sur la ville de Paris*.[1]

THE HYGIENISTS AND THEIR "LABORATORY": CHOLERA IN PARIS

Paris made a good "laboratory" because of the 1832 cholera epidemic.[2] Cholera was different from earlier epidemics: First, it was a "new" disease,

---

1 *Recherches statistiques sur la ville de Paris et le département de la Seine*, 5 vols. (Paris: Imprimerie municipale, 1821–9, 1844).
2 William Coleman, *Death Is a Social Disease: Public Health and Political Economy in Early Industrial France* (Madison: University of Wisconsin Press, 1982). Coleman

believed to be the first occurrence of Indian cholera in France, indeed in Western Europe; second, hygienists, physicians, and administrators had a long lead time to try to prevent its importation; and, third, by the time cholera appeared on French soil, the public health movement was at the height of its activity, preventive measures were widespread, and hygienists were prepared to study the disease. Of major importance was that cholera hit Paris, the center of public health activity, the city with a reputation for a greatly improved public health administration, where the board of health was becoming a model for others to emulate; a city possessing wide-ranging hospital facilities, where medicine was reputed to be the most advanced in Europe.

When cholera invaded Paris in the spring of 1832, French hygienists adhered to three principal theories of disease causation: the traditional miasmatic theory, a contagionist theory, and a social theory of epidemiology. The social theory predominated among leading French hygienists by the late 1820s, owing to Villermé's studies of mordibity and mortality among the rich and poor. Thus, by 1832, many French hygienists were predisposed to believe that cholera would take more lives among the poor than among the wealthy. Observation teams sent to northern and eastern Europe reported that – with few exceptions – this had been the case. When cholera invaded the hygienists' "laboratory," it provided a perfect case study for sociomedical investigators, an opportunity to apply their scientific methodology to the investigation of epidemic disease.

The story of the cholera in Paris has been told several times, first by George Sussman, and most recently by François Delaporte, Patrice Bourdelais, and Jean-Yves Raulot.[3] There is no need to repeat the historical account here. The point to be made is that public hygienists used cholera to test the three main theories of disease causation, using the same scientific methodology they employed for investigating any public health problem. The final report by the public hygienists, *Rapport sur la marche et les effets du choléra-morbus dans Paris*, is a masterpiece of sociohygienic investigation, ranking in importance with the other classics of the period, such as Villermé's *Tableau physique et moral des ouvriers* and Parent-Duchâtelet's *De la prostitution dans la ville de Paris*. Many of these investigating hygienists were physicians who served on health commissions in their *quartiers*, took care of cholera patients, and participated in door-to-door sanitary investigations. They were not just scholars in libraries; rather,

referred to Paris as a "laboratory," but this is a concept developed by the hygienists themselves.

3 George Sussman, "From Yellow Fever to Cholera: A Study of French Government Policy, Medical Professionalism, and Popular Movements in the Epidemic Crises of the Restoration and July Monarchy" (Ph.D. dissertation, Yale University, 1972); François Delaporte, *Disease and Civilization: The Cholera in Paris, 1832* (Cambridge, MA: MIT Press, 1985); Patrice Bourdelais and Jean-Yves Raulot, *Une peur bleue: Histoire du choléra en France* (Paris: Payot, 1987).

they were intimately involved with the cholera effort at several levels: investigation, prevention, management, and care. The conclusions they reached supported the social theory of epidemiology, which held that inequality in life was correlated with inequality in the face of death.[4] In his recent study of cholera, Delaporte has emphasized, however, that the only strong correlation with high mortality was the population density of individual dwellings rather than of quartiers or arrondissements.[5] The primary contributing factor in the spread of cholera seemed to be crowded buildings inhabited by people living in destitution. The conclusion, then, was what hygienists had expected: Wealth diminished mortality; poverty increased it. The cholera report confirmed the earlier and by now widely accepted findings of Villermé's studies of the 1820s on the rich and poor areas of Paris.

The hygienists concluded by calling for solutions to alleviate poor living conditions. Poverty, social reformers had asserted, could be dealt with only by major socioeconomic reform, which few Establishment hygienists could support, or by individual moral reform, which all advocated. As William Coleman emphasized in his study of Villermé and the hygienist-economists, this approach led to a dead end, given the socioeconomic and political climate of Louis-Philippe's France.[6] Thus, in terms of practical health reform, the conclusions of the cholera investigating committee led nowhere, and hygienists turned to more practical, manageable problems. Whether poverty was the major predisposing cause of disease or not, the reality of day-to-day public health reform in Paris was *assainissement*, or sanitary reform. Thus, although cholera was extremely important as a case study for hygienists testing the etiology of the disease, the conclusions of the investigating team had little direct influence on the day-to-day practice of public health in Paris. Hygienists functioned much the same way before, during, and after the cholera epidemic. Whatever theoretical disagreements they may have had over disease causation, most hygienists adhered strongly to no particular theory, judging each case on its own merits. The Paris cholera epidemic is undeniably of great interest for epidemiologists and was the major public health event in early-nineteenth-century Paris. But it did not substantively affect the routine practice of public health in Paris.

The main focus of early-nineteenth-century public health in Paris was sanitary reform, based on the belief that most diseases were spread as a result of harmful miasms from garbage heaps, sewers, dumps, badly kept dwellings, and polluted water. Proponents of the miasmatic theory of

4 Coleman, *Death Is a Social Disease*, pp. 172–3.
5 Delaporte, *Disease and Civilization*, pp. 73–86.
6 Coleman, *Death Is a Social Disease*, pp. 237–8.

disease causation advocated *assainissement,* or cleaning up the city, as the best preventive measure against disease and epidemics. Although the movement for sanitary reform was already underway in Paris by the early 1830s, fear of cholera was an important motivating factor in sanitary reform in particular and the public health movement in general. During these years, numerous books and articles were published on cholera, with the general consensus that the best preventive measure was cleanliness. This meant that improving the sanitary condition became the focal point of Parisian public health reform. The attention of public hygienists and municipal administrators was drawn to unhealthy and dirty situations, such as the dump, sewers, cesspools, dirty streets, infected dwellings, dissection rooms, and anatomy amphitheaters, as well as prisons and hospitals with inadequate sanitary facilities.

A major clean-up campaign was an important part of the cholera program that went into effect in the first months of 1832. In spite of all precautions, however, the epidemic hit Parisians with a vengeance in the spring and summer of that year. By the time it was over, more than 18,000 Parisians (out of a population of 785,000) had died. In retrospect, then, it would seem that the sanitary reforms had failed, and indeed, some of the assumptions of the hygienists were later proved wrong. Yet, at the time, sanitary reformers and public hygienists believed that, although their efforts had not prevented the epidemic, they had lessened its impact; and, if they had failed, it was because the clean-up campaign had not been vigorous enough and because the poverty in which many Parisians lived had complicated the evils of filth. Thus, the movement for sanitary reform continued, and hygienists remained convinced that by cleaning up the city, disease and epidemics would be thwarted.

Their ideas were confirmed by the findings of Villermé, Benoiston de Châteauneuf, and others, who demonstrated the relationship between poverty, unsanitary living conditions, and high mortality and morbidity rates.[7] Villermé's hypothesis on the relation of poverty to disease received quasi-official sanction by the cholera commission after their investigations showed that the areas hardest hit by the cholera were crowded, unsanitary streets, primarily inhabited by the poor.[8] Even though Villermé asserted that the underlying cause of disease was poverty, reformers believed that by improving the city's sanitary conditions, an important cause of disease would be eliminated.

---

7 Louis-René Villermé, "Mémoire sur la mortalité en France dans la classe aisée et dans la classe indigente," *Mém. de l'Acad. Roy. de Méd.* 1 (1828): 51–98; "De la mortalité dans les divers quartiers da la ville de Paris," *Annales d'hygiène publique* 3 (1830): 294–341.
8 Louis-François Benoiston de Châteauneuf et al., *Rapport sur la marche et les effets du choléra-morbus dans Paris...*(Paris: Imprimerie royale, 1834).

PARENT-DUCHÂTELET: HYGIENIST OF PARIS

Alexandre Parent-Duchâtelet stands out as the champion of public health reform in Paris. His primary interest was urban health, especially occupational hygiene. Parent-Duchâtelet was recognized during his lifetime as the leading French urban hygienist, noted for his rigorous investigative techniques, his unwillingness to accept consensus opinions without researching a topic for himself, and his debunking of commonly held beliefs concerning public health. Rejecting armchair philosophy, Parent-Duchâtelet spent much of his time in the city dump, sewers, boarding houses, and brothels in order to test firsthand hypotheses that had long been taken as truth.

Like many public hygienists, Parent-Duchâtelet subscribed to no one theory of disease causation. His research caused him neither to accept nor to reject miasmatic theories, for he could neither prove nor disprove them. For example, it was commonly believed that dangerous miasms coming from unclean places were an important cause of disease. But in his research on the city dump Parent-Duchâtelet did not find that those who habitually breathed the smelly emanations from the dump developed any health problems, and he therefore doubted whether such odors caused disease. He also investigated the influence of the air from the dirty Bièvre River on people who lived in the vicinity and could find no correlation between the air and the bad health of the inhabitants. Nor did he find that these emanations had any harmful effect on food.[9]

Nevertheless, Parent-Duchâtelet was an an advocate of sanitary reform. He believed that even though he was unable to establish the harmful effects of noxious emanations on health, this in itself did not prove the case, or that such effects might not prove hazardous in the future. He agreed with his colleagues that filth, dirty water, and the city dump must be in some way injurious to health and should be cleaned up. He particularly advocated a much enlarged and improved sewer system for Paris. Parent-Duchâtelet's untimely death in 1836 cut short his productive public health career. Yet his influence was tremendous. More than any other individual, he can be credited for increasing awareness of public health problems in Paris and for encouraging municipal authorities to undertake sanitary reform by enlarging and improving the sewer system and cleaning up the

---

9 A. J. B. Parent-Duchâtelet, "Les chantiers d'équarrissage de la ville de Paris...," *Hygiéne publique*, 2 vols. (Paris: Baillière, 1836), 2: 227–41; "Recherches et considèrations sur la rivière de la Bièvre...," ibid., 1: 128–33; "Recherches pour déterminer jusqu'à quel point les émanations putrides provenant de la décomposition des matières animales peuvent contribuer à l'altération des substances alimentaires," ibid., 2: 85–127.

Bièvre River, the dump and horsebutchering industry, dissection rooms, and anatomy amphitheaters.[10]

ASSAINISSEMENT, OR SANITARY REFORM

The sanitary situation in Paris was typical of most early-nineteenth-century cities, with an inadequate water supply and underground sewers used primarily for draining rainwater. Most waste water ran through open sewers or gutters; human and household wastes were collected in cesspools, if not just thrown out the window. Public urination and defecation were part of the cultural tradition, as was lack of personal hygiene. Paris was smelly if the wind blew in the wrong direction, being polluted by various nuisance industries and by the infamous city dump at Montfaucon. The sanitary situation in early-nineteenth-century Paris deteriorated due to the influx of immigrants from the countryside, who increased the pressure on existing facilities. Even before the cholera epidemic, it was becoming obvious to public hygienists, urban reformers, administrators, and contemporary observers that public health reform was mandatory if Paris was to be livable.

The prerequisite for *assainissement* was an adequate water supply, for sanitary reform and water were interrelated at all levels. An increased water supply and an improved system of distribution necessitated more underground sewers through which to dispose of waste water. At the same time, an increased water supply created problems with the traditional cesspool (septic tank) system: It made cesspools impractical and made desirable their ultimate suppression and replacement by sanitary sewers. More water was the key to a cleaner Paris, and the antiquated system of cesspools was the major stumbling block to an increase in the water supply and its better distribution. As long as cesspools were the primary means of human waste disposal, the water supply could not be increased without major problems. But cesspools could not be suppressed until there was an adequate sanitary sewer system, which required copious amounts of water to dilute wastes and keep sewers clean. Thus reform in one area necessitated accompanying reforms in related areas. The sanitary revolution in waste disposal was bound to involve a long and tedious period of transition.

The effects of a sanitary revolution would be many, hygienists believed.

---

10 On Parent-Duchâtelet, see Ann Fowler La Berge, "A. J. B. Parent-Duchâtelet: Hygienist of Paris, 1821–1836," *Clio Medica* 12 (1977): 279–301. See also Alain Corbin, "Présentation" to Alexandre Parent-Duchâtelet, *La Prostitution à Paris au XIXe siècle*, texte présenté et annoté par Alain Corbin (Paris: Seuil, 1981), pp. 9–47; Jill Harsin, *Policing Prostitution in Nineteenth-Century Paris* (Princeton, NJ: Princeton University Press, 1985), ch. 3.

Once a sanitary sewer system replaced cesspools, the city dump could be suppressed. Once there was plenty of water and a way to dispose of it, bathing would become cheap and convenient. Once cesspools were eliminated and replaced by sanitary sewers, water could be distributed directly to private dwellings. *Assainissement* would eventually be achieved by a revolution in waste disposal, a sanitary revolution encompassing an enlarged water supply and a modern distribution system, suppression of cesspools and dumps, and the enlargement and construction of a storm and sanitary sewer system.

Public hygienists were at the forefront of the Parisian sanitary reform movement. Working alongside the administration on investigations and projects, either as health council members or on municipal commissions, hygienists created an awareness of public health problems and the necessity of sanitary reform. Reforms were made in many areas, although the sanitary revolution had barely started by the end of the 1840s. The revolution in waste disposal had to await the transformation of the city under Prefect of the Seine Haussman in the 1850s and 1860s and additional reforms and changing attitudes in the latter part of the century. In accounting for the tardiness of the French to implement sanitary reform, cultural attitudes were as important as, if not more important than, economic and administrative considerations.

WATER SUPPLY AND SANITARY REFORM

At the beginning of the nineteenth century the Parisian water supply was notoriously inadequate. Claude Rambuteau, Prefect of the Seine, estimated that about 8 liters of drinkable water were available for each person per day. The water came from the Seine (7,000 cubic meters a day), distributed by means of pumps at Chaillot, Gros-Caillou, Notre-Dame, and Pont Neuf (the Samaritaine pump); from the Ourcq River via a canal (10,000 to 12,000 cubic meters); and from the Arceuil source via an aqueduct that brought water in from Rungis (1,000 cubic meters). Additional water came from sources at Belleville and Pré-St.-Gervais. By 1815 approximately 20,000 cubic meters of water were available daily from all sources, excluding private wells. The amount of well water is unknown, but indications from hygienists are that much of it had been infected by cesspool seepage and was unusable. Many wells were not maintained by proprietors, perhaps for this very reason.[11]

11 Claude Rambuteau, *Mémoires du Comte de Rambuteau publiés par son petit-fils* (Paris: Calmann-Lévy, 1905), p. 378. For a history of the Parisian water supply, see Louis Figuier, *Les Eaux de Paris. Leur passé, leur état présent, leur avenir* (Paris: Michel Lévy, 1862), esp. pp. 124–56, and Jean-Pierre Goubert, *The Conquest of Water: The Advent of Health in the Industrial Age* (Princeton, NJ: Princeton University Press,

A major increase in the Parisian water supply took place in the 1820s when Gilbert Chabrol, Prefect of the Seine, completed the project launched by Napoleon in 1802 to bring water via canals from the Ourcq River. The first canal, opened in 1809, generated an additional 10,000 to 12,000 cubic meters of water. Under Chabrol, the St.-Martin and St.-Denis canals were opened, bringing additional water from the Ourcq into Paris, thereby increasing the water supply by 105,000 cubic meters. By the 1830s, then, Parisians had available to them an average of 100 liters of water per person per day, although an outmoded distribution system denied most of them access to such water.[12]

In early-nineteenth-century Paris most water was distributed by fountains and water carriers. Only a few people had water piped directly into their homes, and as late as 1850 a mere 20 percent of the Parisian population enjoyed such a convenience. Three types of fountains were used: commercial or merchant fountains (*fontaines marchandes*), of which there were about fourteen by 1832, for the use of professional water carriers; public fountains (*fontaines publiques*) for the use of individuals and free of charge; and short, or street, fountains (*bornes-fontaines*), intended primarily for cleaning streets and gutters but also used by the poor as a source of water.[13]

For those who could afford it, water could be bought from water carriers who, having obtained a concession from the city government, fetched the water from the merchant fountains and delivered it to their customers' homes. British traveler Frances Trollope described the way many Parisians got their water: "Nearly every family in Paris receives this precious gift of nature doled out by two buckets at a time, laboriously brought to them by porters, clambering in *sabots*, often up the same stairs which lead to their drawing rooms."[14] There were two principal types

1989). See the memoirs of Haussmann in Louis Réau, Pierre Lavedan, et al., *L'oeuvre du Baron Haussmann, préfet de la Seine (1853–1870)* (Paris: Presses universitaires de France, 1954), pp. 134–6; Jean Tulard, *Nouvelle histoire de Paris: Le Consulat et l'Empire* (Paris: Hachette, 1970), pp. 228, 238; Guillaume de Bertier de Sauvigny, *Nouvelle histoire de Paris: La Restauration* (Paris: Hachette, 1977), p. 92.

12 Rambuteau, *Mémoires*, p. 378; Maxime Du Camp, *Paris. Ses organes. Ses fonctions et sa vie dans la seconde moitié du XIXe siècle*, 6 vols. (Paris: Hachette, 1868–75), 5: 315. None of the figures indicate whether this figure included water for industrial use and cleaning the city, or simply personal use. It was probably the former. The hygienist Michel Lévy stated that in 1844 each inhabitant had forty liters of water a day, compared with ninety liters a day in Glasgow. He was probably referring to personal use. Note that the figure of available water per person might be much higher than what many people actually had at their disposal. See Michel Lévy, *Traité d'hygiène publique et privée*, 2 vols. (Paris: Baillière, 1844), 2: 545–6.

13 David Pinkney, *Napoleon III and the Rebuilding of Paris* (Princeton, NJ: Princeton University Press, 1958), p. 21; Rambuteau, *Mémoires*, p. 380. Rambuteau says that by 1840, 5,300 houses had water piped in.

14 Frances Trollope, *Paris and the Parisians in 1835*, 2 vols. (London: Richard Bentley, 1836), 1: 231–2.

of water carriers: those who carried buckets of water – usually drinking water – on their shoulders (*à bretelles*), and those who used carts equipped with big barrels to distribute large amounts of water for drinking and cleaning purposes.[15]

It was up to Rambuteau to distribute the new supply of water from the Ourcq. He was partially successful, but by 1850, only half of the 100 liters per day theoretically available for every person could be used because of the outmoded distribution system.[16] Once additional water became available, various companies offered to establish a modern distribution system for Parisians. The administration never accepted these offers because of the cost, because the companies were English, and because they judged the sewerage system inadequate to handle additional water. Furthermore, serious opposition was mounted by proprietors who feared the increased expense of additional cesspool cleaning, as well as by various interests that benefited from the status quo, notably the water carriers, whose livelihood was threatened by progress in water distribution. In addition, the issue was complicated not only by economic considerations and propertied interests but by a cultural tradition of uncleanliness. Demand was not sufficient, and many citizens did not want more water enough to pay for it. In order to make it economically feasible, both the city and the water company had to be certain of a sufficient number of subscribers. Individual subscribers were not numerous, since most Parisians rented apartments in multifamily dwellings. Proprietors did not want to make more water available to renters when it would necessitate more frequent emptying of cesspools and additional expense. Increased expenses would then have to be passed on to renters in the form of higher rents.

Most hygienists assumed that if workers had enough water, they would bathe and keep their living quarters clean. Some, however, disagreed. Pierre S. Girard, chief engineer of the municipal service of Paris, even though he was probably rationalizing the status quo, asserted in 1831 that Parisians needed on the average only seven and a half liters of water a day, and if they had four times that much (as one company was proposing), they would not know what to do with it.[17] In spite of his vested interest (for he was former chief engineer of the water service of Paris), Girard's explanation is plausible. Comparing the water situations in London and Paris, he contended that although, in theory, Londoners required no more water for personal use than Parisians, in practice they did, because their lifestyle was different. In London there were fewer people per household,

---

15 APP, Da69, Ville de Paris, Compte de recettes et dépenses de 1832 et Budget de l'Exercice de 1834.
16 Pinkney, *Rebuilding of Paris*, p. 21.
17 Pierre S. Girard, *Eaux publiques de Paris* (Paris: Carilian-Goeury, 1831), pp. 47–79; see also Goubert, *The Conquest of Water*.

and it was more practical to have water piped right into the house. The sewer system was more extensive in London than in Paris, so that all waste water ended up in sewers, thereby cleaning them. In London, household waters used for bathing, cooking, and water closets were disposed of directly through sewers. In Paris, however, it was not practical to have water piped in, because of the high population density and the continued widespread use of cesspools. In addition, most houses were not connected to sewers. Sewers and gutters were cleaned directly by water from street fountains, for household waste water that in London flowed directly into sewers went into cesspools in Paris.

Rambuteau considered himself a *"préfet voyer,"* a prefect whose main concern is public works, and he claimed that when he came to office his main goal was to supply Parisians with "shade, light, and water." In his memoirs Rambuteau took credit for improving water distribution in Paris. He claimed to have built 200,000 meters of underground pipes and six great reservoirs, each holding 10,000 cubic meters of water. He also had the older steam pump at Pont-Neuf replaced with a turbine installation. The number of dwellings with piped-in water increased; by 1848 over 5,000 dwellings paid seventy-five francs a year to have 100 liters of water available per day. Rambuteau was also proud of the proliferation of street fountains (*bornes-fontaines*), from 124 in 1828, to 700 by the late 1830s, to 1,840 by 1848. The Paris health council had encouraged increasing the number of street fountains for street and gutter cleaning as the best way to use the additional water for public health purposes.[18] The proliferation of street fountains was a direct contribution to the hygienists' goal of *assainissement*.

As health council members, public hygienists devoted little attention to the Parisian water supply. At first glance this is surprising, given the fact that sanitary reform of Paris was dependent on an adequate water supply. The reason was mainly administrative: Water supply and distribution were specific duties of the Prefect of the Seine, not of the Prefect of Police, whom the health council advised. The prefect of police and the health council were in charge of public health and *assainissement*, but their duties did not include water supply, only inspection of the water service and testing of water samples for purity. Public hygienists were, therefore, mainly interested in how best to use the existing water supply for street and sewer cleaning and bathing and how to ensure its quality. Prior to

---

18 Rambuteau, *Mémoires*, pp. 378–81; *Moniteur universel*, December 2, 1828, p. 1777; APP, Da207, Service des bornes-fontaines dans les 4 inspections des eaux de Paris. Itinéraire général; The hygienist Jean Boudin gives the figure of 1,784 for 1851. See Jean Boudin, "Etudes sur le pavage, le macadamisage et le drainage," *Annales d'hygiène publique* 45 (1851): 275; *R. G., Paris*, 1829, p. 36. See also APP, Da208, Lettre de Lappey, de l'établissement royal des eaux clarifiées et depurées de la Seine, au préfet de police, le 15 décembre 1841.

1848 the Paris health council had only three major discussions concerning the Parisian water supply: in 1810, 1829, and 1841. In 1829, for example, the health council discussed how additional water from the Ourcq could best benefit public health, suggesting that more street fountains would keep streets and gutters clean. Their suggestions were effected, the number of street fountains multiplying dramatically after 1830.[19]

Prefects of the Seine Chabrol and Rambuteau made considerable progress in increasing the water supply and improving the distribution system. The water supply had been quintupled since the beginning of the century, and distribution had been improved by the construction of numerous fountains, especially street fountains, and underground pipes that made water available from the tap in at least one-fifth of the private dwellings. Yet Paris still lagged far behind London and Glasgow, the cities most often cited for comparison by hygienists and contemporary observers. Distribution was an even greater problem than the total amount of water available. Parent-Duchâtelet considered the cesspool system the principal stumbling block to adequate water distribution in Paris, and it could not be replaced without a major extension of the sewer system. Nor could additional water supplies be made available without some means of disposing of the additional water. The increase in the Parisian water supply and its improved distribution went hand in hand with the extension of the underground sewer system.

THE SEWERS OF PARIS

Parisian sewers were primarily storm sewers, whose principal function was rainwater drainage; nevertheless, they were also used for the disposal of waste water, both household and industrial. They were, however, never intended for disposal of human or animal wastes, which went into cesspools (*fosses d'aisance*). Sewers were of three types: underground; open sewers or gutters; and absorbent pits, or drains that absorbed fluids. The number of covered (underground) sewers increased significantly from the 1820s to the 1840s; still, many areas of Paris had no underground sewers, and open gutters running between buildings and down the centers of streets were commonplace. Liquid wastes flowed through open gutters into an underground sewer, then into a larger sewer, and finally into the Seine. Frances Trollope found these open gutters one of the most disgusting aspects of Parisian life in the 1830s. She spoke of "that monstrous barbarism, a gutter in the middle of the streets expressly formed for the reception of filth."[20]

19 Moléon, *R. G. Paris*, 1810, pp. 42–3; 1829, p. 36; 1841, pp. 112–17.
20 Trollope, *Paris and the Parisians*, 1: 116.

There was little uniformity in the construction of Parisian sewers. Some were built of *pierre de taille*, a paving made of small stones and cement, which produced a rough surface, therefore making cleaning difficult, as mud and sand clung to the sides. Most of the principal sewers built after 1830 were of *meulière* – or tiled with large, smooth stones – a material that greatly facilitated their cleaning. The diameter of the sewers varied from fifty centimeters to two meters. In heavy storms the smaller sewers were virtually useless, since they filled up in five minutes. The lengths of the sewers varied from a few meters to over 6,866 meters for the largest sewer in Paris, the *égout de ceinture*, which encircled the whole right bank of the Seine. The sewer drains were covered with iron grills, but there were not enough drains, so much water ran through open gutters instead of draining into sewers.[21]

The authority on sewers was Parent-Duchâtelet, whose early reputation as an urban hygienist came from an 1824 work on the sewers of Paris, in which he discussed their history, construction, layout, and related problems (see Figure 1).[22] Parent-Duchâtelet's biographer, François Leuret, commented on his interest: "It is not surprising that Parent-Duchâtelet did not have the repugnance for sewers that these places naturally inspire. I would almost say that he liked them."[23] In his article, the only major early-nineteenth-century work on sewers, Parent-Duchâtelet pointed out the necessity of an adequate sewer system in large cities, without which they would be virtually uninhabitable. Although many hygienists had done research on cesspools, he noted that they had paid little attention to sewers and sewer workers, which were as important to the public health as cesspools.[24]

---

21 *R. G. Paris*, 1829, pp. 33–5.
22 "Essai sur les cloaques ou égouts de la ville de Paris, envisagés sous le rapport de l'hygiène publique et de la topographie médicale de cette ville," *Hygiène publique*, 1: 156–307. On sewers in general, see also A. J. B. Parent-Duchâtelet, "Egouts" (Hygiène), *Dictionnaire de l'industrie manufacturière* (DIM) 10 vols. (Paris: Baillière, 1833–41), 4 (1835): 360–5, and Gourlier, "Egouts" (Construction), *Dictionnaire de l'industrie manufacturière*, 4 (1835): 365–9.
23 François Leuret, "Notice historique sur A. J. B. Parent-Duchâtelet," *Hygiène publique*, 1: v–xxi. The quotation is from xii. This same notice also appeared in the *Annales d'hygiène publique* 16 (1836): v–xxi, as well as in the introduction to Parent-Duchâtelet's *De la prostitution dans la ville de Paris*, 2 vols. (Paris: Baillière, 1836), 1: v–xiii.
24 Alphonse Chevallier did a general article comparing the sewers of Paris, London, and Montpellier. See "Mémoire sur les égouts de Paris, de Londres, de Montpellier," *Annales d'hygiène publique* 19 (1838): 366–424. Much of the work on sewers and sewer construction was done by civil engineers at the Department of Bridges and Roads (*Ponts et Chaussées*). Two such works, done by H. C. Emmery, chief engineer of the Department of Bridges and Roads, were *Ville de Paris. Egouts et bornes-fontaines* (Paris: Carilian-Goeury, n.d.), extract from *Annales des ponts et chaussées*, mai et juin, 1834; and *Statistique des égouts de la ville de Paris* (année 1836) (Paris: Carilian-Goeury, 1837), extract from *Annales des ponts et chaussées*.

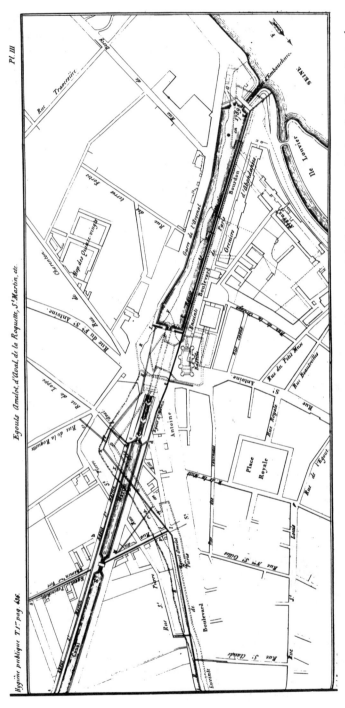

Figure 1 Part of the Paris sewer system in the 1820s showing some of the major right bank sewers: the Amelot, Roquette, and St.-Martin sewers and the St.-Martin canal. From Parent-Duchâtelet, "Rapport sur le curage des égouts Amelot, de la Roquette, Saint-Martin et autres," *Hygiène publique*, I: 436.

Parent-Duchâtelet's detailed description of the Paris sewer system included some of the longest and most important covered sewers in Paris, such as the *égout de ceinture*, which encircled the right bank, starting at St. Paul and emptying into the Seine beyond the steam pump below the Marbeuf garden. Many branch sewers emptied into this sewer. Other major right bank sewers were the Amelot sewer, 3,905 meters long, which also emptied into the Seine; the Carrousel sewer (2,706 meters); and the sewer of the Place Louis XV (2,278 meters).[25] The sewer system on the left bank was less developed than that on the right, with the two longest sewers being the wine market sewer (1,050 meters) and the Champ de Mars sewer (1,350 meters), which served the Ecole Militaire. The total length of the underground sewers in 1824 was 35,846 meters, or just about 20 miles. The most important open sewers ran through the most industrialized and populous areas of the city. Located in the Faubourg St. Antoine were the Traversière and Rambouillet sewers, and in the Faubourg St.-Marceau, on the left bank, the Bièvre River. Absorbent pits (*puisards*) were more common in the rural communes surrounding Paris than in the city, because the rural communes lacked paved and covered sewers.[26]

In the 1820s two specific problems of the sewer system were inadequate drainage, due to too few underground sewers, and the difficulties and dangers of cleaning sewers. By the 1830s the main problem was the insufficient number of sewers. Poor drainage and cobblestone paving contributed to the habitually dirty streets of Paris and the surrounding rural communes. It was customary for mud, often infected with human and animal wastes, to accumulate between the stones, giving off a fetid odor. Drainage problems were worst, of course, during and after a heavy rainstorm. Rambuteau described in his memoirs how pedestrians had to cross streets on boards after a heavy rain, since streets became virtual rivers and sidewalks were uncommon. Water pouring off roofs was also a hazard for pedestrians, and because of bad drainage, household waters stagnated in pools in front of houses.[27] Streets were built so that the sides were more elevated than the center to allow water to flow to gutters in the centers of streets, accumulating there. Many Parisian streets had little incline, so

25 Cleaning the Amelot sewer had caused public health problems since the eighteenth century. See the discussion later in this chapter and in Chapter 4.
26 Under Rambuteau the Place Louis XV was rebuilt and became the Place de la Concorde. Parent-Duchâtelet, "Essai sur les cloaques et égouts," pp. 212–15. For an example of the inconveniences of absorbent pits, see Alphonse Chevallier, "Notice historique sur l'égout dit le grand puisard de Bicêtre: ses inconvéniens; moyens de les faire cesser," *Annales d'hygiène publique* 40 (1848): 110–21. Although absorbent pits were still used in certain instances in Paris, they were not the preferred method of drainage.
27 Rambuteau, *Mémoires*, pp. 375–6; Maxime Du Camp gives a similar description in *Paris*, 5: 432–5.

water stagnated in gutters. Even where there were covered sewers, they often could not serve their intended purpose due to their inability to handle large amounts of water. Some sewers had entrances that were too small, and others were too short or narrow and quickly overflowed. Still other sewers, clogged with filth, had no capacity for water.

Drainage in the rural communes was even worse than in Paris, owing to the lack of any paved and covered sewer system. Guttters and absorbent pits prevailed. As late as 1842 and 1847, the health council noted that improper drainage and stagnant water were major health problems in the rural communes. The members commented that absorbent pits were inadequate and emphasized the need for a sewer system. The situation was so bad that hygienist Alphonse Chevallier reported that streets in the rural communes were cluttered with garbage, vegetable debris, and animal matter, which turned to a half-liquid state when it rained, making streets practically impassable.[28]

Keeping sewers clean was the second major problem (see Figures 2 and 3), since those built before 1830 were constructed of rough stone to which

28 R. G. Paris, 1842, p. 170; 1847, p. 105; Alphonse Cheval[l]ier, *Considérations pratiques sur les moyens d'assainir les communes rurales de France* (Paris: Everat, 1832), p. 2.

Figure 2 Methods and tools used for sewer cleaning in the 1820s. Figures 1 and 2 are proposed models of carts for the transport of wastes. The cart in figure 1 was supposed to sit right over the manhole so that waste material would be deposited directly into the cart. It didn't work. Figures 2 and 3 (end view) show another proposed cart for waste disposal. The barrel would be filled from the top and then rotated so that the waste matter could be emptied out from the bottom. Figure 7 shows the cart in common use in the 1820s. The main problem was its height. A man stands on a stool to deposit solid wastes into the cart, while another man (not shown) stands on the side platform by the wheel to spread out the wastes. The wastes were then covered by a layer of powdered bleach to eliminate odors as these carts traveled through Paris on their way to the city dump. In figures 9 and 11, sewer workers are shoveling and scraping solid waste and putting it in buckets. In figures 8 and 9 the buckets are hoisted up by a pulley, and then the solid waste is deposited in the cart. Figures 4, 5, 9, and 10 demonstrate attempts to block off segments of sewer so that ventilation could be controlled. Figures 4, 9, and 10 show the use of sandbags to limit circulation of noxious air. Figure 5 shows a hanging drop cloth, one way to try to control the escape of noxious gases. In figure 6 a small fire is used to create a draft to force noxious air out of the sewer. A hazard of this method was the spread of the fire or explosion. From Parent-Duchâtelet, "Rapport sur le curage des égouts Amelot, de la Roquette, Saint-Martin et autres," *Hygiène publique*, 1: 436.

Appareils pour le curage des fosses.

Pl. IV

Fig. 1.

Fig. 2.

Fig. 3.

Fig. 4.

Fig. 5.

Fig. 6.

Fig. 7.

Fig. 8.

Fig. 9.

Fig. 10.

Fig. 11.

Pl. V page.

Appareils pour le Curage des Égouts.

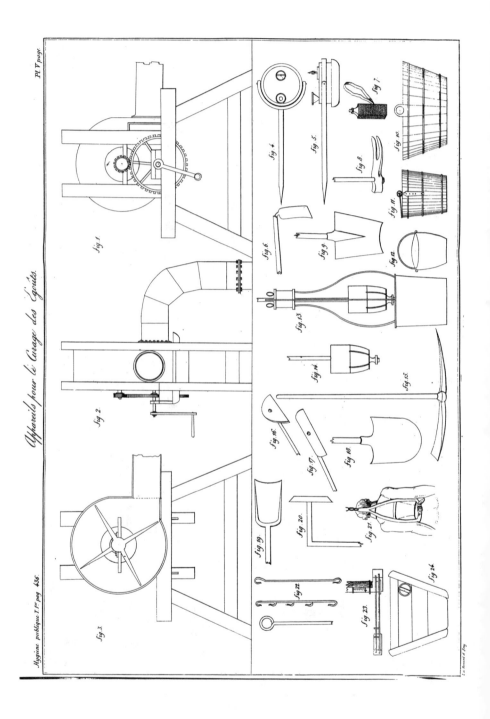

Fig. 1.
Fig. 2.
Fig. 3.
Fig. 4.
Fig. 5.
Fig. 6.
Fig. 7.
Fig. 8.
Fig. 9.
Fig. 10.
Fig. 11.
Fig. 12.
Fig. 13.
Fig. 14.
Fig. 15.
Fig. 16.
Fig. 17.
Fig. 18.
Fig. 19.
Fig. 20.
Fig. 21.
Fig. 22.
Fig. 23.
Fig. 24.

solid matter, sand, and mud clung. Many sewers clogged up rapidly because of their small diameter, which also made them difficult to clean. Additionally, many sewers lacked sufficient incline, so that matter stagnated in them until a good rainstorm washed it out. Finally, and most important, before the 1830s the system of water distribution in Paris was inadequate to flush out sewers, since during dry spells there was not enough water to keep them clean. Cleaning sewers was hazardous to sewer workers, with the major health problems being asphyxiation (*plomb*) and severe eye irritation (*mitte*), from which cesspool cleaners also suffered. Attention had been drawn to the problem of asphyxiation in 1782, when eight workers were asphyxiated in the Amelot sewer, prompting hygienists Antoine Cadet de Vaux and Jean-Noël Hallé to investigate and publish reports on the subject. In 1826 the Paris health council reported that it had been so long since some of the sewers had been cleaned that they had actually been lost. Therefore in June 1826, the prefect of police named a commission, including some health council members, to determine the hygienic precautions to be taken before the sewer could be cleaned. The commission recommended adequate ventilation, along with thorough disinfection of the sewers with chloride of lime. Hygienists judged the job, begun the next month and completed in January 1827, a great success, because an examination of sewer workers following completion of the work found them in good health. All totaled 3,000 cubic meters or 2,150 barrels of solid matter and two and one-half times that much liquid matter were extracted. The solids were deposited at the city dump at Montfaucon, and the liquids were dumped into the Seine. The cleaning of the Amelot sewer set an important public health precedent, showing that

Figure 3 Figures 1, 2, and 3 are proposed ventilating systems to alleviate the danger of asphyxiation in sewer cleaning. Lamps for use in sewers are shown in figures 4 and 5. Figures 6, 8, and 15 are picks; figures 9, 18, and 19 are shovels for removing solid wastes; and figures 16 and 17 are instruments for scraping solid wastes off the bottom of the sewers. Figures 10, 11, and 12 are buckets, and figure 22 shows hooks. Figures 20, 23, and 24 illustrate pipes and a wooden barrier with a pipe running through it, the idea being to pipe out the liquid wastes. Figure 21 shows how a sewer worker can be lowered into and removed from a sewer. Figure 7 is a bottle containing powdered bleach that can be hung from the worker's neck in an attempt to purify the air. Figures 13 and 14 are apparati developed in an effort to trap noxious sewer gases. From Parent-Duchâtelet, "Rapport sur le curage des égouts Amelot, de la Roquette, Saint-Martin et autres," *Hygiène publique*, 1: 436.

with proper precautions sewer cleaning need not be hazardous to health, thereby encouraging more frequent cleaning of sewers in the future.[29]

Uncovered sewers also caused public health problems. The Bièvre River, one of the most important uncovered Parisian sewers, was a much discussed public health issue in the 1820s (see Figure 4). Sometimes called the Gobelins river after the Royal Tapestry Manufacture of the Gobelins located on its banks, the Bièvre was a small, shallow river about eight to ten feet wide that emptied into the Seine. More than 150 workshops and factories, primarily laundries, tanneries, and dyeing and degreasing establishments, were situated on the banks of the Bièvre. Long regarded as hazardous to those living in its vicinity, it ran through the St.-Marceau quarter on the left bank, which was one of the most heavily industrialized areas of Paris. As early as 1789, when physicians attributed various types of fevers and sore throats to emanations from the river, the government had asked the hygienist Jean-Noël Hallé to do a report on the sanitary state of the Bièvre and to suggest ways to clean up the air in the vicinity. As a result of the Hallé report, some improvements had been made by the 1820s. Nevertheless, problems and complaints persisted. Industries located along the banks of the Bièvre used its water supply while dumping industrial wastes into the river. Laundries used river water for washing clothes, and the health council pointed out in 1822 that customers complained of big yellow spots left on their clothes by the water. Animal carcasses were thrown into the river, and smaller open sewers emptied human and household wastes into the Bièvre. To make matters worse, the course of the river was natural, not embanked, with a sluggish current. The bottom and banks were a slimy, muddy mass that, when churned up by factory waterwheels, spread offensive odors throughout the area. Odors were particularly bad in summer, when the water level was low and the river practically stagnant. Parent-Duchâtelet described the Bièvre as "a veritable sewer filled with water charged with animal matter, habitually exhaling a

29 Parent-Duchâtelet, "Essai sur les cloaques ou égouts," pp. 260–1; see Jean-Noël Hallé, Recherches sur la nature et les effets du méphitisme des fosses d'aisance (Paris: Pierres, 1785); Antoine-Alexis Cadet de Vaux, Observations sur les fosses d'aisance, et moyens de prévenir les inconvéniens de leur vidange (Paris: Pierres, 1778). Cadet de Vaux's work was done in collaboration with Laborie and Parmentier. Moléon, R. G. Paris, 1826, pp. 365–71; see the report of the commission, written by the reporter, Parent-Duchâtelet, "Rapport sur le curage des égouts Amelot, de la Roquette, Saint-Martin et autres, ou exposé des moyens qui ont été mis en usage pour exécuter cette grande opération, sans compromettre la salubrité publique et la santé des ouvriers qui y ont été employés," Hygiène publique, 1: 308–437. The other members of the commission were Joseph d'Arcet, Pierre Girard, and Henri Gaultier de Claubry, members of the Paris health council; R. E. Devilliers, chief engineer of the St. Martin canal; Pierre Cordier, division inspector of mines and professor of geology at the Museum of Natural History; and Parton, general inspector of salubrity for Paris.

detestable odor, especially during the heat of summer," and Claude Lachaise spoke of the "thick, gooey mud several feet deep upon either side."[30]

The Royal Academy of Medicine and the Paris health council debated the problems of the Bièvre in 1821–2, discussing whether the river was a health hazard or not, and if so, what should be done about it. The health council made some general recommendations, but the best research on the topic was the joint report of Parent-Duchâtelet and Charles Pavet de Courteille, submitted to the Royal Academy of Medicine and read there in January 1822. This report launched Parent-Duchâtelet's career as a public hygienist and earned for him praise from colleagues.[31] The hygienists' examination of those living near the river did not support the commonly held view that unsanitary conditions in the neighborhood of the Bièvre caused bad health and general weakness. Using methods of on-site observation as well as analysis of hospital and dispensary records, Parent-Duchâtelet and Pavet de Courteille concluded: "Even though [we were] prejudiced against the river when we began our research, it has been impossible to find the slightest difference in the health and physical constitution of those who inhabit its banks and those who live in other quarters."[32] All workers questioned said that even though the river's odors were foul, their health did not suffer. The records of the local dispensary showed no difference in Bièvre inhabitants and those from other areas, and Parent-Duchâtelet and Pavet de Courteille suggested – to account for the difference of opinion – that residents had become acclimated to the river, since most of those questioned had lived there all their lives. Personnel at the Hôtel-Dieu, however, claimed that residents of the St.-Marceau quarter had more serious cases of disease, taking longer to recover than other Parisians. Although Parent-Duchâtelet and Pavet de Courteille found this opinion to have some foundation, they believed that if these workers suffered from poor health, the cause was not emanations from the river, but workers' physical constitutions and their type of work. From their on-site investigations, the hygienists concluded that bad air was not the

30 Hallé's report was presented at the Royal Society of Medicine in 1790. See Claude Lachaise, *Topographie médicale de Paris* (Paris: Baillière, 1822), p. 200. Quotation, p. 198. See pp. 198–210 for Lachaise's discussion of the Bièvre. Quote from A. J. B. Parent-Duchâtelet and Charles Pavet de Courteille, "Recherches et considérations sur la rivière de Bièvre...," *Hygiène publique*, 1: 128. For a history of odors with particular reference to France, see Alain Corbin, *Le miasme et la jonquille: L'odorat et l'imaginaire social, 18–19e siècles* (Paris: Aubier Montaigne, 1982), esp. part 2.
31 Moléon, *R. G. Paris*, 1821, pp. 185–8. The report on the Bièvre was first published in 1822: *Recherches et considérations sur la rivière de Bièvre* (Paris: Crevot, 1822). The report on the Bièvre was also published in *Hygiène publique*, 1: 98–155.
32 Parent-Duchâtelet and Pavet de Courteille, "Recherches et considérations," p. 130.

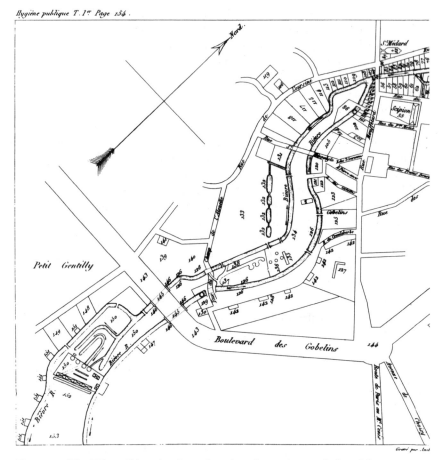

Figure 4 The Bièvre River in 1822, showing the numerous industrial establishments located on its banks and in the vicinity. Industrial establishments included distilleries, laundries, tanneries, dying and degreasing establishments, starch works, and leather shops. The following points of interest are identified: 3, the quai de l'Hôpital; 4, the quai St.-Bernard; 5, the mouth of the Bièvre, emptying into the Seine; 11, the hospice de la Salpêtrière; 12, the old Salpêtrière sewer; 13, the new Salpêtrière sewer; 14, the Villejuif abattoir; 15, the sewer from the Villejuif abattoir; 16, restaurants and private houses; 31, hospice de la Pitié; 32 dissection amphitheater at the Pitié; 42, Austerlitz fountain; 98, large building housing many laundries; 125, Gobelins tapestry works. From Parent-Duchâtelet and Pavet de Courteille, "Recherches et considérations sur la rivière de Bièvre," *Hygiène publique*, 1: 154.

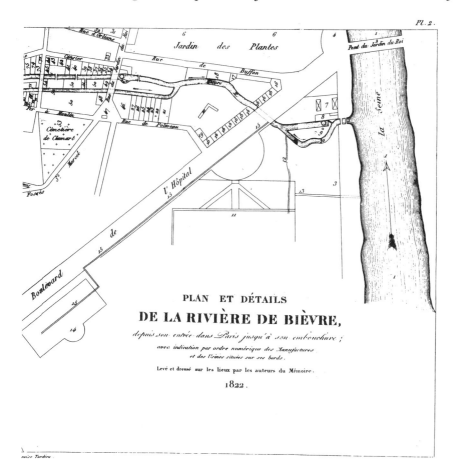

PLAN ET DÉTAILS

DE LA RIVIÈRE DE BIÈVRE,

depuis son entrée dans Paris jusqu'à son embouchure ;

avec indication par ordre numérique des Manufactures
et des Usines situées sur ses bords.

Levé et dressé sur les lieux par les auteurs du Mémoire.

1822.

only factor that caused bad health, but other work- and constitution-related conditions as well.

In order to improve the quality of air in the vicinity of the Bièvre, Parent-Duchâtelet and Pavet de Courteille recommended an increased water supply so that the river would flow more quickly, embankment of the river to facilitate cleaning, and removal of high structures and trees from its banks in order to improve air and water circulation. The hygienists argued that the cost of the improvements, estimated at 300,000 to 400,000 francs, should be borne by rich manufacturers whose establishments were located along the river. Some of the hygienists' suggestions were taken. Under Rambuteau, the Bièvre was embanked and cleaned out, improving for a while the general situation on the left bank. But as late as the 1870s, the river still functioned as an open sewer, because numerous workshops crowded along its banks continued to use it as a receptacle for their industrial wastes.[33]

Some sewer drainage problems were solved by the 1840s, when the construction of new underground sewers proceeded rapidly. In 1824 Paris had only 35,846 meters of underground sewers, but by 1837 this figure had doubled. Rambuteau claimed that annually from 1833 to 1848 he built 7,000 to 8,000 meters of cement sewers, which added to existing sewers totaled – by 1848 – about 140,000 meters of underground sewers. Sewers built after 1830 were better constructed than earlier ones, since they were paved and large enough to clean. In addition, the increased water supply, the improved water distribution through pipes into some establishments and homes, and the proliferation of street fountains made it possible to keep sewers cleaner. More water ran continuously through the sewers, virtually eliminating the problem of asphyxiation. Sewers were easily washed out and cleaned regularly two or three times weekly. Finally, more widespread use of disinfectants made sewer cleaning less obnoxious and less hazardous.[34]

In his 1824 study Parent-Duchâtelet advocated the complete reconstruction of the Paris sewer system, envisaging the connection of each dwelling and factory with sewers by underground pipes. He suggested one set of pipes to carry fresh water directly into each establishment and dwelling, and another to carry household and human liquid wastes directly to the sewers. There were no immediate practical results of his recommendations, however. Although he was not officially consulted on the immense underground sewer works undertaken between 1824 and 1835, his suggestions were taken into consideration. Parent-Duchâtelet later noted that when improvements were finally made, the engineers had faithfully followed his indications.[35]

33 Parent-Duchâtelet and Pavet de Courteille, "Recherches sur la rivière de Bièvre," pp. 137–53; Rambuteau, *Mémoires*, p. 371; Pinkney, *Rebuilding of Paris*, p. 19; Archives de Paris et de l'ancien département de la Seine, V. I⁵3, Mémoire de l'inspecteur général des Ponts et Chaussées, directeur des eaux et des égouts. Undated, but probably 1871.

34 Parent-Duchâtelet, "Essai sur les cloaques ou égouts," pp. 207, 210; Parent-Duchâtelet reported that by 1830 there were 40,000 meters in service; that between 1830 and 1834, 21,960 meters were built; and that in 1835, 5,028 meters were built. Alphonse Chevallier, "Mémoire sur les égouts de Paris, de Londres, de Montpellier," p. 382; Rambuteau, *Mémoires*, p. 376. Maxine Du Camp said Rambuteau had built 78,675 meters of new sewers. See *Paris*, 5: 431; Boudin, "Etudes sur le pavage," p. 270. Boudin said there were 130,000 meters of sewers in Paris, 5,900 meters outside the walls but serving for the *assainissement* of Paris, and 4,500 meters of individual sewers kept up by the administration, giving a total of 140,000 meters, which comes very close to Rambuteau's figure. Boudin reported that by 1851 sewers were cleaned twice a week, some major ones every other day, by washing and extraction. See Boudin, "Etudes sur le pavage," p. 270.

35 Parent-Duchâtelet, "Des cloaques ou égouts," p. 299; Parent-Duchâtelet, "Rapport sur les améliorations à introduire dans les fosses d'aisance," *Hygiène publique*, 2:

In 1847 the Paris municipal council debated a vast sewer project that would have included building two large main sewers paralleling the banks of the Seine to carry water from all existing sewers down below the Pont d'Iéna, where all matter would be dumped into the river. The sewer project was part of a master plan that Rambuteau proposed, but that was never implemented, because of the 1848 revolution. Rambuteau commented in his memoirs that the sewer project was in a sense his "last will and testament." A major overhaul of the sewer system was not undertaken in the first half of the nineteenth century, so many problems persisted, such as uncovered sewers and gutters and the notorious Bièvre. The drainage situation in the rural communes was not solved, even as late as 1847. And the sewer system, although it had been significantly extended and improved, was still inadequate for a city the size of Paris.[36]

It is important to note that even reform-minded Parent-Duchâtelet did not have a complete sanitary sewer system in mind when he envisioned the total overhaul of the Paris sewers. One individual who did advocate multipurpose sewers for Paris and the total abolition of cesspools had his ideas rejected by a commission of which Parent-Duchâtelet was a member. It was the opinion of the commission that such a system would be impractical in Paris because of insufficient incline and inadequate water.[37] The underlying assumption of most French hygienists and administrators was that human wastes were too valuable as fertilizer and ammonia products to be washed away through sewers. Parent-Duchâtelet was one of the first to suggest the radical idea of disposing of liquid wastes through sewers. But even he never suggested sending solid wastes through sewers. In the early nineteenth century the prevailing French idea was waste conservation, not waste disposal, and for this purpose the cesspool system, which had been widely adopted, had some merit.

CESSPOOLS AND SANITARY REFORM

Parent-Duchâtelet believed cesspools were the main stumbling block to major sanitary reform in Paris. The suppression of cesspools and the disposal of human wastes through sewers was a revolution that did not come easily or quickly. At stake were a number of interest groups, economic considerations, and the underlying philosophy of waste collection and disposal, which was based on cesspools and waste conservation. French

370–89, 392–402; Parent-Duchâtelet, "Introduction," *De la prostitution dans la ville de Paris*, 3rd ed. (Paris: Baillière, 1857), p. 17.
36 Rambuteau, *Mémoires*, pp. 292–3. R. G. *Paris*, 1847, p. 105.
37 "Rapport fait au préfet de police sur une modification proposée dans le système des égouts de Paris," *Annales d'hygiène publique* 32 (1844): 326–50.

hygienists and the public thought in terms of the collection and *conservation* of wastes instead of the collection and *disposal* of wastes. Human wastes were usually disposed of in cesspools, which were large underground tanks, built of impermeable material, in which liquid and solid human wastes accumulated.[38] A pipe connected the cesspool with the latrine, and in some dwellings a small stream of water washed waste matter down the pipe. When cesspools were introduced in Paris in the sixteenth century, they promised to be a vast public health improvement over the then-common habit of throwing wastes into streets and gutters. Enforcement of regulations regarding cesspool construction was lax until the eighteenth century; then, when cesspools came into widespread use, there were some unexpected and unfortunate consequences. Many were not carefully built, so that liquid wastes seeped into the ground. Waste seepage polluted the water supply, which came mainly from private wells, with the result that much private well water became unfit for drinking and even for cleaning purposes. In addition, without liquids to dilute the solid matter in cesspools, solid wastes fermented, and many cesspools became infected, making cleaning a major public health problem, since cesspool cleaners were quickly asphyxiated. This unanticipated development motivated eighteenth-century hygienists to focus on the problem of cesspool cleaning, but it was not until the nineteenth century that effective measures were taken to improve cesspool construction.[39]

Nineteenth-century regulations on cesspool construction helped eliminate some problems, but they also created new ones. Ordinances of 1809 and 1819 prescribed the size, shape, type of material, and ventilation requirements for new cesspools, as well as guidelines for the reconstruction and repair of existing ones. An ordinance of 1834 regulated the method of cleaning and the service of both fixed and movable cesspools.[40] Improved construction kept liquid wastes from leaking out, thereby making cleaning easier and asphyxiation less of a problem. When liquids no longer seeped out, however, the cesspools had to be emptied more frequently, an onerous charge for proprietors. Parent-Duchâtelet noted that by 1835 many cesspools had to be cleaned once or twice annually, whereas before, when liquids seeped into the ground, they were cleaned only once every eight or ten years.

38 Parent-Duchâtelet, "Rapport sur les améliorations," pp. 381–2; Parent-Duchâtelet, "Essai sur les cloaques ou égouts," p. 215. The exceptions were the Ecole Militaire, the Hôtel des Invalides, and the hospice of Salpêtrière, which did not have cesspools and so emptied wastes directly into sewers.

39 On the history of cesspools, see A. J. B. Parent-Duchâtelet and Henri Gaultier de Claubry, "Latrines" (Hygiène et technologie), *Dictionnaire de l'industrie manufacturière* 7 (1838): 105–19; see also the article that follows by Gourlier, "Latrines" (Construction), pp. 119–26.

40 A.N., F¹³986 (1809); A.N., F⁸175 (1919); A.N., F⁸186 (1834).

Thus, by the 1830s, improvements in cesspool construction and an increasing water supply temporarily made the situation worse than ever. Better-built cesspools no longer allowed liquid wastes to seep into the ground; whereas before only solid wastes had to be cleaned out and removed, now liquids did too. Increased water supply and better water distribution further complicated the situation, for more water meant more frequent cesspool cleaning. The growing popularity of at-home bathing also added to the problem, as leftover bath water was most conveniently thrown into the latrine, ending up in the cesspool. Many cesspools that had formerly been cleaned every four or five years now had to be cleaned two or three times a year, with 90 percent of the extracted matter being liquid. By the 1830s cesspools were becoming outmoded in Paris, even though their use continued into the twentieth century.

The main problem with cesspools was cleaning them (see Figure 5). Many hygienists, physicians, and laymen associated bad smells with disease-causing agents, so cleaning cesspools always constituted a public health problem. Figures from the 1840s illustrate the magnitude of the problem. Between 200 and 250 cesspool cleaners, or *vidangeurs*, cleaned an estimated 30,000 cesspools in Paris in 1842, and hygienist Alphonse Guérard estimated that in 1846 about 100 cesspools were cleaned each night. Cesspool cleaners, who obtained the concession from the city government, paid the city a given amount per cubic meter of liquids and solids extracted, and then could exploit the resources as they wanted. At the same time, proprietors paid the cesspool cleaners for the cleaning operation. New methods of cleaning cesspools were developed during the period, the most popular of which consisted of using a pump to extract liquid wastes. Once the liquids were removed, cesspool cleaners descended into the cesspool, shoveled the heavy wastes into barrels, and scraped and cleaned the bottom and sides of the cesspool. Both liquid and solid wastes were put into closed barrels, which were then transported on wagons to the city dump at Montfaucon. Before the discovery and use of disinfectants, cleaning cesspools was a horrible spectacle by all accounts.[41]

Before the 1830s, when the situation came to a head with the increased water supply, hygienists devoted their attention to improving the existing cesspool system. Hygienist and industrial chemist Joseph d'Arcet

---

41 Treatises on cesspools include Alexandre Bottex, *Des améliorations à introduire dans la construction et le curage des fosses d'aisance* (Lyon: Extrait des *Annales des sciences physiques et naturelles d'agriculture et d'industrie*. Publié par la Société royale d'agriculture de Lyon, 1838); Martin jeune, *Mémoire sur le curage des fosses d'aisance dans la ville de Lyon* (Lyon: Rusand, 1829); and of course, Parent-Duchâtelet, "Rapport sur les améliorations à introduire dans les fosses d'aisance." Isidore Bricheteau, Alphonse Chevallier, and Furnari, "Note sur les vidangeurs," *Annales d'hygiène publique* 28 (1842): 48; Alphonse Guérard, "Note sur un nouveau système de vidanges des fosses d'aisance," *Annales d'hygiène publique* 35 (1846): 77–8.

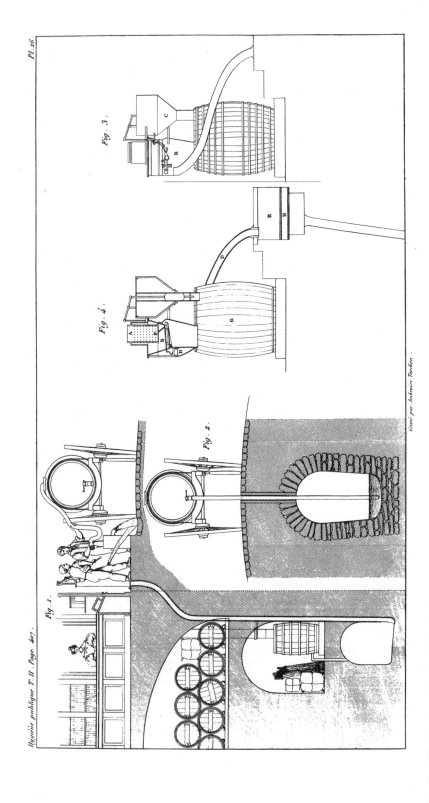

Pl. 26.

Fig. 1.

Fig. 2.

Fig. 3.

Fig. 4.

Gravé par Imbroise Tardieu.

emphasized improved ventilation and developed a system of forced ventilation, whereby noxious gases would be blown off into the air above the house through a tall chimney. He believed this improvement, along with the use of disinfectants, would make the cesspool acceptable and modern. A more popular solution, advocated by most hygienists, was the movable cesspool (*fosse mobile*) (see Figure 6), developed in 1818 by J. Martin Cazeneuve.[42] The movable cesspool consisted of two barrels, one for liquids and one for solids, instead of the usual permanent underground pit. The waste matter flowed through a pipe into one barrel, with the liquids flowing down into a pipe leading to another barrel. The barrels were closed and therefore theoretically odorless. When full, they could simply be carted off and replaced by an empty barrel. The main advantages of the movable cesspool were that it eliminated the dangers and inconveniences associated with cesspool cleaning (see Figure 7), and it separated wastes, making it easier to convert solid matter into fertilizer. Although movable cesspools offered obvious advantages, they were expensive, the barrels had to be removed often, and hence they were not widely adopted by the 1830s. They were mainly used in public buildings and in the homes of the wealthy. They became fairly common in Paris, but in Lyon, according to

42 Bottex, *La construction et le curage des fosses d'aisance*, p. 6; J. P. Joseph d'Arcet, "Instruction du Conseil de salubrité sur la construction des latrines publiques, et sur l'assainissement des latrines et des fosses d'aisance" (1822), in *Collection de mémoires relatifs à l'assainissement des édifices publics et des habitations particulières*, 2 vols. (Paris: Mathias, 1843), 1: 144–59; A. N., F[13]986, dossier Fosses d'aisance, 1806–21; *Des Fosses d'aisance mobiles inodores* (Paris: aux Bureaux de l'Entreprise générale, 1818) accompanied by Dubois, Jean-Baptiste Huzard, and Héricart de Thury, *Rapport sur les fosses mobiles et inodores de MM. Cazeneuve et Cie.*, fait à la Société royale et centrale d'Agriculture, dans sa séance du 19 août 1818. This dossier also contains several letters on movable cesspools that are of great interest. Hygienists in other cities took up the innovation for consideration. For example, Archives Municipales de Lyon, I¹267, Grognier, Terme, and Tissier, *Rapport sur les fosses d'aisance mobiles et inodores, fait à la Société de Médecine de Lyon, 16 avril 1819.*

Figure 5 Cesspools and cesspool cleaning. Figure 1 shows a cross section of a building with three underground levels, the bottom one being reserved for the cesspool. This arrangement, common in Parisian buildings, made cleaning very difficult, and Parent-Duchâtelet proposed converting the cesspool into a receptacle for liquid wastes and placing a barrel for solid wastes on the second level. The drawing shows the liquid wastes being pumped out and either poured into the street, along with water from a street fountain, or being put in a barrel to be disposed of elsewhere. Figure 2 shows the contents of the barrel in figure 1 being piped into a sewer. Figures 3 and 4 show one of several types of movable cesspools available at the time to separate liquid from solid wastes, this being the apparatus of Burand and Payen. This type of movable cesspool was being used at the Bicêtre hospital. From Parent-Duchâtelet, "Rapport sur les améliorations à introduire dans les fosses d'aisances," *Hygiène publique*, 2: 407.

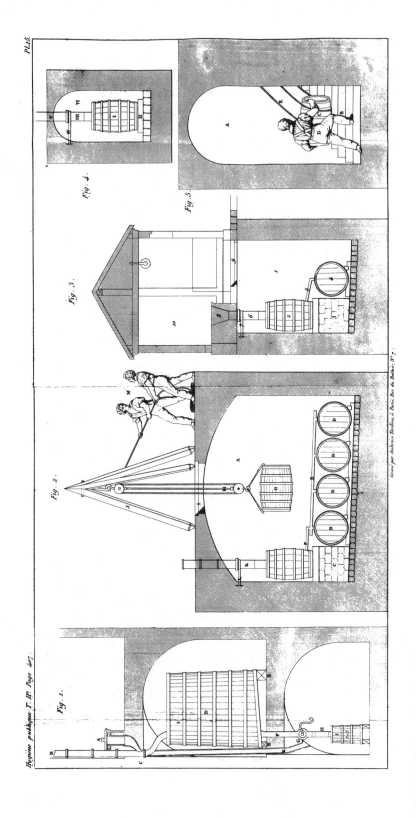

Fig. 1.

Fig. 2.

Fig. 3.

Fig. 4.

Fig. 5.

Pl.15.

Lyonnais hygienists Jean-Baptiste Monfalcon and Isidore Polinière, they were hardly in use by 1846, except in some public buildings.[43] By the mid-1830s, with the continually increasing amounts of water flowing into cesspools, the question of cesspool cleaning came to a head.

In 1835 a health council commission composed of Parent-Duchâtelet (chairman) and pharmacist-chemists A. G. Labarraque and Alphonse Chevallier published a report on the public health problems associated with cesspools and dumps. The commission proposed the adoption of movable cesspools so that liquids could be separated from solids, which could then be converted into fertilizer. The liquids, they suggested, could be thrown into sewers or the river, as was the practice in London and other cities. The commission argued that the proportion of water to urine would be great enough – due to increasing amounts of water flowing through the sewers – that this new method would not pose a public health problem. With a cheap, convenient way to dispose of liquid wastes, proprietors would be more inclined to favor increasing the water supply, hygienists contended. The commission blamed cesspools and the archaic system of cesspool cleaning for the outmoded water distribution system in Paris, suggesting that proprietors were reluctant to provide more water to renters because of the difficulty and expense of cleaning cesspools. The commission suggested that liquid wastes be sent through gutters, for if they were diluted with water, they would be no more foul than other household wastes already flowing through open sewers. If necessary, disinfectants could be used. The commission foresaw a time when all houses

---

43 Parent-Duchâtelet, "Améliorations des fosses d'aisance," pp. 357–63; Bottex, "Fosses d'aisance," pp. 17–20; Jean-Baptiste Monfalcon and A. P. Isidore de Polinière, *Hygiène de Lyon* (Paris: Baillière, 1846), p. 395; Jean-Baptiste Monfalcon and A. P. Isidore de Polinière, *Traité de la salubrité dans les grandes villes* (Paris: Baillière, 1846), pp. 71–2, 76; Parent-Duchâtelet, "Latrines," pp. 109–11. Several other systems for immediate separation of liquids and solids were available, but hygienists believed the movable cesspools to be most advantageous.

Figure 6 *Fosses mobiles*, or movable cesspools. Figure 1 shows Gourlier's movable cesspool system, whereby the wastes from the water closet (A) flowed to a large barrel (D), where the solids were collected, and the liquids flowed on to a movable cesspool or barrel (I). Figure 2 shows an ordinary cesspool with a movable apparatus. The barrel for solids is between K and C, and the four barrels marked D are for liquids. Workers are removing one of the barrels for disposal. Figure 3 shows a cesspool like that in figure 2, but with room for only one barrel for liquid wastes. (10) is the water closet, (2) is the barrel for solid wastes, and (4) is the barrel for liquid wastes. Figure 4 gives the detail of a barrel for solid wastes. Figure 5 shows a different method of removing a movable cesspool. From Parent-Duchâtelet, "Rapport sur les améliorations à introduire dans les fosses d'aisances," *Hygiène publique*, 2: 407.

MASQUES POUR PÉNÉTRER DANS LES LIEUX INFECTÉS.

Pl. 1.

Fig. 6.

Fig. 21.

Fig. 20.

Fig. 10.

Fig. 9.

Fig. 5.

Fig. 18.

Fig. 17.

Fig. 4.

Fig. 16.

Fig. 19.

Fig. 11.

Fig. 12.

Fig. 13.

Fig. 14.

Fig. 15.

Fig. 3.

Fig. 2.

Fig. 7.

Fig. 1.

Fig. 8.

Gravé par Ambroise Tardieu.

and other establishments would be connected to underground sewers by underground pipes, and then only solid wastes would have to be collected in cesspools.[44]

The commission's proposals constituted what Parent-Duchâtelet called a "veritable revolution" in waste disposal: the suppression of permanent cesspools made possible by eventual conversion of storm sewers into multipurpose sewers for disposal of liquid wastes, collection of solid wastes in movable cesspools, conversion of solid wastes into fertilizer by the use of disinfectants, and decentralization of the fertilizer industry by the establishment of many small processing factories.[45] Parent-Duchâtelet, Labarraque, and Chevallier still did not advocate a complete sanitary sewer system, however, for in the first half of the century the conversion of solid wastes into fertilizer was an important industry that yielded substantial municipal revenues as well as individual profits. Some hygienists questioned the wisdom of disposing of liquid wastes through sewers, not only for public health but also for economic reasons, since liquid wastes were

44 Even as late as 1873, out of about 85,000 cesspools in Paris, only about 19,000 were movable. See Du Camp, *Paris,* 5: 471, note 1; Parent-Duchâtelet, "Rapport sur les améliorations."
45 Parent-Duchâtelet, "Rapport sur les améliorations," pp. 387–8, 392.

Figure 7 Masks for protection against infected air. Figure 1 shows a plague outfit worn by Marseillais physicians during the 1720 plague epidemic, and figures 2 and 3 show outfits worn by quarantine officials who managed the Marseilles lazaretto in 1819 (at the time of the Spanish yellow fever scare). Each holds a fumigating apparatus. An apparatus containing a cotton filter is pictured in figure 4. Air breathed in passed through a cotton filter that was supposed to purify it. An ordinary sponge is shown in figure 5, and in figure 6 it is used as an air filter. Figure 7 shows a man carrying a leather air tank with enough air for thirty minutes. In figure 8 a man descends into a sewer or cesspool to rescue an asphyxiated worker. He's breathing outside air through a tube, but if he forgets and takes a breath, he will be instantly asphyxiated. A major problem with this breathing apparatus is that the rescue worker doesn't have the use of his right hand to carry out the asphyxiated worker. The apparatus was judged not suitable for the job. The apparatus shown in figure 9 improved upon some of the inconveniences of that in figure 8, because it freed the hands and arms, but the wearer could still be asphyxiated if he breathed through his mouth. A safer model is shown in figure 10. The nostrils are pinched shut, and the wearer breathes in pure air through the mouth. Figures 11, 12, 13, 14, 15, 16, 17, and 18 show cross sections of parts of the equipment in figure 10, and figure 19 shows pincers for keeping the nostrils shut. In figure 20 Robert's mask is illustrated. Robert was a physician at the Marseilles lazaratto. Figure 21 is a modified version of figure 20 as developed by Parisian firemen. From "Mémoire sur un moyen mécanique nouvellement proposé pour respirer impunément les gaz délétères et pénétrer avec facilité dans les lieux qui en sont remplis," *Hygiène publique,* 1: 92.

used to make ammonia products. Reformers argued that increased dilution of urine resulting from increased water use meant that the industry was being displaced anyway, so there was no economic reason for opposing the proposed plan.

Not until 1850 were liquid wastes disposed of by sewers, as Parent-Duchâtelet and the health council commission had recommended. The practice did not prove as odorless as had been anticipated, however. Sewers were not used for the disposal of solid wastes until the late nineteenth century. The monumental sewer system of Haussmann was primarily a storm sewer system, designed to solve the city's drainage problems and clean up the Seine. Cesspools continued to be in common use through the third quarter of the century, their cleaning problems becoming more acute with the increasing water supply. As late as 1873 there were more than 85,000 cesspools in Paris, of which 52,000 still required the traditional *vidange*.[46]

THE DUMP AT MONTFAUCON

One of the most widely publicized public health problems was the city dump at Montfaucon (see Figure 8), whose odors, wafting over the city, made Paris smell horrible if the wind blew in the wrong direction. The dump was composed of two parts, one that served as the receptacle for human wastes and the other – considered even more disgusting by contemporary observers – the horsebutcher yards. Since the late eighteenth century the dump had attracted the attention of administrators and hygienists who demanded its suppression, but by the 1830s there was still no suitable alternative. Fear of cholera focused renewed attention on the dump when sanitary commissions singled it out as a likely foyer of infection. Although hygienists had asserted the harmlessness of its putrid

---

46 Du Camp, *Paris*, 5: 471, note 1; Pinkney, *Napoleon III and the Rebuilding of Paris*, pp. 129, 144–5.

Figure 8 Overview of the Montfaucon dump, where the horsebutcher yards were located. The dump also served as a depot for wastes from the city of Paris. This is the view from Butte-Saint-Chaumont, with the hill of Montmartre in the background. In the lower left-hand corner are the old horsebutcher yard of Dusaussois and three gut workshops. To the right are kilns and, a little in front of them, another horsebutcher yard. In the background are houses in the commune of La Villette and, to the far left, Poissonnière. Between the houses in the background and the horsebutcher yards are two thirty-feet-deep basins where wastes were deposited. Liquid wastes drained off into lower basins and solids were left to dry out, later to be used as fertilizer. From Parent-Duchâtelet, "Les chantiers d'équarrissage de la ville de Paris," *Hygiène publique*, 2: 256.

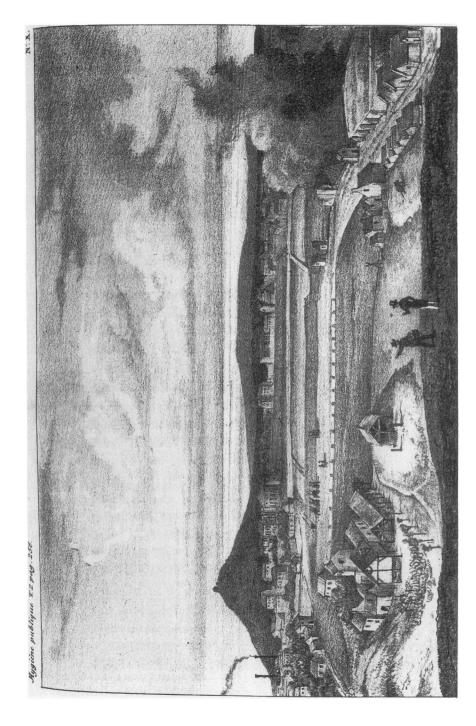

emanations, common sense dictated that such a foul place must cause disease.[47]

The area where the dump was located, at the foot of the hills of Belleville, had centuries earlier been quarried, with the result that huge basins had been dug. These basins, used for the deposit of human wastes, were more than 32,800 square meters in area. In the 1820s between 230 and 244 cubic meters of waste products from cesspools were brought to Montfaucon daily, to be deposited in the two basins, which were each thirty feet deep. There solids were separated from liquids, which flowed into lower basins, eventually traveling via canals and sewers back into the Seine. The solid matter was deposited to dry on some eighteen acres of land and was then transported into the rural communes surrounding Paris, where it was piled in heaps to ferment into fertilizer. After 1823 liquid wastes flowed first to the canal St.-Martin, thereby crossing the city, then into the Seine. Hygienist Henri Gaultier de Claubry called the situation a state of barbarism, pointing out that wastes flowed into the Seine below the Pont d'Austerlitz, where some of the public baths were located.[48]

In earlier times the dump had not been a major problem for Parisians, for it was located away from the center of the city. However, by the late eighteenth and early nineteenth centuries, Paris had expanded outward toward Montfaucon, so that the dump became surrounded by dwellings. In addition, as the population grew, the amount of cesspool matter deposited at Montfaucon increased, with the result that recently populated

47 A. J. B. Parent-Duchâtelet, "Les chantiers d'équarrissage de la ville de Paris envisagés sous le rapport de l'hygiène publique," *Hygiène publique*, 2: 224–41. Parent-Duchâtelet had become intimately acquainted with the dump in the early 1820s while completing his first hygienic investigation, which dealt with the health hazards to sailors of transporting fertilizer by ship: "Recherches pour découvrir la cause et la nature d'accidens très graves développés en mer, à bord d'un bâtiment chargé de poudrette," *Hygiène publique*, 2: 257–85. He presented this report to the Royal Academy of Medicine in 1821; the first investigation set the tone for his public health works and won for him praise by Charles C. H. Marc and Jean-Baptiste Huzard, who lauded his zeal and perseverance, as well as his rigorous observational method. Marc, a physician, and Huzard, a veterinarian, were both members of the Paris health council.

48 Parent-Duchâtelet, "Essai sur les cloaques ou égouts," p. 234. The figures refer to 1824. The whole group of five basins was called Loiseau's pond (*l'étang de Loiseau*), after Loiseau, an old horse flayer who made a name for himself in the trade. Prefect of Police Gisquet (1831–6) estimated that daily about 220 cubic meters of liquid wastes (*eaux vannes*) flowed into the Seine. Gisquet, *Mémoires*, 4: 229–301. See H. Gaultier de Claubry, "De la suppression de la voirie de Montfaucon comme consé-quence des procédés perfectionnés de désinfection des fosses d'aisances," *Annales d'hygiène publique* 40 (1848): 311–12. Before the opening of the St.-Martin canal, sewage wastes from Montfaucon flowed into the Seine above Chaillot, below the most inhabited area of the city. See Parent-Duchâtelet, "Des chantiers d'équarris-sage," p. 252. This practice caused many complaints, and the health council dealt with the problem. See Moléon, *R. G. Paris*, 1823, p. 265; 1827, pp. 36–8; 1828, pp. 329–30; 1839, pp. 254–5.

areas – and sometimes even the city center – were subjected to increasingly insupportable odors coming from the dump. The foul emanations were, however, only partially caused by the deposits of human waste matter. Montfaucon served a dual purpose, housing one of the main workshops of the Parisian horsebutchering industry. As far as contemporaries were concerned, the horsebutcher yards were much more offensive than the basins filled with human wastes.[49] The horsebutchering (*équarrissage*) industry, an old, established industry in Paris, was generally viewed as distasteful, disgusting, and unhealthy. What to do with old, sick, and dead horses was a major public health concern in the early 1830s, when Parent-Duchâtelet estimated the Parisian horse population to be about 20,000. Rambuteau estimated that in 1848 there were 70,000 horses circulating in the city of Paris, whereas historian David Pinkney put the figure at only 37,000 by 1850.[50] Nearly all parts of the horse were worth money: The hide was sent to tanners, the blood was used both by refineries and as animal food; the flesh was eaten by both people and animals; the insides were used for fertilizer; the tendons, for glue; the oil, by industry, as it made good burning oil; the horse shoes were reused; the bones were used for ammonia, to make gelatin, and for fertilizer. Horsehair, surprisingly, was not an important product, much of the hair having been lost by old and sick horses.

Two of the most important Parisian horse slaughteryards (*clos d'équarrissage*) were located at the Montfaucon dump (see Figure 9), which made even more serious the supposed disease-causing odors emanating from the

49   Parent-Duchâtelet, "Les chantiers d'équarrissage," pp. 222–41. See also Corbin, *Le miasme et la jonquille*, pp. 141–2; Prefect of Police Gisquet commented, for example, that the human waste matter at the dump smelled like perfume in comparison with the emanations from the horsebutcher yards. Gisquet, *Mémoires*, 4: 307. Although the situation in Paris was bad enough, in some places it was worse. Parent-Duchâtelet reported that in Paris the horsebutchering industry had been practiced along these lines since the sixteenth century. Monfalcon and Polinière stated that until late in the eighteenth century in Lyon, horses and other animals were just thrown into the Rhône River, where they putrefied in the mud along the banks. See Monfalcon and Polinière, *Hygiène de Lyon*, pp. 395–6.

50   Parent-Duchâtelet, "Les chantiers d'équarrissage," pp. 167–213, p. 160, note 1. On the question of whether the cutting up and flaying of animals that had died of contagious diseases constituted a public health problem, see Parent-Duchâtelet, "Notice sur cette question: Peut-on sans inconvénient laisser tomber en desuétude l'art. 6 de l'arrêt du Conseil d'Etat du 16 juillet 1784, relatif à l'enfouissement des animaux morts de maladies contagieuses," *Hygiène publique*, 2: 332–49. The commission of the Academy of Medicine, which dealt with the problem (Louis-René Villermé, Jean-Pierre Barruel, Joseph Pelletier, Nicolas Adelon, Pierre Girard, and Alexandre Parent-Duchâtelet), concluded that the practice was not dangerous to the public health. Parent-Duchâtelet, "Les chantiers d'équarrissage," pp. 159–62. Pinkney, *Napoleon III and the Rebuilding of Paris*, p. 19. Rambuteau, *Mémoires*, p. 369. The discrepancy between Rambuteau's and Pinkney's figures cannot be explained for certain. Perhaps Pinkney referred to the permanent horse population, whereas Rambuteau included transients as well.

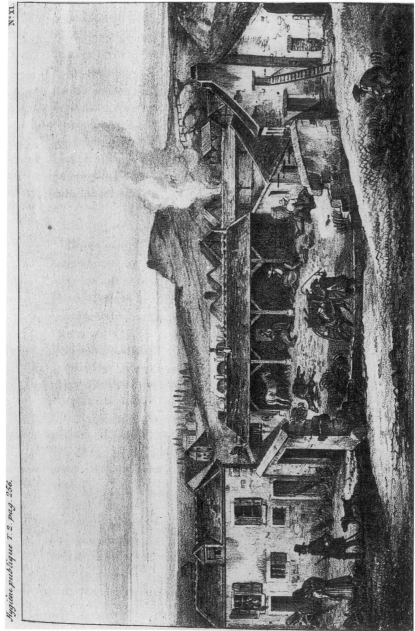

dump. Parent-Duchâtelet described the horsebutcher yards at Montfaucon, which were situated in the highest and most remote part of the dump. The first yard consisted of a paved court with a covered hangar that was attached to a stable and a large storehouse. Nearby was a foundry. These buildings were surrounded by walls and solid doors. Beneath the yard were two small houses where the horseflayer and his family and the gutmaker lived. A deep pit absorbed the liquid residue. If this enclosure did not present too disgusting an aspect, the second one did. In the second yard the flaying and butchering of horses and other small animals was done in the open air (see Figures 10 and 11). There were no buildings, except one containing horsemeat to be sold later as food. The courtyard had some partial paving beneath the soil, so that liquids were not easily absorbed, but instead stagnated. Since blood and intestinal debris were constantly underfoot, a few paths were shoveled out so that the workers could get to the places where the various processes were carried out. A wall that had formerly surrounded the second yard had been destroyed by rats, so it was replaced by horse carcasses stacked one on top of the other. There were no wells or any adequate water supply, so cleaning the yard was impossible. Nor were there containers for gathering and saving rainwater.[51]

The horsebutcher yards located at the city dump at Montfaucon offered a perfect opportunity to subject the miasmatic theory of disease causation to scientific scrutiny, since there was considerable disagreement about the public health dangers of the yards. On the occasion of the impending cholera epidemic of 1832, sanitary commissions were established to investigate sources of infection and areas in need of sanitary reform. The horsebutcher yards were a prime target of investigation. Even though some hygienists like Parent-Duchâtelet had questioned the harmful effects of the horsebutcher yards, the sanitary commission expressed the majority opinion: "As for us, in spite of all the reasoning of men of art, and all the logic of

---

51 Parent-Duchâtelet, "Les chantiers d'équarrissage," pp. 155–9. Parent-Duchâtelet recounted (p. 159, note 1) the story of some men who were at the yard doing physiological research. When they asked for water to wash their hands, it was brought to them in a large horse intestine that had been tied together at one end.

Figure 9 Detail of part of the old horsebutcher yard of Dusaussois. On the right, a worker is gathering maggots. On the left a man, a woman, and a dog are carrying horsemeat. The small dwelling on the right is the workshop of the gutmaker; the building on the left is occupied by a worker and his family, who live on the first floor. The ground floor contains a large room where dogs and cats are butchered. In the center are horses that have died in Paris. Since they are fleshy, it takes longer to degrease and dry them out. From Parent-Duchâtelet, "Les chantiers d'équarrissage de la ville de Paris," *Hygiène publique*, 2: 256.

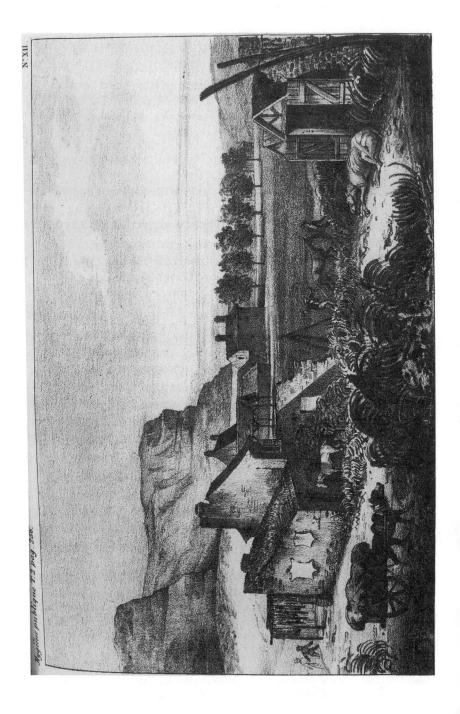

science, our spirit refuses to believe that establishments as infected as those at Montfaucon offer no cause for insalubrity."[52]

After the cholera epidemic was over, Parent-Duchâtelet talked with workers in the vicinity of the dump and examined hospital records to determine the incidence of cholera in the area. If the miasmatic theory was correct, then the number of cholera cases in and around the dump should have been among the highest in the city, but during the epidemic not one horse flayer had died. Nor one was even sick. Among the workers employed in related industries in the vicinity, such as fertilizer preparation and gutmaking, mortality was very low compared with the rest of the city.[53]

In a later article on the horsebutcher yards, Parent-Duchâtelet reiterated his earlier findings and took the opportunity to lash out against those physicians and hygienists who refused to apply the scientific method to public health.[54] The specific case was the proposed relocation of the horsebutcher yards, which for centuries had been located at the city dump at Montfaucon. A number of physicians voiced their opposition to the plan, asserting that the yards would be a foyer of infection, giving rise to miasma. Horsebutcher yards were a public health hazard, they maintained, because bad smells caused disease. Parent-Duchâtelet's task was to determine if the horsebutcher yards constituted a health hazard and whether the miasmatic theory could be tested scientifically. By this time Parent-Duchâtelet had been carrying out observations at the housebutcher yards for about fourteen years. Based on his observations and on statistical data gathered after the cholera epidemic, he asserted that in spite of the putrid gases and smelly emanations, he found no evidence to indicate that the yards harmed the health of those who habitually breathed the vapors. He challenged physicians who made contrary assertions to examine the

52 Ibid., p. 237.
53 Ibid., pp. 237–41.
54 Parent-Duchâtelet, "Des obstacles que les préjugés médicaux apportent," *Hygiène publique*, 1: 12–58.

Figure 10 The interior of a horsebutcher yard. In order to do this drawing the artist had to remove many of the horse carcasses, which were stacked like a wall as high as the top of the building on the left. On the far left is a dog-drawn cart. Although in the past such carts had been used by ragpickers, they had by this time been outlawed in Paris. On the wall of the little building behind them, cat and dog skins are stretched out to dry. To the left, tendons hang to dry. In the middle, a horse is pulling a carcass. After having transported the carcass outside the yard, this horse will be butchered. In the background to the left are the summits of Saint-Chaumont. From Parent-Duchâtelet, "Les chantiers d'équarrissage de la ville de Paris," *Hygiène publique*, 2: 256.

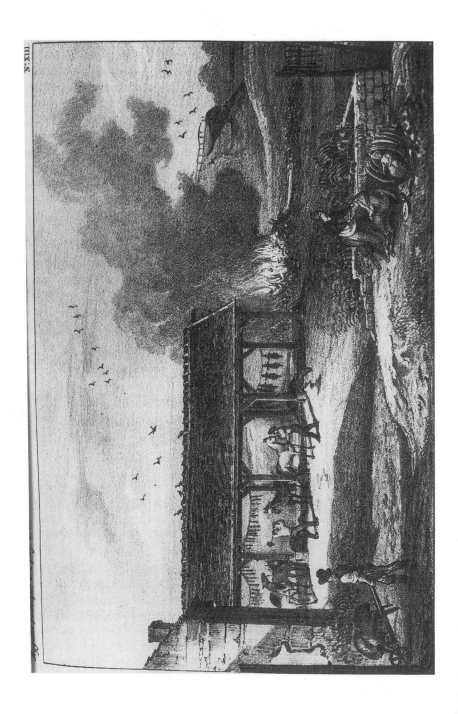

comparative mortality figures for cholera and to account for the increasing population of the vicinity. According to Parent-Duchâtelet, if the physicians who opposed public health and industrial reform had carried out observational and statistical research, they might have acquired sufficient knowledge to speak intelligently on the matter. As a result of sustained scientific inquiry, physicians would realize, if he was right, that traditional assertions about the health dangers associated with the horsebutcher yards did not hold up under scientific investigation.

Still, the sanitary commissions held to their convictions, urging immediate suppression of the dump. Yet the findings of the cholera commission suggested that Parent-Duchâtelet had been correct in his contentions. Parent-Duchâtelet, himself a member of the commission, after having examined the effects of cholera in the vicinity of the dump, found that no horsebutchers had died of the disease; nor had the adjacent Montfaucon and La Villette areas been affected by it. The mortality in areas near the horsebutcher yards was low compared with that of Paris in general. Parent-Duchâtelet's data suggested that the miasmatic theory, which associated bad smells with seats of infection, did not offer a convincing explanation of disease causation in the case of cholera.[55] Not all hygienists subscribed to a miasmatic theory of disease causation. Parent-Duchâtelet was neither a convinced contagionist not an anticontagionist, but in his investigations he did not find bad smells to be a cause of disease.

Although the emanations from the dump were not a proven health hazard, public opinion opposed the dump and demanded its immediate suppression. It had been a source of embarrassment to the city for too long. Alternatives for both parts of the dump had to be found, however, before the final suppression of Montfaucon could take place. Various efforts were made to get rid of the part of the dump that served as the receptacle for human wastes. Before the use of disinfectants became commonplace, a new location for the dump seemed to be the best solution,

---

55 Ibid.; Benoiston de Châteauneuf et al., *Rapport sur la marche et les effets du choléra-morbus*....

Figure 11 Interior of a horsebutcher yard. A separate hangar built by the horsebutcher Dusaussois. Two methods of killing horses are shown: bleeding, on the right, and clubbing, on the left. Cat skins hang on the line in the hangar. The fire to the right of the hangar shows the old method of disposing of horse carcasses. From 500 to 600 were accumulated, then set on fire; sometimes the fire burned for two to three weeks and gave off a terrible stench. By the 1830s, this method of disposal had become outmoded, for the bones had become too valuable. In the lower right-hand corner a child plays in a horse carcass. From Parent-Duchâtelet, "Les chantiers d'équarrissage de la ville de Paris," *Hygiène publique*, 2: 256.

but none could be found. After the opening of the Ourcq canal, a piece of land was purchased in the Bondy forest, about ten miles from Paris, where a new dump was to be dug at considerable cost to the municipal government. The plan – that cesspool products would be sent to Bondy on barges via the Ourcq canal – went into effect briefly, and dumping at Montfaucon was forbidden. However, because drainage problems made it practically impossible to eliminate liquid wastes, Bondy was declared unsuitable. Some cesspool matter could be handled by Bondy, but most of it continued to go to Montfaucon; so, during the Restoration and the July Monarchy, dumping wastes at Montfaucon continued.[56]

Parent-Duchâtelet argued that closing the dump permanently required long-range administrative planning. Meanwhile, he proposed using the newly discovered disinfectants to render waste matter odorless, then transporting it by canal and railroad to departments surroundings Paris, where it could be used as fertilizer. With improved navigational and railroad transport, Parent-Duchâtelet envisaged sending wastes 70 to 100 miles away from Paris. The major weakness of his plan was that it would take too long. Suppression of the dump had been under discussion for almost forty years, and quick solutions were mandated.[57]

In the mid-1830s, two chemists, Anselme Payen and L. J. Salmon, discovered a process that used a carbon powder to render solid wastes odorless while absorbing liquids, thereby turning wastes into odorless powder. A dump where solid wastes were spread over a large surface to dry out, such as Montfaucon, was thus no longer necessary. In addition, by the 1840s, some of the earlier problems associated with the Bondy dump had been solved, so that the final suppression of Montfaucon was at last feasible. The engineer Louis-Charles Mary solved the problem of transporting the wastes from Paris to Bondy by proposing the construction of a vast depository at the suburb of La Villette, where steam power in underground pipes would help transport liquid wastes. The solid wastes could then be sent in closed barrels by boat to Bondy. Rambuteau solved the drainage problem at the Bondy dump by having an aqueduct built from Bondy to the Seine near St.-Denis, along which liquids flowed, finally emptying into the river at St.-Denis. The depository itself consisted of fourteen quadrilateral reservoirs used to separate the liquid from the

---

56 Gisquet, *Mémoires*, 4: 302–4; Parent-Duchâtelet, "Les chantiers d'équarrissage," p. 144; Parent-Duchâtelet, "Rapport sur les nouveaux procédés de MM. Salmon, Payen et Compagnie, pour la dessication des chevaux morts et la désinfection instantanée des matières fécales; précédé de quelques considérations sur les voiries de la ville de Paris," *Hygiène publique*, 2: 285–9. Commenting on the insufficiency of the Bondy dump, Parent remarked that it was against the advice of the prefecture of police and the Paris health council that the dump at Bondy had been built in the first place.

57 Parent-Duchâtelet, "Rapport sur les nouveaux procédés," pp. 292–3.

solid matter. Slanted bottoms allowed the liquid wastes to run from one reservoir to another, and at the end of the last one there was a pipe to transport the matter to Bondy.[58]

As early as 1815 projects for moving the Montfaucon horsebutcher yards were being discussed. The success of the municipal slaughterhouses that had been built under Napoleon had led municipal administrators to consider building a central slaughterhouse for horses. At that time the Paris health council favored moving the industry to a central location and combining into one central slaughterhouse the horsebutcher yards from Montfaucon, other small slaughteryards, and industries associated with animal debris. The health council believed that centralization would eliminate many of the inconveniences associated with the horsebutchering industry and would facilitate government surveillance. The health council continued to favor the construction of a central slaughterhouse until the mid-1820s. An 1825 commission of which Parent-Duchâtelet was chairman drew up a plan for a model slaughterhouse (see Figure 12), but the expense was so great that nothing came of it. In addition, by the mid-1820s, major improvements were being made in the industry. Provided that the government would grant them a monopoly, various individuals offered to clean up the horsebutchering industry by the application of new processes involving the use of steam power. For fear that progress would be thwarted, however, the government consistently refused to grant a monopoly.[59]

In his 1831 investigation Parent-Duchâtelet reiterated the health council's earlier recommendation, providing for centralization of the horsebutchering industry in a monumental slaughterhouse whose construction would take advantage of the most recent developments in terms of cleanliness, ventilation, adequate water supply, and disinfection. His recommendations were not effected, however, and no central establishment was built. By the mid-1830s when the administration again began considering

58 Parent-Duchâtelet, "Rapport sur les nouveaux procédés," pp. 290–308. For his development of the disinfectant "noir animalisé," Salmon received the Montyon prize given by the Royal Academy of Sciences in 1834 for the invention of a process capable of rendering a trade less unhealthy. See "Variétés," *Annales d'hygiène publique* 13 (1835): 505; Rambuteau, *Mémoires*, p. 370. R. G. *Paris*, 1848, pp. 218–19; Gisquet, *Mémoires*, 4: 302.

59 There were other small establishments for the flaying and cutting up of horses and small animals, but the large enclosures at Montfaucon, which had been there in one form or another since the late sixteenth century, attracted the most attention. Moléon, R. G. *Paris*, 1815, p. 89; the health council continued to favor this project until major improvements rendered such a plan unnecessary. See, for example, ibid., 1824, p. 299; see the report of the commission: Parent-Duchâtelet, chairman, *Recherches et considérations sur l'enlèvement et l'emploi des chevaux morts, et sur la nécessité d'établir à Paris un clos central d'écarrissage* (Paris: Bachelier, 1827); Parent-Duchâtelet, "Les chantiers d'équarrissage," pp. 143–5; R. G. *Paris*, 1835, pp. 104–6.

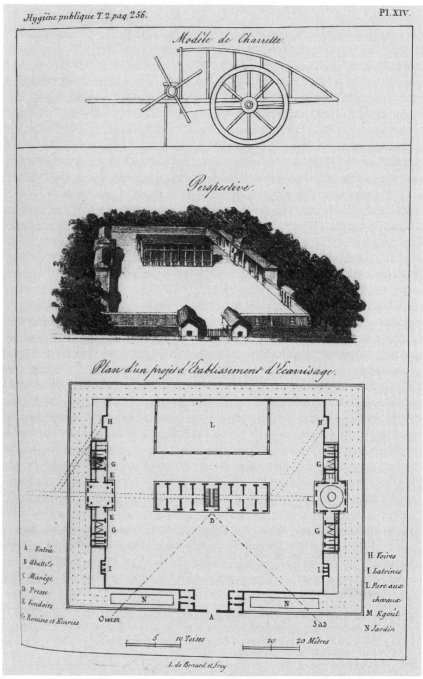

Modèle de Charrette.

Perspective.

Plan d'un projet d'Etablissement d'Ecarrisage.

A *Entrée*
B *abattoir*
C *Manège*
D *Presse*
E *Fondoirs*
G *Remises et Ecuries*

H *Voirie*
I *Latrines*
L *Parc aux chevaux*
M *Egout*
N *Jardin*

Ouest   A   *Sud*

5   10 *Toises*   10   20 *Mètres*

L. de Bernard et frey

Figure 12 The plan for the new abattoir proposed by the 1825 commission. It was never built. From Parent-Duchâtelet, "Les chantiers d'équarrissage de la ville de Paris," *Hygiène publique,* 2: 256.

the construction of a slaughterhouse, Parent-Duchâtelet's model had become outmoded due to improvements in the industry. Payen's discovery of a method of instantaneously disinfecting solid wastes and transforming them into fertilizer and a new steam-powered process acted as catalysts for solving the industry's problems. In 1835 the company of Payen, Buran, and Cambacérès sought authorization from the prefect of police for a horsebutchering establishment incorporating the new processes, which, they claimed, would render the material odorless and enable them to use all parts of the horse profitably. In a one-and-a-half- to two-hour process, the cadaver would be cut into pieces and placed in an iron container that could accommodate four horses simultaneously. Steam from a boiler would act on the pieces, skinning the flesh and bleaching and removing grease from the bones. The bones would then be removed and the remains put under a hydraulic press that extracted all oil. What was left over could be used as fertilizer, and no odor remained. The resulting matter could kept indefinitely and was easily transported.[60]

The Paris health council was impressed by the Payen process, noting that were it adopted, the horsebutchering industry could be practiced in the interior of the city without posing public health problems. The horsebutchering industry could be reclassified second class, thereby eliminating the need to establish an elaborate central slaughterhouse. Convinced of the effectiveness of the new process, the Paris health council ceased advocating the central slaughterhouse, which had been under consideration since 1815. Instead, the council advised the administration to purchase a vast tract of land for a slaughteryard where individual proprietors could set up their businesses. Centralization could thus be accomplished with only a modest outlay of money. By 1839 the administration had completed its plan for the establishment of a horse slaughteryard like the one the council had recommended. Adequate water supply, good drainage, the new steam processes, and adequate waste disposal were all included in the plans. The suppression of the horsebutcher yards at Montfaucon was at last realized in 1841 with the opening of the new horse slaughteryard at Aubervilliers.[61]

60 Parent-Duchâtelet, "Les chantiers d'equarrissage," p. 147; Parent-Duchâtelet's opinion, based on numerous interviews and observations, was that these emanations were not harmful to health. See ibid., pp. 227–41. Opinion among many hygienists and physicians was generally that the emanations gave rise to disease. Parent-Duchâtelet, "Rapport sur les nouveaux procédés de MM. Salmon, Payen et Compagnie," pp. 294–6; *Journal des Débats*, January 30, 1835, p. 3, and February 2, 1835, p. 3.

61 *R. G. Paris*, 1835, pp. 104–6; Parent-Duchâtelet, "Rapport sur les nouveaux procédés," pp. 300, 305. On classification of industrial establishments, see Chapter 5; Parent-Duchâtelet, chairman, "Projet d'un rapport demandé par M. le préfet de la Seine sur la construction d'un clos central d'équarrissage pour la ville de Paris," *Hygiène publique*, 2: 309–26; *R. G. Paris*, 1839, pp. 233–5; 1841, pp. 101–2. For an examination of this whole question from the point of view of the Paris health council, see Chapter 4.

GARBAGE DISPOSAL AND PUBLIC LATRINES

The system of garbage and mud collection and the common habit of citizens of using any part of the city as a public latrine contributed to the habitually filthy Parisian streets. Disposal of garbage and mud collected from the streets was a major public health problem. Garbage was collected daily by wagons that picked up heaps deposited at frequent intervals along the streets, a system in use since the eighteenth century. One observer, William de Blaquière, writing in 1826, described the filthiness of the streets, with heaps of fuel and garbage stacked along the pavement. The garbage heaps were usually dissected by dogs and ragpickers, so that by the time the garbage collectors arrived, much of the refuse was spread all over the pavement. Blaquière wondered why Parisians did not adopt the London system, whereby garbage men rang the doorbell to notify inhabitants to bring down their garbage. Some Parisians did not even bother to stack their garbage in heaps along the pavement, but simply threw it out the window into the streets.[62] Police ordinances forbade this practice, but Parisians paid little heed. Speaking of the scorn of Parisians for such ordinances, Claude Lachaise, author of a major medical topography of early-nineteenth-century Paris, noted that as soon as night fell, Parisians emptied all sorts of filth out the windows into the public thoroughfare, and Frances Trollope, reported that the life of a pedestrian in Paris was quite hazardous because of this practice.[63]

Once garbage and mud were collected, they were sent out to the communes surrounding Paris, where they were deposited along roads in big heaps to ferment into fertilizer. Alphonse Chevallier noted that in the early 1830s about 230 barrels of mud and garbage were carted off daily. The health council deplored this practice, stating that the land surrounding Paris was becoming a major source of infection. The council had received numerous complaints from inhabitants of the rural communes about the bad odors emanating from the garbage heaps, and members also lamented that visitors approaching Paris smelled the stench of the city before they saw its monuments. The council claimed it was self-defeating to have the interior of the city clean and beautiful if it was surrounded by piles of garbage, noting in their 1828 report that most of the roads leading out of the city had heaps of mud and garbage piled along their sides. A continual complaint of hygienists was that the administration spent too much money

---

62 Louis-Sébastien Mercier, *Tableau de Paris*, 2 vols. (Hamburg, Virchaux; Neufchâtel, Fauche, 1781), 1: 46, 93; William de Blaquière, *Mémoire concernant diverses améliorations urgentes à apporter au système de police de la ville de Paris...* (Paris: Berlin, 1826), pp. 7–9. For comments on Blaquière's brochure and some others, see Bertier de Sauvigny, *La Restauration*, p. 86.

63 Lachaise, *Topographie médicale*, p. 194; Trollope, *Paris and the Parisians*, 1: 116–18.

on showy monuments and too little on practical things like sewers. Rambuteau justified such expenditures by arguing that monuments were as necessary to the population as sewers.[64]

Problems of garbage disposal and collection were not solved before 1848, although reforms were proposed. In 1823 the Paris health council proposed a plan in which garbage would be picked up daily and sent out of the city on barges, to be deposited and eventually used as fertilizer. The administration rejected the plan, ostensibly because it was too expensive, although resistance from ragpickers and garbage collectors may also have accounted for the administration's decision. Heaps of rotting garbage continued to line the roads of the rural communes. By the late 1830s disinfectants had come into common use, and it became possible to render garbage heaps odorless. The health council changed its recommendation to enforcement of disinfection, rather than encouraging the administration to eliminate the heaps altogether. The garbage problem was only temporarily allayed, however, since there was no major renovation of the system before 1850.[65]

Nineteenth-century Parisians were in the habit of using any area of the city as a latrine. Urinating and defecating in gutters, on sidewalks, in streets, on buildings, and off bridges into canals and the river were common practice, to the chagrin of many hygienists. In fact, there was little practical alternative when one was away from home, for public conveniences were few. The only mention of public latrines in Paris dates from an 1817 health council report in which latrines located in the Rue Neuve St.-Augustin were mentioned. Ordinances against public urination and defecation were on the books, but Prefect of Police Gisquet (1831–6) commented that these had not changed the habits of Parisians. Hygienists and observers advocated the proliferation of public latrines and public

---

64 This was also the traditional system. Mercier, *Tableau de Paris*, 1: 46, 93. The mud deposit problem was an old one. A lengthy report had been prepared on the problem in 1802, but the recommendations had not been acted on. See A.N., F¹³739, Voiries de Dépôt, 9 prairial an 10. In 1820 Prefect of the Seine Chabrol suggested that perhaps once Montfaucon was suppressed as the receptacle for human wastes, the mud could be deposited in the basins there. In A. N., F¹³739, Chabrol à M. Le Conseiller d'Etat, Directeur des Travaux de Paris, 5 avril 1820. Chevallier, *Considérations pratiques*, p. 7; Moléon, *R. G. Paris*, 1827, pp. 36–8. *Mémoires*, pp. 269–70; *R. G. Paris*, 1828, pp. 329–30; *R. G. Paris*, 1837, pp. 186–7.

65 Moléon, *R. G. Paris*, 1823, p. 265; 1839, pp. 253–5. Edwin Chadwick, ed., M. W. Flinn, *Report on the Sanitary Condition of the Labouring Population of Great Britain, 1842* (Edinburgh: Edinburgh University Press, 1965), pp. 162–3; Sussman, "Yellow Fever to Cholera," pp. 290–303. Chevallier, who opposed the health council's plan as being a waste of good fertilizer, had a proposal for cleaning up the rural communes by digging special ditches in which the mud and garbage could ferment. His research was done at the request of the administration in 1832 in an attempt to clean up the city as a preventive measure against cholera. See *Considérations pratiques*.

urinals (*pissotières*) to improve the city's sanitary state. Gisquet endorsed a plan to provide the city with 200 free public latrines and urinals equipped with running water, estimating a construction cost of 400,000 francs with a yearly maintenance charge of 50,000 francs.[66] No evidence exists, however, to show that his successor, Gabriel Delessert, carried out his plan.

FROM SANITARY REFORM TO SANITARY REVOLUTION:
THE FIRST PHASE: 1850s

The first phase of the sanitary revolution, which began with the suppression of the Montfaucon dump, would not be completed until the underlying philosophy of waste disposal underwent further transformation later in the century. In the meantime, the dump had been replaced by a new waste depository at La Villette, from which liquid wastes traveled through underground pipes to the new dump at Bondy. By the 1850s a plant had been built at Bondy to convert liquid wastes into ammonia salts, which had important industrial uses. Bondy also functioned as a primitive treatment plant for solid waste, which were converted into a fertilizer known as "la poudrette de Montfaucon."

Major changes in cesspool cleaning and disposal of cesspool wastes were also effected. An ordinance of 1850 made on-the-spot disinfection of cesspool matter mandatory at the time of cleaning so that liquid wastes could be disposed of through gutters.[67] For a short while, an experiment was tried in which disinfected solid wastes were transported to private dumps, but the practice caused many complaints and was quickly abandoned. Solid wastes were again carted to Bondy. Sending liquid wastes through gutters and sewers was an innovation that Parent-Duchâtelet had suggested as early as the 1830s, but his suggestion was realized only in the 1850s following the introduction and widespread use of disinfectants coupled with the increased water supply. Whereas in 1845 only 27,000 cubic meters of liquid

66 Monfalcon and Polinière, *Traité de la salubrité*, pp. 110–11; Gisquet, *Mémoires*, 4: 429; Moléon, *R. G. Paris*, 1817, p. 115. On the lack of public toilet facilities, see Monfalcon and Polinière, *Traité de la salubrité*, pp. 110–11; Blaquière, *Mémoire concernant diverses améliorations*, pp. 15–16; Pierre Dutertre, *Considérations sanitaires sur la ville de Paris* (Mans: Monnoyer, 1822), p. 5; Félix Hatin, *Essai médico-philosophique sur les moyens d'améliorer l'état sanitaire de la classe indigente* (Paris: Didot le jeune, 1834), p. 3; Gisquet, *Mémoires*, 4: 430–1; Monfalcon and Polinière noted the establishment of a few public urinals and latrines in Lyon by 1846, in *Traité de la salubrité*, p. 395; Gisquet, *Mémoires*, 4: 430–1.

67 Ordonnance concernant les fosses d'aisance. "Revue administrative," *Annales d'hygiène publique* 46 (1851): 453–7. "Mémoire de l'Ingénieur Mille sur le service des vidanges," *Annales d'hygiène publique* 2e série 2 (1854): 448–58. It is interesting that the author noted (p. 454) that principles put forward long ago by the Paris health council were finally being applied.

Table 6. *Changes in waste disposal*

Year	Liquids transported to Bondy	Solids carted off by boat[a]	Liquids disposed of through gutters[a]	Total[a]	Comments
1849	127,000	16,000	—	143,000	Nine months only
1850	231,000	26,000	—	257,000	For the whole year
1851	210,000	28,000	27,000	265,000	For the whole year
1852	174,000	32,000	88,000	294,000	For the whole year
1853	163,000	39,000	152,000	354,000	For the whole year

[a] Quantities in cubic meters.
Source: "Mémoire de l'ingénieur Mille sur le service des vidanges," *Annales*, 2nd series 2 (1854): 453. The lease for *voirie* had decreased from 500,000 francs in the late 1840s to 130,000 francs in 1854, reflecting the reduction in the amount of liquid wastes transported to Bondy. (The author noted on p. 454 that principles put forward long ago by the health council were finally being applied.)

wastes flowed into gutters, by 1853 the figure was up to 152,000 cubic meters (Table 6). This innovation did not mean that liquid wastes flowed from dwellings directly into sewers, but rather that cesspool cleaners had the right, once they had removed the liquid wastes from the cesspools, to dump them directly into the gutters. By the early 1850s there were also improvements in the underground sewer system because of the increased water supply. Throwing household waste waters into open gutters was no longer permitted, and proprietors were given ten years to open underground junctions between each dwelling and the public sewer.

The long-range goal of sanitary reformers in the early 1850s was *écoulement direct*, or a system in which water was piped directly into houses, with liquid wastes flowing from each household through underground pipes into sewers. With this system, immediate separation of liquids and solids in cesspools occurred. The complete suppression of cesspools and sending solid wastes through sewers were not yet envisaged, since waste conservation rather than waste disposal was still the aim. Since, however, 90 percent of the matter in cesspools was liquid, its disposal through sewers was a major reform. Cesspool cleaning would be greatly simplified and costs lowered.

Critics of *écoulement direct* feared that liquid wastes sent through sewers would become infected, whereas proponents claimed that urine would be diluted in such a proportion (1/100) that it would not be a health problem. Opponents charged that products of liquid wastes would be lost by *écoulement direct*, but hygienists countered that this was inevitable, since liquid wastes were becoming more diluted by increasing amounts of water. Although about half of all liquid wastes were being eliminated through sewers by the 1850s, only one-third of the streets of Paris had underground sewers. Total *écoulement direct* was a proposal for the future, with massive sewer construction necessary for its attainment.

The public health advantage of *écoulement direct* was the salubrity of houses and streets. One obvious benefit was that it would remove major obstacles to a further increase in the water supply and better water distribution. Cesspools were incompatible with increased amounts of water, since more water made frequent cleaning necessary. Proprietors opposed increased water supply, therefore, because of the expense and inconvenience of cesspool cleaning. Any proposed change in the habits of domestic water use threatened to complicate the problem of cesspool cleaning. For example, if Parisians adopted the habit of using water in their latrines as the English did – two or three liters per flush – the result would be an additional financial burden for proprietors. Proprietors would be reluctant to subscribe to city water as long as liquid wastes accumulated in cesspools. A direct connection between sewers and cesspools – *écoulement direct* – promised to eliminate these problems, making proprietors more willing to provide water in their dwellings. In summary, the advantages of the sanitary revolution proposed in the early 1850s were the simplification of cesspool cleaning, economy for proprietors, an increase in water, and improved water distribution.

SANITARY REVOLUTION: THE INTERMEDIATE AND
FINAL PHASES: 1870S

Twenty years later, the goals of the sanitary reformers of the early 1850s had not been attained. Although massive construction had taken place under Haussmann, these sewers were primarily storm sewers. By the early 1870s, only a small number of Parisian houses had direct waste disposal through sewers. In these households solid and liquid wastes were separated by a dividing apparatus, the filtering barrel (*tinette-filtre*), through which liquids ran directly into the sewer, with solids collected in the barrel. This disposal system had been available since 1867, with approximately 6,444 in use by the early 1870s. This was still comparatively few, considering the number of households being served by permanent and movable cesspools. Dossiers kept on each household by the cesspool cleaning service at the prefecture of police showed that in 1871 there were

    6,444 filtering barrels
    85,776 permanent cesspools
    19,203 movable cesspools
    12,520 dividing apparati (liquids flowed into reservoirs)

123,942 total cesspool apparati for
60,310 households registered with the cesspool cleaning service.[68]

Out of an estimated 68,000 houses, 60,310 had cesspool-cleaning dossiers registered with the administration. The rest had no dossier on record; hence, cesspool cleaning was presumably done illicitly. Clandestine cleaning was a problem for the administration, because waste disposal was closely regulated by the prefecture of police in terms of cesspool construction, maintenance, and cleaning. Each cleaning operation was recorded at the prefecture of police, constituting the dossiers kept for each household. The 7,690 households with no dossier may have had leaking cesspools, or they may have deposited cesspool matter illegally in gardens or courtyards. These households may have used barrels to deposit cesspool matter in ditches and gardens, or they may have had their cesspools cleaned illegally without prior authorization. Most of these irregular operations took place in the former suburbs, the recently annexed zones of the city.

The sanitary revolution moved to an intermediate phase by the 1870s as hygienists advocated the abolition of permanent cesspools and suppression of the Bondy dump, to be replaced by disposal of all wastes through underground sewers. This goal – *écoulement direct* or *vidange à l'égout* – could not be attained, however, until the length of sewers was sufficient, until all individual dwellings were connected with sewers, and until the apparati to replace permanent cesspools had been perfected. During this intermediate phase, solid wastes were still not sent through sewers, but collected in barrels, or movable cesspools. The prerequisite for this phase of the sanitary revolution was the construction of additional sewers. Paris had 536,000 meters of underground sewers in 1871, or almost fifteen times as many as in 1824, when Parent-Duchâtelet had first investigated the sewer system. The administration projected 350,000 additional meters of underground sewers for completion within fifteen years, with construction to begin immediately. Branch sewers to connect individual dwellings with public sewers were also proposed, so that liquid wastes could be sent directly from households to main sewers. During this intermediate stage solid wastes would still be collected in barrels, to be carted off periodically by the cesspool cleaners, who had the privilege of taking them to private dumps. If this plan worked, it meant that the municipal dump at Bondy could be suppressed. Ridding Paris of permanent cesspools would be a major sanitary reform: The equipment for ordinary cesspool cleaning would no longer be necessary, and Paris could be delivered from the fetid emanations that accompanied cesspool cleaning.

68 Archives de Paris et de l'ancien département de la Seine, V I⁵3, Mémoire de l'inspecteur général des Ponts et Chaussées, directeur des eaux et des égouts. Undated, but probably 1871 or 1872.

Reformers cited major advantages to be obtained from *écoulement direct*. Waste disposal directly through sewers would make the use of water in latrines obligatory, thereby converting them into water closets and improving the sanitary state of workers' dwellings. As late as 1871 almost no workers' houses had water piped in. Since cesspool cleaning was so expensive, proprietors wanted as little water as possible. Apparently some proprietors actually forbade the use of water in latrines. The situation was so grave that in most workers' dwellings the annual capacity of the cesspools was about 300 cubic liters per inhabitant, or the same as the normal volume of wastes without any additional water. The resulting filthy situation defied the imagination. Hygienists suggested that the habitual uncleanliness of workers was due to this disgusting situation alone. Having no water to keep clean and becoming accustomed to filth, workers had no motivation to cultivate habits of cleanliness. Reformers maintained that one of the most important effects of the sanitary revolution would be the change that would take place in workers' dwellings. Customarily several families shared one latrine, but hygienists hoped that if workers were given their own individual water closets, they would be motivated to keep their dwellings clean. Distribution of water into each dwelling and conversion of latrines into water closets were dependent upon the conversion of the cesspool system to the system of liquid waste disposal directly through underground sewers.

There were serious problems connected with the intermediate phase of the sanitary revolution. The construction and layout of many Parisian houses made it difficult or even impossible to connect each house directly with a public sewer. Filtering barrels were expensive, and many proprietors were reluctant to install them; furthermore, their frequent removal made them unpopular. Barrels would only have to be removed annually in households of fewer than ten persons, but in larger buildings with many inhabitants, removal might have to be done as often as twenty-four times a year. In barracks and hospitals, barrels would have to be changed every three or four days. Reformers pointed out that objections to filtering barrels could be resolved by sending solid and liquid wastes through sewers. This final phase of the sanitary revolution would represent a major shift in thinking: from waste conservation and exploitation, which had prevailed, to waste disposal. Major obstacles stood in the way: First, sending solid wastes through sewers seemed to pose a public health hazard, because the filth theory of disease was still dominant. Second, there were construction problems because of the difficulty of connecting some houses with sewers. And finally, the Paris sewer system was still inadequate for the job.

Opponents argued that sending solid wastes through sewers was a health hazard. Hygienists countered that if the quantity of water washing through sewers was sufficient, there was no problem. Nor was a health hazard posed by the discharge of solid wastes into the river if they were diluted by enough water.[69] A more difficult problem was sewer construction and connection of sewers with houses: Many buildings were separated from the street by courtyards, and in some cases, the difference in the level between the lowest latrine and the sewer was not sufficient for the fall pipe, which connected the latrine to the sewer, to function properly.

The key to the final phase of the sanitary revolution was the completion of the projected sewer construction. Since new sewers would take many years to build, in the interim, reformers had to be content with suppression of permanent cesspools and their replacement by dividing apparati and filtering barrels. This reform would permit liquid wastes to run into sewers, and solid wastes would be collected in filtering barrels, ridding the city of permanent cesspools, cesspool cleaning, and the Bondy dump and improving the dwellings of the poor and workers by better water distribution. The final phase would include a complete system of sanitary sewers in which filtering barrels would be discontinued and all wastes would be sent directly through sewers. In 1871, Paris had 535,691 meters of underground sewers, with 490,809 additional meters projected. The construction of four main collectors was also planned, one of which would help close at last the Bièvre, the uncovered sewer that had caused so many complaints for almost 100 years.[70]

By the 1870s a change in the philosophy of waste disposal made the sanitary revolution a likely possibility. The sanitary reform movement was finally achieving practical results. The actual sanitary revolution proposed in the 1870s took a long time and is not within the scope of this book.[71] Indications are that some aspects of waste disposal were slow to change. For example, permanent cesspools were still undergoing the traditional nightly cleaning as late as the 1930s. As one observer described the spectacle:

> In spite of the law, there were still thousands of cesspools and the cleaning industry was one of the most lucrative; it was the only one that didn't have to buy its raw material, and the only one that earned money at both ends, collecting and selling the same thing.

69 Estimates were 200 cubic meters of solid waste a day into the sewers. The volume of water discharged by the main sewer was expected soon to reach 300,000 cubic meters a day, or 150 times as much water as solid wastes. As for the Seine, even when the water was low, there was twenty times as much water as the amount discharged by the main sewer; thus the solid wastes were further diluted by the river.

70 All the information on the 1870s comes from Archives de Paris et de l'ancien département de la Seine, V I⁵3, Mémoire de l'inspecteur général des Ponts et Chaussées, directeur des eaux et des égouts. Undated, but probably 1871 or 1872.

71 On the sanitary revolution of the latter part of the nineteenth century and the implementation of *tout à l'égout*, see Gérard Jacquemet, "Urbanisme Parisien: La bataille du tout à l'égout à la fin du XIXe siècle," *Revue d'histoire moderne et contemporaine* 46 (1979): 505–48.

The arrival of the cesspool cleaners was far from subtle. Several macabre wagons drawn by white horses would advance in a lugubrious column through the narrow streets, and the squeak of the axles, the creak of the wheels, and the clatter of iron-shod hoofs on the cobblestones would jar the sleeping citizens awake.[72]

CONCLUSION: SANITARY REFORM AND SANITARY REVOLUTION

Early-nineteenth-century hygienists and administrators launched a movement for sanitary reform in Paris. Their program was influenced by the prevailing filth theory of disease, concern for working-class welfare, fear of cholera, and a philosophy of urbanism, or creating a clean and more beautiful Paris. Although some hygienists were content with piecemeal reform, others, such as Parent-Duchâtelet, were already envisaging a sanitary revolution as early as the 1830s. Ultimately it would take a revolution to accomplish the sanitary reform that hygienists and administrators advocated. The main ideas of the late-nineteenth-century sanitary revolution – with the exception of solid waste disposal through sewers – had all been espoused and publicized by early-nineteenth-century public hygienists. The completed sanitary revolution was the fruition of their program. This does not mean that hygienists and administrators achieved no practical results before 1850. Major reforms in water distribution, sewer extension, suppression of the dump, sewer cleaning, and improvements in street cleaning were all made between 1820 and 1848 during the administrations of Chabrol and Rambuteau. Nevertheless, one wonders why the ideas and programs of the sanitary reformers were so slow in being adopted, why the Parisian sanitary revolution took so long, and why the Parisian sanitary program lagged behind those of London and other English cities at midcentury.

Parisian sanitary reform was slow because of vested interests that thrived on the status quo and played a major role in blocking reforms. This was the case with garbage collectors, ragpickers, water carriers, and proprietors. The water carriers of Gros-Caillou, for example, complained to the prefect of police in 1843 about the establishment of street fountains in their quarter, asserting that the availability of free water was destroying their industry.[73] The costs of massive reform also acted as a major stumbling

---

72 Brassai (Gyula Halasz), *The Secret Paris of the 30's*, trans. Richard Miller (New York: Pantheon Books, 1976). The book is not paginated, but the quotation is from the section entitled "A Night with the Cesspool Cleaners."

73 APP, Da208. Letter from the water carriers of Gros-Caillou to the prefect of police, March 19, 1843. How the vested interests of cesspool cleaners, ragpickers, street cleaners, garbage collectors, horseflayers, water carriers, and proprietors slowed down and in some cases determined the course of sanitary reform promises to be an interesting and potentially fruitful area of further investigation.

block to large programs such as sewer extension and water distribution. Financing such programs was difficult – if not impossible – given the outlook of the municipal and national governments of the July Monarchy. It took the broad vision and massive financing programs of Napoleon III and Baron Haussmann to effect major transformations in these areas.

The nineteenth-century French philosophy of waste disposal was another factor retarding sanitary reform, since money could be made off wastes. Economic considerations were more important than public health and aesthetic considerations for many French citizens. By the 1830s and 1840s, however, public health problems began to be taken more seriously in response to the publicity of hygienists and the stark reality of cholera. There was also the practical consideration that as more water diluted the wastes, they were no longer as valuable. Popular displeasure with traditional sanitary practices also increased as the tolerance level for filth and bad odors decreased, at least at certain levels of society. A modern sanitary sewer system became theoretically possible by the second half of the century as prevailing attitudes began to shift from waste conservation to waste disposal.[74]

Cultural attitudes were as important as, if not more important than, economic considerations in explaining the slowness of Parisians to adopt many of the practical sanitary recommendations of the hygienists and reformers. There was a long French tradition of uncleanliness, or disregard for personal hygiene, at all levels of society. The average nineteenth-century French citizen used little water and rarely took a bath. He or she did not seem to require or desire them. One student of the subject, Guy Thuillier, in his work on the Nivernais, found that many of these ideas of personal hygiene changed slowly; in fact, many did not change until the second half of the twentieth century. Nineteenth-century hygienists were reluctant to admit the French preference for uncleanliness, and they consistently argued that if people had enough water, they would stay clean; that if workers had private water closets, they would keep their houses clean; that if cheap, plentiful baths were available, people would bathe. Perhaps. However, it appears that cleanliness did not have top priority in nineteenth-century France, for whatever reasons. In their fight against disease-causing filth, hygienists realized that personal habits would be hard to change. Public health reforms such as sewer extension and improved water distribution were the prerequisites, but even then, private habits and private filth would be a much thornier problem. One could make facilities available, but private hygiene could hardly be legislated.

---

74 The classic French work on the conservation of wastes or the use of human manure in agriculture is Jean-Baptiste Boussingault, *Economie. rurale considérée dans ses rapports avec la chimie, la physique, et la météorologie*, 2 vols. (Paris: Baillière, 1843–4); Corbin, *Le miasme et la jonquille*, part 1.

The repeated laments of prefects of police and hygienists about the unwillingness of Parisians to obey street-cleaning ordinances is testament to the difficulty of changing habits and attitudes.[75]

Public hygienists were central to the early-nineteenth-century program of sanitary reform and to the eventual sanitary revolution that resulted from that program. At the administrative level, they made major contributions by their work on the Paris health council and on municipal commissions, as well as by their own individual investigations of public health problems. The great influence of the Paris health council as the advisory board to the prefect of police on public health matters has been documented. Close collaboration between the health council and the administration greatly facilitated public health reform.

The work of the leading hygienists was widely known at the professional and administrative levels from the published health council reports, from published commission reports, and from the *Annales d'hygiène publique*, where most of the major hygienic investigations of the era appeared. Their work also became widely known by well-educated citizens who read periodicals and newspapers that carried news of public health problems and investigations. Not only was the work of hygienists widely publicized, it was also influential. Parisian hygienists like Parent-Duchâtelet, Villermé, and Alphonse Chevallier were respected and convincing. The professional, scientific nature of their research made them authorities, and their influence was great not only in Paris, but throughout France and abroad. During the second half of the century, many of the reforms they had advocated were effected as part of the sanitary revolution.

Although many of the problems associated with *assainissement* remained unsolved by the middle of the century, the contributions of the early-nineteenth-century Parisian public hygienists should not be underestimated. Their investigations and the solutions they offered contributed to a growth of awareness of urban health problems among hygienists, administrators, and reformers in Paris and in other large cities in Western Europe and the United States. Some of their solutions were put into effect and helped improve the sanitary situation in Paris. Others, although not tried before 1848, later became models for sanitary reform. The foundation for the reforms engineered by Haussmann had been laid by 1848. Much of the credit for Haussmann's later successes must go to the municipal administration and to the urban hygienists of the Restoration and the July Monarchy.[76]

75 Guy Thuillier, *Pour une histoire du quotidien au XIXe siècle en Nivernais* (Paris: Mouton, 1977), pp. 11–30, 50–70; Goubert, *The Conquest of Water*, pp. 219–36.
76 This opinion is shared by Pierre Lavedan in *La question du déplacement de Paris et du transfert des Halles au Conseil Municipal sous la monarchie de juillet* (Paris: Imprimerie municipale, 1969), p. 9. Lavedan sums it up nicely:" une bonne part, peut-être la meilleure, de l'oeuvre d'Haussmann est la réalisation des idées formulées par tout un ensemble de recherches urbaines et sociales sous la monarchie de Juillet."

Public health in Paris: Investigation, salubrity, and social welfare

Sanitary reform included much more than improving water and sewer systems. The salubrity of private dwellings and public establishments, such as hospitals and prisons, was critical to the healthfulness of Paris. Personal cleanliness and the purity of food and drink were also areas of major hygienic concern. The scope of early-nineteenth-century public health interests was so broad that hygienists also considered social welfare concerns part of their domain. Indeed, many of these problems were intimately related to public health. In their dual concern over morals and health, hygienists investigated prostitution, which they considered the primary cause of venereal disease. Because of the high infant mortality rate, they also took an interest in the wet-nursing business and the foundling question. Many of these problems had earlier been handled by charitable institutions and would in the second half of the century fall into the domain of social welfare or public assistance, but in the early nineteenth century they were public health problems.

THE SALUBRITY OF PRIVATE DWELLINGS

Claude Lachaise, physician and author of the principal medical topography of Paris, presented a report to the Royal Academy of Medicine in 1840 that described the influence of crowded living conditions on urban mortality.[1] Lachaise noted that although there had been many public health reforms in Paris since 1815, improvements in private dwellings were negligible. Construction had not kept pace with the population increase, and new dwellings were small and badly built. Many Parisians lived in substandard, unsanitary dwellings. Although some quarters of Paris were sumptuous and healthful, others were filthy and filled with hovels – virtual slums, inhabited by the working classes and the dregs of society. Statistics showed little decrease in mortality rates, which were the barometer public

---

1 Claude Lachaise, "De l'influence de l'entassement de la population sur la mortalité des grandes villes; prouvée par les registres mortuaires de Paris de 1820 à 1840," *Bull. de l'Acad. Roy. de Méd.* 5 (1840–1): 570–80; communication verbale, présentée dans le séance du 1 Septembre 1840.

hygienists used to measure the health of a society. Thus from 1817 to 1838, in spite of public health reforms, the average mortality rate had not changed. The mortality rate in eighteenth-century Paris had been 1/28 (one death for every twenty-eight people); from 1804 to 1817 it was 1/31; and from 1817 to 1832 it was 1/32. Lachaise suggested that this improvement was in part due to public health reforms; however, the trend did not continue. By 1831 the rate had increased to 1/30. By 1838 it was back down to 1/32, the same figure as for 1817. Furthermore, Paris had a higher mortality rate than many of the departments. Some departments had a mortality rate as low as 1/41 and 1/42, and the average mortality for France as a whole was about 1/40. According to Lachaise, Parisians had an average life span only three-quarters of that of other French citizens, although more public health improvements had been made in Paris than elsewhere.[2]

Public hygienists had consistently maintained that public health reform, a decreasing mortality rate, and the advance of civilization were concomitant. Therefore, they were at a loss to explain why the city with the best application of public health measures had one of the highest mortality rates in the nation. Lachaise and Villermé attributed high mortality to crowded and insanitary living conditions in the poor areas of Paris. Villermé had presented statistics demonstrating that crowded conditions alone were not necessarily a cause of bad health unless accompanied by poverty.[3] During the cholera epidemic, the mortality rates were higher in crowded areas with narrow streets, quarters inhabited by the poor.[4] Pathological anatomist and public health advocate Pierre-Adolphe Piorry later pointed out that observations on cholera did not prove that it was the result of bad housing, but he argued that crowded living conditions gave the epidemic its serious and fatal character.[5]

The findings on cholera and mortality supported the prevalent environmentalist belief that disease was a direct result of insanitary conditions. Therefore hygienists argued that insalubrity in private dwellings was a major cause of disease. In trying to pinpoint the factors that made narrow, crowded dwellings hazardous to health, Piorry contended that lack of air due to bad ventilation was a principal factor.[6] Lyonnais hygienists Jean-

---

2 Ibid., pp. 572–5.

3 Ibid., pp. 575–9; Louis-René Villermé, "De la mortalité dans les divers quartiers de la ville de Paris," *Annales d'hygiène publique* 3 (1830): 305–7, 322–4. There was a distinction between high population density, which was not necessarily related to high mortality rates, and overcrowdedness, which was usually related to high mortality rates.

4 Lachaise, "De l'influence de l'entassement," p. 44; Louis-François Benoiston de Châteauneuf et al., *Report on the Cholera in Paris* (New York: Samuel S. and William Wood, 1849), p. 164; François Delaporte, *Disease and Civilization: The Cholera in Paris, 1832* (Cambridge, MA: MIT Press, 1986).

5 Pierre-Adolphe Piorry, *Des habitations et de l'influence de leurs dispositions sur l'homme, en santé et en maladie* (Paris: Pourchet, 1838), p. 75.

6 Ibid., pp. 83–5.

Baptiste Monfalcon and Isidore de Polinière also suggested that an inadequate supply of fresh air was the main health hazard of crowded living conditions, noting that both animals and people in overcrowded situations quickly used up the oxygen supply and vitiated the air. Foul emanations from garbage and excrement helped explain why crowded conditions constituted a health hazard, they claimed. Monfalcon and Polinière cited other physicians and health councils who argued that the main cause of serious diseases (such as phthisis, scrofula, chronic gastritis, and rheumatism) that afflicted the poor in large cities was the alteration of the air by deleterious emanations. To illustrate their claim, the two hygienists described the interior of a working-class dwelling in Lyon, noting that physicians who treated the poor at home could hardly stand the fetid odors. Latrines were insufficient and filthy, often located in kitchens and stairwells, and floors were covered with the excrement of babies and animals. Good ventilation was practically nonexistent, and the water supply was insufficient: One pump served several households, and water sold by carriers was too expensive for the poor. Without adequate water and toilet facilities, the poor could keep neither their persons nor their dwellings clean. Their bodies were dirty and smelly, and their houses were filled with mud, excrement, and garbage.[7]

The most crowded and poorly ventilated Parisian dwellings were the lodging houses (*hôtels garnis, maisons garnies*) inhabited by the poorest members of society. Honoré A. Frégier, an administrator at the Prefecture of the Seine and author of an oft-cited work on the dangerous classes of Paris, provided a vivid description of some of the worst of the *hôtels garnis*: The rooms looked out onto corridors without air and light, and the latrines on each floor gave off suffocating odors. Stairs were permanently covered with mud, and the courtyard, only 4 feet square, was filled with garbage. Latrines on the top floor leaked, so that waste matter ran down the stairwell to the street floor. The inhabitants were swindlers, thieves, pimps, and the filthiest of prostitutes – the most abject men and women in society.[8]

The Paris health council was quick to take up the housing problem. In an 1824 report entitled *Des nouvelles bâtisses entreprises dans la capitale* the members viewed the new construction in Paris with alarm. The council noted that most of the recently constructed buildings contained small apartments that, because of poor ventilation and lack of sunlight, were unhealthier to live in than many prisons. Two years later the council again

---

7   Jean-Baptiste Monfalcon and A. P. Isidore de Polinière, *Traité de la salubrité dans les grandes villes* (Paris: Baillière, 1846), pp. 41–5, 87–90.

8   Honoré Frégier, *Des classes dangereuses de la population dans les grandes villes et les moyens de les rendre meilleures*, 2 vols. (Paris: Baillière, 1840), 1: 140–1. On the dangerous classes, see also Louis Chevalier, *Classes laborieuses et classes dangereuses à Paris pendant la première moitié du XIXe siècle* (Paris: Plon, 1958).

considered the housing situation, observing that new streets and buildings were constructed without any attention to public health. Some administrative solution was necessary, council members asserted, in order to clean up and improve private dwellings and *hôtels garnis* so that they would not constitute a health hazard.[9]

The housing problem could not be solved by public health measures alone, for the provision of adequate dwellings for a growing population was as much a socioeconomic as a public health concern. Nevertheless, hygienists proposed several solutions. Lachaise suggested that industrial establishments be required to move out of the city center, the legal height of houses lowered, and the width of courtyards and the height of interior constructions regulated.[10] The Paris health council called for government intervention and regulation to direct new construction, maintaining – to cite one example – that the old law regulating the width of streets in proportion to the height of houses was no longer adequate. The council called for an ordinance requiring that street widths equal the height of the highest building, with no building to be built higher than the street was wide. The members believed this regulation would result in improved ventilation, greater cleanliness, and less population accumulation.[11]

In 1829 the health council called for a law regulating urban construction to protect the health of the poor. Citing differences in mortality rates from one quarter to another, the council asserted that misery was the main cause of unhealthy conditions. Monfalcon and Polinière concurred with the recommendation of the Paris health council and urged a law to regulate urban construction, asserting that until the passage and enforcement of such a law, citizens' health would be at the mercy of builders. They contended that unless builders were constrained by regulations, they would not construct healthful dwellings, since they were more interested in money than health. Monfalcon and Polinière believed improved health would result from regulating the number of rooms per building and requiring adequate ventilation, construction to discourage humidity, clean, well-lighted, large courtyards and stairwells, and latrines and cesspools connected by pipes. Piorry and the physician-hygienist Henri Bayard both recommended governmental surveillance of boarding houses to limit the number of beds in relation to the amount of space and to help ensure clean

9 Moléon, R. G.... *Paris*, 1824, pp. 308–11; 1826, pp. 357–62.
10 Lachaise, "De l'influence de l'entassement," pp. 379–80. For a good discussion of the complicated issue of urban housing, see Ann-Louise Shapiro, *Housing the Poor of Paris, 1850–1902* (Madison: University of Wisconsin Press, 1985).
11 Moléon, R. G.... *Paris*, 1824, pp. 308–11; 1826, pp. 357–62. A law of 1792 had prescribed measures relative to the width of Parisian streets in relation to the height of houses. The height of houses was fixed at fifty-four feet on streets with a width of five fathoms; if the street was narrower, the height was fixed at forty-five feet. See Piorry, *Des habitations*, p. 44.

latrines, whitewashed walls, and the admittance of no more people than could be adequately lodged, given the number of beds and the amount of air.[12]

In 1848 a health council commission addressed two reports to the prefect of police on the salubrity of private dwellings. After investigating housing in several quarters of the city, the council isolated the main causes of the vitiation of air: too many animals and people who used up the oxygen supply and emitted carbon dioxide. Adhering to the miasmatic theory, commission members believed that harmful emanations were the cause of most epidemics. They observed that general uncleanliness prevailed in working-class dwellings: lack of air and light, humid conditions, stagnating household waters, and badly kept latrines. Investigators found some people living in dwellings with no windows at all. The health council urged a police ordinance regulating the salubrity of private dwellings and placing the responsibility for maintaining general cleanliness on proprietors. Responding to the health council's recommendations, on November 20, 1848, the municipal administration issued an ordinance regulating the salubrity of dwellings. Although hygienists considered the 1848 ordinance a minor victory, the measure did not solve the problem. In the second half of the century, public hygienists and municipal administrators continued to focus much attention on unhealthy dwellings and working-class housing.[13]

THE SALUBRÍTY OF PUBLIC ESTABLISHMENTS

Hygienists also investigated the impact of public establishments on health, turning their attention to heating, ventilation, water, and toilet facilities, and, in general, the preservation of clean air and surroundings. Hospitals especially came under hygienic scrutiny. Physicians had studied sanitary conditions in hospitals since the late eighteenth century, and by 1815 many reforms had been made. Yet problems of heating and ventilation persisted. Although high ceilings, large rooms, and numerous windows allowed improved air circulation, heating was almost impossible. Hygienists believed the best temperature for hospitals was 59°F, but it was colder than that in many hospitals. David Johnston, a Scottish physician who visited

---

12 R. G....*Paris*, 1829, pp. 38–9. See, for example, Jean-Baptiste Monfalcon and A. P. Isidore de Polinière, *Hygiène de Lyon* (Paris: Baillière, (1846), p. 386; Monfalcon and Polinière, *Traité de la salubrité*, pp. 49–71; Frégier also called for government intervention in *Des classes dangereuses*, 2: 145–7; Piorry, *Des habitations*, pp. 85–93; Henri Bayard, "Mémoire sur la topographie médicale des Xe, XIe, et XIIe arrondissements," *Annales d'hygiène publique* 32 (1844): 282–5, Bayard became an editor of the *Annales d'hygiène publique* in the late 1840s.

13 R. G....*Paris*, 1848, pp. 172–92. For a full discussion of this issue in the second half of the century, see Shapiro, *Housing the Poor of Paris*.

France in the 1820s, reported that many patients died at the Hôtel-Dieu in Lyon, where the winter temperature could be as low as 32°F. In winter, adequate ventilation was incompatible with heating the hospital, and on still summer days, natural ventilation failed to keep the hospital cool.[14]

Hygienists investigated similar concerns related to ventilation, heat, and light in prisons. In 1829 the Paris health council investigated health conditions at the recently built model prison of La Roquette. The primary consideration in its construction had been surveillance of prisoners, which was achieved, council members asserted, at the expense of sanitary conditions. Ventilation was unsatisfactory, and cesspools were inconveniently located. The health council contended that high mortality rates in prisons were directly related to insanitary conditions.[15] In an 1829 article in the *Annales d'hygiène publique*, Villermé demonstrated statistically that the mortality rate of prisoners was considerably higher than that of the general population. Although he attributed part of the difference to the prisoners' impoverished state before imprisonment, he still argued that their high mortality rate was a direct result of insanitary prison conditions.[16] Many hygienic improvements were made after the establishment of the Royal Society for the Improvement of Prisons in 1819. During the 1820s and 1830s the physical state of prisons improved, and by the late 1830s sanitary conditions were so much better that hygienists and reformers turned their attention to rehabilitation of prisoners – or *moral improvement*, as it was then called.[17]

Heating and ventilation were the main causes of public health problems in theaters. The Paris health council declared in 1820 that there was not

14 David Johnston, *A General, Medical, and Statistical History of the Present Condition of Public Charity in France* (Edinburgh: Oliver and Boyd, 1829), pp. 169–70. On the early-nineteenth-century Lyonnais hospitals, see Olivier Faure, *Genèse de l'hôpital moderne: les hospices civils de Lyon de 1802 à 1845* (Lyon: Presses universitaires de Lyon, 1985).

15 R. G....*Paris*, 1829, pp. 29–33. For the organization of prisons to make surveillance of prisoners easier and the implications of such an arrangement, see the now classic work of Michel Foucault, *Discipline and Punish: The Birth of the Prison*, trans. Alan Sheridan (New York: Random House, 1979).

16 Louis-René Villermé, "Mémoire sur la mortalité dans les prisons," *Annales d'hygiène publique* 1 (1829): 1–100; see esp. pp. 39–41. See also L. R. Villermé, "Note sur la mortalité parmi les forçats du bagne du Rochefort," *Annales d'hygiène publique* 6 (1831): 113–27.

17 Villermé, "Mémoire sur la mortalité dans les prisons," pp. 36–8; Pierre Colombot, *Manuel d'Higiène et de Médecine pratique des prisons* (Chaumont: Cousot neveu, 1824), pp. 21–5; Edouard Ducpétiaux, "Questions relatives à l'hygiène des prisons et des établissements de bienfaisance," *Annales d'hygiène publique* 9 (1833): 272–9. Ducpétiaux noted that many improvements were still necessary, especially with regard to ventilation and cleanliness (291); he also noted that in some places new prisons had been built with little attention given to the practical aspects of heating, lighting, and cooking facilities (273). For the prison situation before many improvements had taken place, see Villermé, *Des prisons telles qu'elles sont et telles qu'elles devraient être* (Paris: Méquignon-Marvis, 1820).

one theater in Paris where the laws of hygiene had been observed. Writing in 1829, industrial chemist and hygienist Joseph D'Arcet stressed ventilation, heating, and proper maintenance of latrines as the three areas that had to be improved to satisfy public health requirements.[18] After the 1820s, hygienists published little on the insalubrity of theaters. There is no indication as to why they abandoned this area of investigation. Their attention may well have been focused on other, more pressing problems associated with urbanization, industrialization, and the cholera epidemic.

Whether it was theaters, hospitals, or prisons, finding better means of heating and ventilation was difficult. The leading nineteenth-century French authority on ventilation and heating was Joseph d'Arcet, the author of numerous articles on ventilation, the improvement of industrial processes, and the salubrity of public establishments. When d'Arcet started his work during the Napoleonic era, the dominant approach was natural ventilation, namely, windows and other openings through which fresh air could enter and stale air exit. Mechanical or forced ventilation, which d'Arcet advocated, was at that time used only in mines. D'Arcet's ventilation theories were based on two principles: (1) natural ventilation alone was insufficient, making forced ventilation necessary; and (2) air had to be regularly distributed and the temperature equalized by gradually increasing openings. D'Arcet contended that good ventilation could not be subject to atmospheric variations but had to be controllable at will, and he argued that the most effective method of power was heat (combustion), which would generate enough force to move air.[19]

Ventilation experts before d'Arcet, who had been primarily concerned with natural ventilation, had conducted research to determine how many cubic feet of air were necessary for healthy and sick people and animals. D'Arcet and ventilation specialist Eugène Péclet popularized the notion of mechanical ventilation. Yet these measures were not widely applied. Another expert, Philippe Grouvelle, pointed out in his introduction to d'Arcet's work that although the French excelled in theories of ventilation, the British and Americans were the experts in practical application. Hygienists maintained that buildings in Britain and the United States were better ventilated than those in France.[20]

18 Moléon, R. G....*Paris*, 1820, pp. 178–9; Joseph d'Arcet, "Note sur l'assainissement des salles de spectacle," *Annales d'hygiène publique* 1 (1829): 152–60.

19 J. P. Joseph d'Arcet, *Collection de mémoires relatifs à l'assainissement des ateliers des édifices publics et des habitations particulières*, 2 vols. (Paris: Mathias, 1843). "Notice préliminaire" par Philippe Grouvelle. For biographical information on d'Arcet, see *Annales d'hygiène publique* 33 (1845): 5–20. Seventy works by d'Arcet on public hygiene are listed in this article. Grouvelle, "Notice préliminaire," pp. i–xxv. On ventilation, see Alain Corbin, *Le miasme et la jonquille: L'odorat et l'imaginaire social, 18–19e siècles* (Paris: Aubier Montaigne, 1982), part 2.

20 Denis I. Duveen and Herbert S. Klickstein, "Antoine Laurent Lavoisier's Contributions to Medicine and Public Health," *Bull. Hist. Med.* 29 (1955): 167–9;

D'Arcet's method of forced air ventilation was successfully used in theaters, in industries, at the mint, and in some private dwellings, but he never had the opportunity to try it in hospitals. A projected new Parisian hospital, where d'Arcet was to install his system, was never built. By the 1840s hygienists began to advocate steam heating in hospitals after its successful installation in the Chamber of Peers and the Chamber of Deputies. But generally speaking, in spite of promotion by hygienists, mechanical ventilation was not in common use in Paris before 1848, and the problems of heating and ventilating public buildings persisted.[21]

Dissection rooms and anatomy amphitheaters – central to the teaching of pathological anatomy – were the subject of much debate among hygienists and administrators, with reports addressed to the Minister of the Interior in 1806, 1807, 1809, and 1810. Hygienists urged the elimination of private dissection rooms and their centralization, along with anatomy amphitheaters, into one central amphitheater. An 1813 order of the prefect of police forbade individual amphitheaters in the city and in hospitals, an exception being made only for the Faculty of Medicine.[22] Dissection amphitheaters at the Faculty of Medicine and the major hospitals were still functioning in 1831, however, when Parent-Duchâtelet and d'Arcet investigated the problem. The received opinion was that dissection rooms were unhealthy, because cadaverous emanations were thought to cause disease. In their investigation, however, d'Arcet and Parent-Duchâtelet found no evidence to support that belief. Nevertheless, complaints about bad odors, disposal problems, and inadequate water supply continued. Parent-Duchâtelet and d'Arcet suggested improvements such as adequate provisions for the deposit, conservation, and dissection of cadavers; for the maceration of anatomical pieces; and proper ventilation and water. While the two hygienists were conducting their study, the municipal administration was

Eugène Péclet, *Traité de la chaleur*, 2 vols. (Paris: Malher, 1828). Cited in Grouvelle, "Notice préliminaire," p. xxv. Grouvelle, "Notice préliminaire," pp. xxv–xxxvi.

21 Grouvelle, "Notice préliminaire," pp. xxv–xxxvi; Jean-Ythier Poumet, "Mémoire sur la ventilation dans les hôpitaux," *Annales d'hygiène publique* 32 (1944): 5–51; Alphonse Guérard, "Observations sur la ventilation et le chauffage des édifices publics, et en particulier, des hôpitaux," *Annales d'hygiène publique* 32 (1844): 52–70; Guérard, "Sur la ventilation des édifices publics et en particulier des hôpitaux," *Annales d'hygiène publique* 38 (1847): 348–66 (this was essentially the same as the earlier article).

22 Parent-Duchâtelet used *salles de dissection* as a general term that included *amphithéâtres d'anatomie*. Anatomy amphitheaters were dissection rooms where anatomy and surgery were taught, built in the traditional design of an amphitheater. A.N. F⁸77, Prefect of Police Pasquier to Minister of the Interior, 9 February, 1813; Minister of the Interior to Chabrol, Prefect of the Seine, February 23, 1813. There is a large dossier of letters on the topic covering the years 1806–14 in A.N. F⁸77.

in the process of closing the remaining private dissection rooms and opening a central establishment on the site of the old Clamart cemetery to
replace the amphitheater and dissection rooms at the Pitié hospital. The
new establishment consisted of four dissection rooms with twenty-five
tables each, an anatomy amphitheater, and a museum for anatomical
curiosities, After 1834, the date slated for completion of the Clamart establishment, dissecting would be permitted only there and at the Ecole de
Médecine. Most of Parent-Duchâtelet's and d'Arcet's suggestions were
implemented at Clamart, where, upon inspection, the health council found
the ventilation adequate, the water supply abundant, and the location
good, a definite improvement, they contended, over the older, private
dissection rooms.[23]

PUBLIC BATHING ESTABLISHMENTS

One public establishment that received much attention from hygienists
was bathhouses. The increased water supply and improved water distribution in early-nineteenth-century Paris had important public health
ramifications, since water became available for domestic use, and bathing,
a practice heretofore restricted to the wealthy, became more commonplace. Still, most Parisians ignored personal cleanliness. One reason was
that bathing was difficult, expensive, and sometimes even dangerous.
Public hygienists consistently advocated the establishment of numerous
free public bathhouses, for they considered private hygiene and personal
cleanliness fundamental to public health. Because of the enlarged water
supply, the number of public baths increased greatly in Paris between 1810
and 1848, and Parisians became more conscious of the benefits of personal
cleanliness. Indeed, when it came to bathing, Parisians were better off than
most French citizens. In many areas of provincial France bathing – except
for river baths – was unknown. Personal hygiene was almost nonexistent among the rural population until the twentieth century. Although
hygienists blamed lack of personal cleanliness on the insufficient water
supply, cultural traditions were probably just as important. A general
indifference to personal hygiene existed even among those who had or
could afford water. Pierre Girard, chief engineer in charge of municipal
service for the city of Paris, may have been correct in his assertion that
even if Parisians had abundant water, they would not have known what

23 J. P. Joseph d'Arcet and A. J. B. Parent-Duchâtelet, "De l'influence et de
l'assainissement des salles de dissection," *Hygiène publique*, 2: 1–70; *Journal des
Débats*, August 25, 1833, p. 2. Erwin Ackerknecht, *Medicine at the Paris Hospital,
1794–1848* (Baltimore: Johns Hopkins University Press, 1967), p. 40. R. G....
Paris, 1847, pp. 119–25. With regard to ventilation, d'Arcet and Parent-Duchâtelet
had advised the use of forced ventilation.

to do with it, that seven and one-half liters of water a day was adequate, given Parisian lifestyles.[24]

In 1810, the health council investigated bathing facilities and found them hopelessly inadequate, noting that only the affluent could afford to patronize public bathing establishments. Bathing at home was not an alternative, the council learned, for most homes did not have an adequate water supply. It was both difficult and expensive to procure enough water for a bath: Some dwellings had wells, but generally, water had to be purchased from a water carrier or hauled from public or street fountains. Additionally, many dwellings were not equipped with permanent bathtubs. Portable bathtubs could be rented, but the time, labor, and expense involved made a bath a major production. Public bathhouses might have provided a suitable alternative, but at the beginning of the century most bathing establishments offered expensive medicinal or steam baths, and were frequented only by the wealthier classes. The poor had to bathe in the Seine or not bathe at all. Bathing boats in the Seine had been popular since the eighteenth century, but many could not afford them either. The river was free, of course, but as the health council noted, this was no real solution, for unless one patronized bathing boats or bathing establishments, bathing in the Seine in the center of the city was forbidden. Anyone who wanted to take a river bath had to go to the outskirts of town, and there, as the council remarked, bathing was often dangerous because of the swift current. Furthermore, weather conditions precluded river bathing for ten months of the year.[25]

Statistical data gathered by Girard document the rarity of a bath: 300 public bathtubs existed in Paris in 1789, increasing to 500 by 1816. In 1817, statistician-hygienist Louis Benoiston de Châteauneuf reported between twenty and twenty-five bathing establishments in the inner city and four bathing boats on the Seine; he estimated that twenty-five baths were taken daily in each of roughly thirty establishments, or 22,500 baths per month,

24 On baths and bathing in general, see Pierre S. Girard, "Recherches sur les établissements de bains publics à Paris depuis le IVe siècle jusqu'à présent," *Annales d'hygiène publique* 7 (1832): 5–59; the articles in the *Dictionnaire de l'industrie manufacturière (DIM)*, 10 vols. (Paris: Baillière, 1833–41): Alexandre Parent-Duchâtelet, "Bains" (Hygiène), *DIM*, 2:24–29; Henri Gaultier de Claubry, "Bains" (Economie industrielle), *DIM*, 2:29–34; Charles Gourlier, "Bains" (Construction), *DIM* 2:34–7; Adolphe Trébuchet, "Bains publics" (Administration), *DIM* 2:37–9; see also Guillaume de Bertier de Sauvigny, *Nouvelle histoire de Paris: La Restauration, 1815–1830* (Paris: Hachette, 1977), pp. 93–6. The principal secondary sources for general comments on bathing and cleanliness are Guy Thuillier, *Pour une histoire du quotidien au XIXe siècle en Nivernais* (Paris: Mouton, 1977), esp, pp. 50–70; Jean-Pierre Goubert, *The Conquest of Water: The Advent of Health in the Industrial Age* (Princeton, NJ: Princeton University Press, 1989); and Pierre S. Girard, *Simple exposé de l'état actuel des eaux publiques de Paris* (Paris: Carilian-Goeury, 1831), pp. 47–9.

25 Moléon, *R. G....Paris*, 1810, pp. 49–50.

and 270,000 baths per year. If Benoiston de Châteauneuf's figures are accurate, then the number of baths in public establishments did not even average one per person per year, since the 1817 Parisian population was 713,966.[26]

Prefect of Police Jules Anglès urged the city to regulate bathing establishments in the interest of public safety and morals. In an 1818 report on public bathing establishments the health council expressed a similar point of view, also emphasizing the importance of baths for the health of the working classes. By 1818 there were approximately thirty-seven public bathing establishments in Paris, which were inversely distributed among the arrondissements according to population, a situation that the health council lamented. For example, in the twelfth, a poor arrondissement with a population of 64,787, there were no bathhouses, while in the wealthy first, with 42,718 inhabitants, there were seven.

There principal types of baths were available at the public establishments: baths for cleanliness (*bain simple ou de propreté*), medicinal baths or showers, and steam baths. Ten of the thirty-seven bathhouses offered baths only for cleanliness, and the rest had two or all three kinds of specialized baths.[27] Seventeen establishments offered medicinal baths that could be taken either by immersion in a bathtub or by shower. Three kinds of medicinal baths were available: Barèges baths, Plombières baths, and oleaginous baths. Medicinal baths varied from place to place: Some establishments used mineral water, whereas others added mineral salts to the water. The oleaginous, or oily baths, quite expensive at four francs, were offered at only a few establishments, one of which was at the workshop of one of the slaughterhouses. (Those were called *tripe baths*; the health council offered no details on how they were administered.) Steam baths, which were popular, were of two types: humid and dry, or fumigating. Humid steam baths were administered with either plain or aromatic water, but the most popular were the sulfur baths. Fourteen bathhouses offered steam baths, but only three had received official authorization. Since steam baths were considered therapeutic, the health

26 Girard, "Recherches sur les...bains publics," pp. 44–8; Louis F. Benoiston de Châteauneuf, *Recherches sur les consommations de tout genre de la ville de Paris en 1817*, 2e partie, *Consommation industrielle* (Paris: Cosson, 1821), p. 141; Claude Lachaise, *Topographie médicale de Paris* (Paris: Baillière, 1822), p. 208. In a budget worked out for the average Parisian, Claude Chabrol, prefect of the Seine from 1815 to 1830, allowed each Parisian two baths a year, one to be taken in the summer in the Seine. See Guillaume de Bertier de Sauvigny. *The Bourbon Restoration*, trans. Lynn Case (Philadelphia: University of Pennsylvania Press, 1966), p. 241. A.N., F⁸77, prefect of police Anglès to Minister of Interior, March 7, 1818; A.N., F⁸77, health council report on public baths, February 4, 1818.

27 A.N., F⁸77, health council report on public baths, February 4, 1818. The report notes that the list was incomplete. For figures on bathing and bathhouses, see Appendix 9.

council contended that quacks abounded and urged regulation to protect the public, guarantee sanitary conditions, and prevent accidents.

The council found the following prices to be standard:

Simple bath (by subscription)	1.25 francs
Simple bath with linen	2.50–3 francs
Oleaginous (oily) bath	4 francs
Showers (with plain or Barèges water)	3 to 8 francs

Most bathing establishments offering simple baths were clean and well kept, the health council discovered, although some were incommodious and unhealthy. Modesty and decency raised other concerns: There were rumors of frequent communications between the sexes and that several bathhouses also functioned as brothels. Recommendations made by the health council in its 1818 report included regulation and surveillance of bathhouses for workers and the provision of free baths by construction of additional establishments. Citing the 1803 law on the practice of medicine, the health council contended that medicinal baths should be administered only by pharmacists, with the bath apparatus built according to a model approved by the health council. Members also urged the construction of working-class establishments, with baths available free of charge or for a nominal charge. If 400,000 baths were taken a year in Paris, the council estimated that only 30,000 to 50,000 persons, or about 14 percent of the population, were bathing. The working classes, who needed baths the most, could not afford them and were therefore deprived of bathing ten months of the year.

The health council outlined both the therapeutic and moral advantages of bathing, noting that the importance of baths was universally recognized by both ancients and moderns. Free baths would benefit the state by decreasing hospitalization for skin diseases and by exerting a good moral influence on the population, the council asserted. Bathing, the members argued, offered moral as well as physical benefits, both of which were related to public health. Echoing the cleanliness-is-next-to-godliness philosophy, the health council suggested:

Uncleanliness, the primary result of misery, degrades man in his own eyes; it discourages him, it accustoms him to rags, to filth and renders him incapable of ideas of order and lofty sentiments. How many people live in debauchery who would change their habits if they had those [habits] of frequent ablutions. It is not without reason that several legislators made it [bathing] an obligation to the people they governed.[28]

The council urged the prefect of police to require factory owners or municipalities to provide free weekly baths for workers and artisans. In its

28 A.N., F[8]77, health council report on public baths.

1821 report the council again stressed the importance of cleanliness, noting the deplorable situation of public baths in Paris. Observing that the poor still had to go outside the city to bathe, the council suggested that the city provide free public baths in the Seine in the middle of the city.[29]

In 1820 the health council investigated the recently opened swimming school (*école de natation*), whose owner had requested authorization. Located near the Gros-Caillou steam pump, the establishment took advantage of an idea that had been suggested earlier by the health council, namely, using hot water from steam engines for its water supply. The swimming school consisted of a pool about 30 meters long by 6.5 meters wide placed under a new one-story building. The pool, which could handle thirty to fifty people at a time, was 2 meters deep in areas designated for swimming but had a shallow one-meter section for non-swimmers. The water was kept at 72°–77°F and was renewed twice a day. The establishment offered showers, swimming lessons, and heated dressing rooms. Favorably impressed, health council members hoped other establishments would open wherever large steam pumps made enough hot water available.[30]

From the 1820s, the increased water supply from the Ourcq permitted the opening of numerous bathing establishments. According to Girard, thirty-seven bathhouses were built in Paris from 1817 to 1831. By contrast with 1816, when Girard found 500 bathtubs in Paris, in 1832 there were 2,374 public bathtubs (*fixes*) and several hundred portable bathtubs (*baignoires mobiles*). There were also five bathing boats along the Seine. Adding together portable and fixed tubs, Girard estimated there were 3,760 public bathtubs in 1832. Not only were there more baths, but they were more affordable, owing to the increased water supply. Thus, by 1832, it was easier and cheaper for even a poor person to bathe occasionally. Frances Trollope, visiting Paris in 1834, criticized the drainage and sewerage system of Paris and the lack of water but was favorably impressed with the cheapness and facility of public baths.[31]

It is no wonder Trollope was impressed. Most bathing establishments were still the preserve of the rich. An example was the Etablissement hygiénique des Néothermes, which opened in 1831. Located in the Chaussée d'Antin, it catered to fashionable society. Elegant and well appointed, it offered a variety of baths and showers, with thirty-seven on

29 Moléon, *R. G.... Paris*, 1821, pp. 198–9.
30 APP, Paris. Health council report, ms., March 17, 1820.
31 Girard, "Recherches sur les...bains publics," pp. 48–56; Trollope, *Paris and the Parisians in 1835*, 2 vols. (London: Richard Bentley, 1836), 1: 232. The *Dictionary of Police* gives the number of bathing establishments in 1835 as seventy-five bathhouses, five bathing boats, and 3,768 bathtubs, not counting portable baths. See Elouin, Adolphe Trébuchet, and Labat, *Nouveau dictionnaire de police*, 2 vols. (Paris: Béchet jeune, 1835), 1: 92.

the price list, ranging from the simple sitz bath to the most expensive Egyptian bath (twelve francs). One observer described the Egyptian bath:

A new thing for the capital is the creation of the Egyptian bath. You can find it at the Néothermes, done completely on the model of those which the rich inhabitants of Africa and Asia possess. The form and the paintings have been copied so faithfully that in entering you will believe you have been transported to Cairo or Alexandria. This bath is composed of four rooms, into which one passes successively and in which the temperature is raised by degrees. In the last, one undergoes a rub-down and massage. This type of bath, marvelous for its effects and for the well-being that it produces for several days afterwards, is known and appreciated by all those who have traveled in Egypt and Asia.

A restaurant, salon/reading room, and billiards room were attached to the establishment. Clearly, this was not a place to go for a simple bath.[32]

An article in the *Moniteur universel* in July 1827 reported that the Seine was covered with public bathing boats, baths in some of them costing so little that even the working class could afford them. Bathing was becoming one of the necessities of life, the article claimed. Yet, in spite of the greatly increased number of public baths by 1832, the supply still did not meet the demand. Seven years later, the health council noted that the number of public baths was still insufficient. That year the council had received only two requests for the authorization of new bathhouses: one for steam baths, the other for Barèges baths. Although new bathing establishments continued to open, the health council reported in 1846 that the number of cheap bathhouses in the city center was insufficient to meet the demand.[33]

France lagged behind England in the number of public bathing facilities, in spite of an 1851 law that made 600,000 francs available for the creation of model baths and wash houses. England had numerous affordable bath and wash houses, whereas in France they were few in number and expensive. Hygienists lamented the situation, claiming that physical and moral improvements would result if workers were able to bathe weekly. A commission formed in the late 1840s under the auspices of the Minister of Agriculture and Commerce found that bathing establishments in Paris provided 2 million baths a year, or approximately two and one-quarter baths per year per capita, but that the poor class did not participate.

32 A.N., F⁸150, Prospectus of the Néothermes; A.N., F⁸150, Bouland to Minister of Commerce and Public Works, October 21, 1831. In the letter to which Bouland attached the Prospectus of the Néothermes, he emphasized the therapeutic advantages of baths and asked the minister to give the prospectus to the Royal Academy of Medicine for its examination. See Appendix 10 for the Néothermes price list. Quote is from the prospectus.
33 *Moniteur universel*, July 12, 1827, p. 1062; A Barèges bath was a sulfur water bath; it was named after a town in the Pyrenees. R. G.... *Paris*, 1839, p. 257; 1846, p. 25.

Whereas in England by midcentury even workers could afford a bath, in France bathing was still the preserve of the comfortable classes.[34]

FOOD AND DRINK ESTABLISHMENTS AND THE SAFETY OF FOOD

Public hygienists and the Parisian administration recognized the importance or pure food and drink for public health. In order to ensure pure food, the municipal government provided administrative surveillance through the office of the prefecture of police. Complaints by individuals about food and drink were handled by the prefect of police or police commissioners, who then usually turned them over to the health council for investigation. Health council members tested samples of the substance in question, but sometimes investigators had to engage in more extensive research involving on-site visits and interviews. The provision of pure food and drink was regulated by means of police ordinances and inspections, and for this purpose the prefecture of police employed both wine tasters and food inspectors who periodically made the rounds of the Parisian eating establishments. Some questions and problems investigated by public hygienists were adulteration of milk, vinegar, bread, wine, salt, and other commodities; the safety of eating pigs fed on horsemeat and of eating meat from diseased cows; and the safety of food colorings and metals used for food containers and counters in wine shops. Many beverages and liquids, such as wine, beer, liquor, coffee, water, and vinegar, were investigated for supposed adulterations, but most complaints concerned milk.[35]

In 1828, the municipal government asked the health council to investigate additives used in milk. The health council found that none were harmful and concluded that consumers could be left to their own devices to deal with merchants of bad faith. That same year pharmacist Jean-Pierre

34 "Revue administrative," *Annales d'hygiène publique* 46 (1851): 457–62; for the commission report itself, see Alphonse Pinède, reporter, *Rapport adressé à M. le ministre de l'agriculture et du commerce sur les bains et lavoirs publics de l'Angleterre* (Paris, 1849).

35 See, for example, Antoine-Germain Labarraque and Pierre-Joseph Pelletier, "Rapport fait au Conseil de salubrité sur un sel de plomb contenu dans l'eau de fleurs d'oranger," *Annales d'hygiène publique* 4 (1830): 55–62; Jean-Pierre Barruel, "Analyse d'une bière que l'on croyait falsifiée. Rapport à M. le Préfet de police," *Annales d'hygiène publique* 10 (1833): 75–9; Jean-Pierre-Louis Girardin, "Rapport sur un café avarié par l'eau de mer et livré à la consommation," *Annales d'hygiène publique* 11 (1834): 96–103; Pierre Boutigny, "L'eau qui coule sur les toitures en zinc, est-elle potable?" *Annales d'hygiène publique* 17 (1837): 281–95; Alphonse Chevallier, Théodore Gobley, and E. Journeil, "Essais sur le vinaigre, ses falsifications, les moyens de les reconnaître, d'apprécier sa valeur," *Annales d'hygiène publique* 29 (1843): 55–82; R. G....Paris, 1843, pp. 232–3; 1844, p. 264; 1845, pp. 311–14.

Barruel, a member of the council, investigated milk, discovering that the most common adulteration was dilution with water. Another substance, often flour, was then added as a thickening agent. Barruel found no harmful additives but believed the authority should require clear labeling and the sale of only pure milk. In the early 1840s, when police received complaints that milk was being adulterated with animal brains, they turned the problem over to the health council, which put pharmacist Henri Gaultier de Claubry in charge. He and his colleague, pharmacist T. A. Quevenne, examined the milk but found no evidence of adulteration.[36]

The most common adulteration of bread was the addition of a starch other than wheat, such as potato or rice flour, and although these were not harmful to health, their nutritional value was uncertain. Some adulterations involved the use of leavening agents such as alum, which was not believed to be a health hazard but whose long-range effects were unknown. In 1842 many suspicious bread samples checked by the police were found merely to be molded.[37] Investigating in the early 1830s, the health council found the adulteration of kitchen salt to be common. The council examined 3,000 samples from salt merchants in Paris and the vicinity and determined that 309 had been adulterated. As a result, a police ordinance issued on July 20, 1832, forbade the adulteration of salt. One year later Alphonse Chevallier noted that the results of the periodic examinations required by the new ordinance were unacceptable. He accused the inspectors of carelessness, for eighteen out of nineteen of them found the salt they examined to be pure, when in fact, Chevallier claimed, it was

36 R. G. ... *Paris*, 1828, pp. 4–5; Jean-Pierre Barruel, "Considérations hygiéniques sur le lait vendu à Paris comme substance alimentaire," *Annales d'hygiène publique* 1 (1829): 404–19; Henri Gaultier de Claubry, "Sur la sophistication du lait au moyen de la matière cérébrale," *Annales d'hygiène publique* 27 (1842): 287–95. This work was originally read at the Royal Academy of Medicine; T. A. Quevenne, "Mémoire sur le lait," *Annales d'hygiène publique* 26 (1841): 5–125; and "Falsification du lait," *Annales d'hygiène publique* 27 (1842): 241–86. On the importance of pharmacists in the public health movement, see Ackerknecht, *Medicine at the Paris Hospital*, p. 124, and Alex Berman, "Conflict and Anomaly in the Scientific Orientation of French Pharmacy, 1800–1873," *Bull. Hist. Med.* 37 (1963): 453–7; see also by Berman "The Pharmaceutical Component of 19th Century French Public Health and Hygiene," *Pharmacy in History* 11 (1969): 5–10.

37 R. G. ... *Paris*, 1835, pp. 116–17; 1838, pp. 255–6; 1840, pp. 72–3; 1841, pp. 121–5; 1842, pp. 174–5; see also Alphonse Guérard, "Note sur une altération singulière du pain," *Annales d'hygiène publique* 29 (1843): 35–9, and Alphonse Chevallier, "Note sur le pain moisi," *Annales d'hygiène publique* 29 (1843): 39–50; for other articles on adulteration of bread, see Jean-Pierre Barruel, "Conseil de salubrité. Rapport sur une prétendue falsification du pain par les sulfates de cuivre et de zinc," *Annales d'hygiène publique* 3 (1830): 342–6; Alphonse Chevallier, "Sur l'emploi d'un sel de cuivre dans la préparation du pain," *Annales d'hygiène publique* 4 (1830): 20–4; Frédéric Kuhlmann, "Considerations sur l'emploi du sulfate de cuivre et de diverses matières salines dans la fabrication du pain," *Annales d'hygiène publique* 5 (1831): 338–56; Alphonse Chevallier, "Pain dans la fabrication duquel on a fait entrer du savon," *Annales d'hygiène publique* 27 (1842): 306–13.

adulterated. Enforcement was lax and the situation worsened, as evidenced by the yearly examination of salt samples in 1840, which revealed that 2,561 of 4,878 samples were adulterated. Chevallier suggested the appointment of one competent person as salt examiner.[38]

The use of coloring in food and food wrapping paper posed yet another problem. In an 1829 examination of liqueurs and colored candies, the health council found lead salt, copper, and arsenic and proposed that no mineral colors be used in food. Abuses lessened subsequent to the police ordinance of 1830 that regulated the use of food coloring and instituted regular visits by inspectors to candy sellers. An 1832 health council report to the prefect of police resulted in modifications of the original ordinance by eliminating certain mineral colors from food and food containers such as candy wrappers. To enforce the ordinance, health council members made regular visits to candy and liquor stores, and in their 1837 report they noted that the ordinance was generally being obeyed. The ordinance was reissued every few years – November 15, 1838, and September 22, 1841, but even though the situation was much improved by 1842, there were still infractions. That year, for example, a man was poisoned following consumption of cheese wrapped in paper tinted with mineral colors. After this incident, the health council posted a public notice warning consumers about possible poisoning, especially from green and blue paper. Sellers were reminded of their legal responsibility for accidents.[39]

The safety of eating meat from pigs fed on horsemeat from both healthy and sick horses raised further public health questions. Veterinarian Jean-Baptiste Huzard and Parent-Duchâtelet, both health council members, investigated the problem, concluding that such pork was not hazardous. Furthermore, they argued that the practice was economically beneficial, since the waste from horse slaughtering (*équarrissage*) could be cheaply

---

38 R. G....*Paris*, 1830–4, pp. 65–6. See also Alphonse Chevallier, "Essai sur les falsifications qu'on fait subir au sel marin, muriate de soude; travaux faits sur ce sujet; dispositions prises par l'autorité par suite de ces falsifications," *Annales d'hygiène publique* 8 (1832): 250–311; Alphonse Chevallier, "Rapport à M. le Préfet sur l'examen du sel vendu à Paris," *Annales d'hygiène publique* 9 (1833): 85–9; the ordinance of July 20, 1832, forbade falsifications and provided for visits from time to time to check on the purity of salt with the assistance of specialists; see Chevallier, "Essai sur les falsifications," p. 306; R. G....*Paris*, 1840, pp. 80–1.

39 "Salubrité. Rapport à M. le Conseiller d'Etat, Préfet de police sur le danger qui peut résulter de l'emploi des bonbons coloriés," *Annales d'hygiène publique* 4 (1830): 48–51; *Annales d'hygiène publique* 28 (1842): 55–72; Henri Gaultier de Claubry, "Rapport à M. le Préfet de Police, sur les visites faites chez les confiseurs, distillateurs, et débitants de bonbons et liqueurs," *Annales d'hygiène publique* 7 (1832): 114–27; R. G....*Paris*, 1837, pp. 177–82; 1841, p. 134; Alphonse Chevallier and F. Habert, "Sur la nécessité d'indiquer légalement aux confiseurs, pastilleurs qui habitent les départemens et à tous ceux qui préparent des sucreries coloriés et des liqueurs; les matières colorantes qu'ils doivent employer pour colorier ces produits," *Annales d'hygiène publique* 28 (1842): 55–72; R. G....*Paris*, 1842, pp. 182–3.

purchased as pig feed. A related problem concerned consumption of meat from diseased animals, a timely question, since many cows in the Parisian area were tubercular. Investigating hygienists concluded that unless the meat looked or smelled peculiar, it could be safely eaten. On a related issue, they contended that eating improperly aged (too young) veal was a health hazard requiring regulation.[40]

Hygienists investigated the potentially harmful effects of metal containers on food and of different types of counters on wine, since spilled wine ran down the counters, was collected, and was sold as a mixture. Parent-Duchâtelet attested to the safety of marble and tin counters as long as wine merchants and others who sold beverages were required to use an alloy of tin containing at most 18 percent lead. Both merchants and hygienists judged copper and lead harmful for food containers. If copper was used, containers had to be tinned, they argued. The 1832 ordinance regulating the use of food coloring, however, did not cover food containers, and in 1837 and 1841 the council proposed that the regulation be extended to them as well.[41]

There were other questions related to the safety of food. Hygienists wanted to know if green fruits were harmful to health and whether merchants should be forbidden to sell them. They also wanted to determine if ingredients used in sausage were safe. They wondered if food that smelled rotten was fit for human consumption.[42] The safety of drinking water was also a public health concern. Not only was the water supply

40 R. G. . . . Paris, 1835, pp. 114–16; Nicolas Adelon, Jean-Baptiste Huzard fils, and Alexandre Parent-Duchâtelet, "Examen de cette question: peut-on sans inconvénient pour la santé publique, permettre la vente, l'abattage et le débit des porcs engraissés avec de la chair de cheval, soit que cette chair leur ait été donnée à l'état cuit ou à l'état de crudité?" Annales d'hygiène publique 14 (1835): 240–57. Also in Hygiène publique 2: 445–59; Jean-Baptiste Huzard fils, "Rapport fait au Conseil de salubrité sur la vente de la chair provenant des animaux morts des maladies," Annales d'hygiène publique 10 (1833): 80–4; Jean-Baptiste Huzard fils, "Rapport à M. le Préfet de police, sur la pommelière ou phthisie pulmonaire des vaches laitières de Paris et des environs," Annales d'hygiène publique 11 (1834): 447–56; R. G. . . . Paris, 1840, pp. 75–6; 1841, pp. 125–34; L. F. Grognier, "De l'usage alimentaire de la chair de veaux trop jeune," Annales d'hygiène publique 2 (1829): 267–77; Etienne Sainte-Marie, Lectures relatives à la police médicale faites au Conseil de salubrité de Lyon et du Département du Rhône pendant les anneées 1826, 1827, et 1828 (Paris: Baillière, 1824), p. 39.
41 This is explained in Alexandre Parent-Duchâtelet, "Observations sur les comptoirs en étain et en marbre dont se servent les marchans de vin de la ville de Paris," Hygiène publique, 2: 460–78; Jean-Pierre Barruel, "Note sur les inconvéniens des vases de cuivre et de plomb employés dans la préparation des alimens," Annales d'hygiène publique 14 (1835): 131–3; R. G. . . . Paris, 1837, pp. 182–6; 1841, pp. 120–1; 1835, pp. 111–12; 1839, pp. 255–6.
42 Alexandre Parent-Duchâtelet, "Recherches pour déterminer jusqu'à quel point les émanations putrides, provenant de la décomposition des matières animales, peuvent contribuer à l'alteration des substances alimentaires," Hygiène publique, 2: 85–127.

insufficient, but the quality of drinking water was poor. The Seine, which furnished a major portion of the city's water before the 1820s, was also the receptacle for the city's sewage. Water quality had generally been ignored up to the 1820s. Historian Jean Tulard reported, for example, that during the Napoleonic era, most people were more concerned with the insufficient quantity than with the bad quality of water. Though contemporaries thought Seine water safe for for drinking, hygienists questioned its purity.[43]

In his 1824 article on the sewers of Paris, Parent-Duchâtelet discussed pure drinking water, questioning whether the mass of water was great enough to render wastes harmless. He reported that chemists had performed experiments on Seine water that showed the composition to be the same both before and after sewage was added. They had concluded that sewage had no influence on the water, because the amount of water was great enough to neutralize any harmful effects of the sewage. Parent-Duchâtelet did not agree, claiming instead that the condition varied with the season. In winter Seine water was safe to drink, because the current was swift and the river high, but he noted that summer storms stirred up the mud and sewage from the Seine, which often looked black and filthy, especially where the Bièvre River emptied into it.[44]

One way to improve the quality of drinking water was to get it from another source, such as the Ourcq, which had not been polluted by sewage; the main drawback to this solution was that Parisians preferred the taste of Seine water. A second solution was to use filtering devices to purify Seine water; carbon, wool, and sand filters, along with sponges acting as grease filters, were used. The health council reported in 1841 that all the filtering methods employed were effective. Filters were located at the various pumping stations and merchant fountains, where water carriers purchased water. Public fountains did not have their own filtering devices; however, some private houses and establishments did.[45] Ultimately pure water was obtained by bringing water to Paris from new sources, one of the major accomplishments of the urban transformation of Paris under Haussmann during the Second Empire.

The hygienists' principal solution to public health problems raised by unhealthy food and drink was regulation and inspection. Although there

---

43 Jean Tulard, *Nouvelle histoire de Paris: Le Consulat et l'Empire* (Paris: Hachette, 1970), p. 228.
44 Alexandre Parent-Duchâtelet, "Essai sur les cloaques out égouts de la ville de Paris," *Hygiène publique*, 1: 235–46. The Bièvre flowed into the Seine below the city, below the Pont d'Austerlitz.
45 *R. G. ... Paris*, 1841, pp. 112–20; Maxime Du Camp, *Paris. Ses organes. Ses fonctions et sa vie dans la seconde moitié de XIXe siècle*, 6 vols. (Paris: Hachette, 1868–75), 5: 346–7; Augustus Kinsley Gardner, *Old Wine in New Bottles, or Spare Hours of a Student in Paris* (New York: Francis, 1848), p. 285.

was no administration specifically in charge of overseeing the safety of food and drink, there were market and shop inspectors and wine tasters employed by the prefecture of police. Additionally, the Paris health council investigated suspicious samples. At the urging of the council, police ordinances were issued to ensure the purity of food and drink, but their effectiveness depended on enforcement, which varied according to the item. (Health council reports indicate that enforcement of ordinances was greater in this area of public health administration than in others.)

PROSTITUTION AS AN URBAN HEALTH PROBLEM

Parent-Duchâtelet, author of the definitive sociohygienic work on prostitution in early-nineteenth-century France, considered prostitution a public health problem, because prostitutes were the primary source of venereal diseases. Parent-Duchâtelet believed that prostitution was as inevitable in big cities as sewers, dumps, and garbage heaps. He argued that there was no way to eliminate prostitution, since it was an "industry against hunger," but active governmental surveillance and regulation could lessen the inconveniences and related health problems. Parent-Duchâtelet's two-volume *Prostitution in Paris* – like his other public health investigations – exemplifies his research methodology and his attempt to practice public hygiene in a scientific manner. He spent eight years researching the topic, using material in the archives of the prefecture of police, making personal visits to brothels, and conducting interviews with prostitutes.[46] The number of prostitutes in Paris was a matter of debate. Estimates from 1762 to 1826 put the number between 15,000 and 30,000. Registration of prostitutes began in 1816, making an accurate count more likely, although many prostitutes refused to register, practicing their trade illegally. In 1832, the number of registered prostitutes was 3,358. Four years later, Honoré Frégier reported 3,800 registered prostitutes, approximately 4,000 unregistered prostitutes, and 186 legally recognized – or "tolerated" – brothels.[47]

Parent-Duchâtelet, Lyonnais physician-hygienist Ariste Potton, and

46 Alexandre J. B. Parent-Duchâtelet, *De la prostitution dans la ville de Paris*, 2 vols. (Paris: Baillière, 1836), 2: 526–8. For a contemporary review of Parent-Duchâtelet's book, see François-Louis-Isidore Valleix, *De la prostitution...par A. J. B. Parent-Duchâtelet* (Paris: au bureau du *Journal hebdomadaire*, 1836). *Extrait du Journal hebdomadaire des progrès des sciences médicales*, notes 41 and 44, 1836; Parent-Duchâtelet, *De la prostitution*, 1: 621. On Parent-Duchâtelet's methodology and the scientific study of prostitution, see William Coleman, "The Scientific Study of Prostitution," essay prepared for Franco Maria Ricci, editore, based upon the Jason A. Hannah Lecture; Alain Corbin, "Présentation" to Alexandre Parent-Duchâtelet, *La prostitution à Paris au XIXe siècle*, texte présenté et annoté par Alain Corbin (Paris: Seuil, 1981), pp. 9–42; Jill Harsin, *Policing Prostitution in Nineteenth-Century Paris* (Princeton, NJ: Princeton University Press, 1985).

47 Parent-Duchâtelet, *De la prostitution*, 1: 28–37; see Frégier, *Des classes dangereuses*, 1: 48. Frégier won a prize given by the Academy of Political and Moral Sciences for this work.

other hygienists endorsed preventive measures against venereal disease. Proposed measures included active governmental surveillance of prostitutes and creation of a sanitary administration to provide early treatment. Paris set the example in the administrative treatment of prostitutes as a public health problem, employing toleration of prostitution, registration, police surveillance, and enforcement of sanitary measures. A prefectoral ordinance of July 1816 prescribed a general registration of all prostitutes, requiring them to register at the prefecture of police and to submit to regular examinations by physicians employed by the sanitary service.[48] Potton contended that the Parisian method should be followed by other large French cities. Henri Gisquet, prefect of police from 1831 to 1836, stated that statesmen from nearly all European countries had written to him asking for a collection of Parisian regulations concerning prostitutes, which he interpreted as evidence that the Parisian system was superior. The Parisian model had its champions in the United States as well. In the 1850s William Sanger, a prominent New York physician, recommended that New York adopt the Paris system of sanitary inspection of prostitutes, and the city of St. Louis tried it in the 1870s.[49]

The Parisian sanitary program had its origins in the eighteenth century, when physicians began to make sanitary visits to prostitutes. Attempts to treat prostitution as a public health problem were made during the Revolution, when a law of July 22, 1791, mandated severe penalties for prostitutes who did not present guarantees of good health. The idea of requiring prostitutes to have physical examinations by physicians dated from 1798, but no program was developed at that time. That prostitution should be treated as a public health hazard was not a compelling argument until the nineteenth century, and even then many criticized the notion. Under Dubois, the first prefect of police of Paris (1800–10), several projects were considered and sanitary visits were formalized: The administration hired physicians to locate prostitutes, examine them, and then charge them for their examinations. It is not surprising, given such an arrangement, that physicians sought out and examined only those who could afford to pay.[50]

The creation of a special center where sick prostitutes could receive free

48 Ariste Potton, *De la prostitution et de la syphilis dans les grandes villes, dans la ville de Lyon en particulier* (Paris: Baillière, 1842); F. S. Ratier, "Mémoire en réponse à cette question: quelles sont les mesures de police médicale les plus propres à arrêter la propagation de la maladie vénérienne," *Annales d'hygiène publique* 16 (1836): 262–97; Potton, *De la prostitution*, pp. 215, 247–8; Parent-Duchâtelet, *De la prostitution*, 1: 369.

49 See Henri Gisquet, *Mémoires de M. Gisquet, ancien préfet de police écrits par lui-même*, 4 vols. (Paris: Marchant, 1840), 4: 366. See 4: 347–66 for his discussion of prostitution in Paris during his time as prefect of police. John C. Burnham, "Medical Inspection of Prostitution in America in the Nineteenth Century: The St. Louis Experiment and Its Sequel," *Bull. Hist. Med.* 45 (1971): 203–18.

50 Parent-Duchâtelet, *De la prostitution*, 2: 50–60.

treatment was realized in 1802 when the Health Dispensary (*Dispensaire de salubrité*) was opened. Prefect of Police Etienne Pasquier reorganized the Dispensary in 1810, establishing a permanent commission to oversee it. At the same time, municipal sanitary authorities began more intensive surveillance of prostitutes, instituting biweekly visits by physicians. Hygienists judged Pasquier's reorganization a success. Active surveillance lowered the incidence and gravity of venereal disease among prostitutes, they claimed, and the advantages of such a sanitary program began to be recognized. Anglès, prefect of police from 1815 to 1821, continued and completed Pasquier's work, making surprise visits routine, in addition to regular semimonthly visits. Registration of prostitutes at the prefecture of police began in 1816, and during the early years of the Restoration, François Becquey, Minister of the Interior, began to study the possibility of a nationwide program of surveillance and a special infirmary for prostitutes. However, no national law regulating prostitution was passed, nor was nationwide surveillance instituted.[51]

There were several problems associated with the Parisian sanitary program for the surveillance and regulation of prostitution: lack of effective treatment for venereal disease, clandestine prostitution, extending the jurisdiction to the rural Parisian communes, and public opinion, which opposed a program of prevention rather than cure. Part of the sanitary program involved treatment of prostitutes infected with venereal disease. Although no effective treatment was available, the sanitary program provided for mercury or potassium iodide therapy, with an average hospital stay of 65 to 70 days. Hygienists wrongly believed that all who were treated were healed, probably because overt symptoms disappeared. The first Parisian hospital for the treatment of prostitutes dated from 1683, when one room at Salpêtrière hospital was allocated for this purpose. To gain admittance, a prostitute first had to be arrested. Upon entering the hospital, she was then punished and beaten, since venereal disease was considered a crime rather than a disease. The mortality rate of afflicted prostitutes was high, probably due just as much to insanitary conditions in hospitals as to the diseases for which patients were being treated. Conditions began to improve, as in most Parisian hospitals, in the late eighteenth century, and the mortality rate dropped from about 1/10–12 (one death for every ten to twelve prostitutes afflicted with venereal disease) to 1/47.[52]

Treatment was difficult and uncertain, because relatively little was known about venereal disease. At the time of Parent-Duchâtelet's research in the early 1830s there was still no positive differentiation between the

51 Ibid., pp. 50–69; 73–81.
52 Ibid., 2: 231, 239–44, 167–201.

various venereal diseases, and it was not until 1837 that physician Philippe Ricord successfully established gonorrhea and syphilis as two distinct diseases. In retrospect, preventive measures against venereal disease were all the more important, since there was no certain cure. Yet the importance of prevention was not widely appreciated, for it was commonly believed that if the symptoms disappeared, the disease was cured. After the publication of Ricord's 1837 work on syphilis, the tertiary symptoms of syphilis were recognized, along with the often lengthy period of latency between the secondary and tertiary stages. Venerealogists began to realize that what had been thought to be a cure actually meant merely that the first stages of syphilis were over.[53]

Clandestine prostitution was the second problem associated with the sanitary program. Registered prostitutes were submitted to sanitary surveillance, and statistical data showed a significant decline in the number infected with venereal disease. In 1800, according to statistics provided by Adolphe Trébuchet at the prefecture of police, examining physicians found one prostitute in nine (1/9) afflicted with venereal disease, but the percentage dropped to 1/26 by 1816 and to 1/60 by 1836. The real problem was prostitutes who did not register with the authorities but practiced their trade clandestinely. Many women practiced prostitution secretly; they did not live in brothels, but worked in small rooms or boutiques. In addition, "kept" women, of a higher social status than the common prostitute, did not register. For others, prostitution was not a permanent way of life, but a passing occupation in times of unemployment. The effectiveness of the sanitary program was further jeopardized by the failure of the municipal administration to extend it to the rural communes surrounding Paris, the justification being the expense of hiring new physicians and opening new dispensaries. The necessity of extending the program to the rural communes was obvious, however, since soldiers garrisoned outside Paris were a bona fide attraction for the poverty-stricken women. In 1840 and 1841, when workers and additional soldiers were sent to build new

53 Erwin Ackerknecht, *History and Geography of the Most Important Diseases* (New York: Hafner, 1965), p. 119. Thomas Parran gives 1837 as the precise date in *Shadow on the Land: Syphilis* (New York: Reynal & Hitchcock, 1937), p. 44; Philippe Ricord, *Traité pratique des maladies vénériennes* (Paris: Rouvier and Le Bouvier, 1838); Philippe Ricord, *Mémoires et observations* (Paris: l'auteur, 1834); Philippe Ricord, *Lettres sur la syphilis* (Paris: Bureau de l'Union médicale, 1851). On the various stages of syphilis and problems of treatment, see Alexandre Bottex, *De la nature et du traitement de la syphilis* (Lyon: Perrin, 1836). Bottex recognized the distinction between syphilis and gonorrhea, as demonstrated by Ricord. Bottex believed that mercury was the most effective antisyphilitic, even though it did not cure all cases. On the treatment of syphilis, see Owsei Temkin, "Therapeutic Trends in the Treatment of Syphilis Before 1900," *Bull. Hist. Med.* 29 (1955): 309–16. For a history of venereal disease, including information on treatment, see Allan Brandt, *No Magic Bullet: A Social History of Venereal Disease in the United States Since 1880* (New York: Oxford University Press, 1987).

fortifications around Paris, hygienists judged the situation critical, as prostitution flourished.[54]

A final problem associated with an effective sanitary program was unfavorable public opinion, which opposed preventive measures. Parent-Duchâtelet and Potton urged prevention, however, arguing that syphilis was worse than epidemic diseases, being both endemic and contagious, and affecting not only those afflicted but their offspring as well. The French national government had traditionally been more concerned with epidemics such as plague and yellow fever than with syphilis and other endemic diseases that affected more citizens but did not provoke a crisis. The sanitary law of 1822 regulated the importation of contagious and epidemic diseases; however, no national law regulating prostitution, the main source of the propagation of syphilis, was passed. Parent-Duchâtelet pointed out that in spite of many attacks on the sanitary administration, citizens still defended the system, regarding it as an important public health measure. He further noted that through the years the national government had spent millions of francs on plague and yellow fever but nothing on syphilis, which had been wrecking lives for three centuries, at least in France. One problem was that people considered prostitution a moral rather than a public health issue. A common opinion held that if it were not for fear of venereal disease, morals would be even worse, since venereal disease was perceived to be a punishment for sexual misconduct. Because prostitutes were considered immoral and criminal, citizens reasoned that money spent on them would be badly spent. Public health advocates dismissed as old-fashioned those critics who did not support a program of regulation and sanitary surveillance, and argued that preventing disease was crucial.[55]

Discussions of prostitution and public health came to a head over taxation of prostitutes. Registered prostitutes had to pay three francs for a medical examination and a two-franc fine if they missed a doctor's appointment. Managers of brothels paid a twelve-franc tax each to have their houses legally recognized, or "tolerated." In the early 1820s, critics of the program argued that it was an unfair tax, asserting that since prostitutes had not asked for sanitary surveillance, they should not have to pay for it. Hygienists and administrators at the prefecture of police, meanwhile, believed the sanitary program benefited the whole community and should be financed by public funds, like the national sanitary administration. Throughout the 1820s, the prefect of police repeatedly asked the Paris municipal council to allocate money to support the sanitary program. Finally, an investigative committee appointed by Prefect of Police Louis

54 Trébuchet's figures are found in F. S. Ratier, "La maladie vénérienne," p. 282, note 1, and p. 284, note 1; Parent-Duchâtelet, *De la prostitution*, 1: 596–609.
55 Parent-Duchâtelet, *De la prostitution*, 2: 37–42.

Debelleyme in 1828 concluded that the tax on prostitutes was illegal, immoral, and contrary to the spirit of the institution, and therefore, the public should pay.[56]

In the final analysis, even Parent-Duchâtelet could not escape the prevailing climate of opinion, which was more concerned with immorality than with public health. Prophylactics, which were effective in preventing the spread of venereal disease, were available, and one authority on syphilis, the physician Félix S. Ratier, advocated their use. Yet Parent-Duchâtelet, fearing the wrath of public opinion, would not propose the use of condoms, noting that the man credited with inventing the prophylactic in England in 1820, Dr. Condom, had had to change his name as a result of public outrage. Parent-Duchâtelet maintained that endorsing prophylactics would cause a negative public reaction, for he believed that when citizens and the government had to choose between public morals and public health, morals had to be chosen. Parent-Duchâtelet argued that once a prostitute had the disease, it was the duty of the government and the physician to treat her and prevent the disease's spread, but he did not advocate specific preventive measures, fearing that to do so might encourage public license. Judged according to the standards of his time, Parent-Duchâtelet was outspoken for investigating brothels and publishing a detailed account on the subject. At a time when two major Parisian newspapers, the *Temps* and the *Débats*, would not even use the word *syphilis* in their columns, at a time when the pope's pastoral letter of 1826 decried prophylactics as interfering with decrees of providence (who wanted to punish God's creatures when they sinned), Parent-Duchâtelet was more public health–minded than most of his contemporaries. But he was not willing to flout ideas of morality even for public health.[57]

Prefect of Police Gabriel Delessert received additional funds from the municipal council to extend sanitary surveillance to the rural communes in the late 1830s. Delessert pointed out in a letter to the municipal council that among prostitutes who were not subject to sanitary surveillance, the incidence of venereal disease was 1/4, much higher than among those under surveillance. In 1842, when the Minister of the Interior made additional money available, the municipal government extended the sanitary program

56 Ibid., 1: 374–87; 2: 392.
57 Ratier, "La maladie vénérienne," pp. 285–6. So also did Valleix, a reviewer of Parent-Duchâtelet's work. See Valleix, *De la Prostitution...par A. J. B. Parent-Duchâtelet*, p. 42. Potton was also favorable; see Potton, *Prostitution*, pp. 287–8; Parent-Duchâtelet, *De la prostitution*, 2: 543. See Henry Alan Skinner, *The Origin of Medical Terms*, 2nd ed. (New York: Hafner, 1970), p. 121. According to Skinner, Dr. Condom (or Conton) was an eighteenth-century London physician credited with inventing the prophylactic. The origin of the term is controversial. Parent-Duchâtelet, *De la prostitution*, 2: 529–44; Ratier, "La maladie vénérienne," p. 266. Ratier also pointed out that the philanthropic and mutual aid societies in France refused all assistance to members afflicted with venereal disease (266).

to the rural communes. The success of the sanitary program was limited, however, because there was no effective way to deal with clandestine prostitutes, who, hygienists believed, were the main carriers of venereal disease. Parent-Duchâtelet attributed the continual widespread existence of syphilis in Paris to the inability of the authorities to regulate these prostitutes. Of course, the continued existence of syphilis was also attributable to the lack of a cure for the disease. Many prostitutes whom physicians found free of the disease when examined did in fact have syphilis after all. Parent-Duchâtelet's solution for prostitution was a national law and a nationwide sanitary administration to enforce it. Such a law would have been aimed at repressing prostitution on a nationwide scale and initiating a system of dispensaries and sanitary programs to prevent the spread of venereal diseases. These facilities would have been assimilated to the other national sanitary establishments. Parent-Duchâtelet argued there were three advantages to such a law: (1) it would give a legal basis to the dispensaries; (2) it would give legal power on the national level for the repression of prostitution; and (3) it would place the sanitary establishments for prostitutes and the control of venereal disease with other establishments of recognized public utility.[58]

Whereas Parent-Duchâtelet's solution was statist and regulatory, placing responsibility for regulating prostitution and public health on the state, Lyonnais venerealogist Ariste Potton proposed a different solution. The ultimate solution, Potton asserted, was the elimination of poverty. Potton did not think prostitution would ever be completely eliminated, but it might be drastically reduced, for he believed women were driven to it by low wages, unemployment, and industrial crises. Discrimination against women was another cause, he argued, for in Lyon women's wages were normally one-third to one-half those of men. Thus Potton contended that prostitution could be eliminated or its incidence greatly reduced by a change in the socioeconomic organization to eliminate misery caused by low wages, industrial crises, and unemployment. Potton asserted that poverty caused disease, and then, in turn, disease caused poverty. He pointed out, for example that syphilis had a debilitating effect on those afflicted with it, especially the working class: Not only could they not afford to quit work to go to the hospital for treatment (typically sixty-five

58 APP, Da122, Conseil municipal. Séance du 5 mai 1837. Demande de la création de sept nouveaux inspecteurs du dispensaire (brigade sanitaire); Préfecture du Département de la Seine. Extrait du Registre des procès-verbaux des Séances du Conseil municipal de la ville de Paris. Séance du 5 mai 1837; APP, Da122, Lettre de Delessert, préfet de police, à MM. les Membres du Conseil Municipal de la ville de Paris. Le 4 juin 1841; APP, Da122, Delessert à MM. les membres du Conseil Général du Département, le 15 Oct. 1841. Also Lettre du Sous-secrétaire d'état au département de l'intérieur à Delessert. Le 29 avril 1842; Parent-Duchâtelet, De la prostitution, 1: 492–9; 2: 516–23.

to seventy-five days), but they passed the disease on to their children. Citing syphilis as an important cause of poverty among workers, Potton advocated the same sanitary measures as did Parent-Duchâtelet, but he went further by urging a reorganization of the social order. Potton's proposed reform was far too radical for the age and hence was never realized. Nor was Parent-Duchâtelet's proposed national law passed. Paris continued to operate a reasonably effective program that other cities copied, but no nationwide program was initiated. Like other public health problems, prostitution continued to be managed on a local level.[59]

WET NURSING

Although social welfare was part of the domain of public health in the early nineteenth century, the Paris health council and leading hygienists devoted little attention to hospitals, hospices, and at-home relief, because their management came under a separate administration, the *Conseil général des hospices*, founded in 1801. Wet nursing and wet-nursing establishments were a different case, however, for although they came under the authority of the *Conseil général des hospices*, hygienists perceived the industry to be a growing public health problem.

The care and feeding of infants was a major public health concern in nineteenth-century France, where infant mortality ranged from about 20 percent (20 percent of those born died before their first birthday) among the general population to about 60 percent among foundlings. Physicians believed infant feeding methods to be the principal cause of high infant mortality. The most common feeding method for Parisian babies and the most abhorrent to hygienists was wet nursing. Evidence suggests that wet nursing was widespread at all social levels in eighteenth- and nineteenth-century France. In his study of French wet nursing George Sussman asserted that nowhere else in Europe in any historical period was the practice conducted on such a broad scale and in such an organized fashion as in nineteenth-century France.[60]

Infant feeding practices varied widely from one part of France to another, with maternal breast-feeding being the norm in some areas, whereas in others, a majority of infants were farmed out to wet nurses. Farming out was the custom in many large cities, but the system reached

59 See Potton, *Prostitution*, pp. 6, 15–30, 164–81, 241–8. For the fate of the Parisian sanitary program for prostitutes in the nineteenth century, see Harsin, *Policing Prostitution*.
60 George D. Sussman, "The Wet-Nursing Business in Nineteenth Century France," *French Historical Studies* 9 (1975): 304–28; George D. Sussman, *Selling Mothers' Milk: The Wet-Nursing Business in France, 1715–1914* (Chicago: University of Illinois Press, 1982). See also Fanny Faÿ-Sallois, *Les nourrices à Paris au XIXe siècle* (Paris: Payot, 1980).

its apogee in Paris and Lyon. Yet in some cities – such as Lille – wet nursing was hardly practiced. Lillois physician Jean-Pierre Thouvenin reported that approximately half of the mothers there – many of whom worked outside the home – breast-fed their babies. In addition, many infants and small children in Lille were cared for at home by *gardes*, usually older children. Common child care practices in Lille included early introduction of cow's milk, baby pap (bouillie), and solid foods. In addition to maternal nursing and wet nursing, artificial feeding (bottle feeding) was practiced among the urban upper classes by midcentury and became more widespread at all levels of society as the century progressed. Physicians had urged an end to wet nursing since the late eighteenth century. Indeed, the practice of farming out babies to rural wet nurses was declining among the upper classes by the early nineteenth century, probably due to the publicity given the issue by Rousseau and other authors of infant hygiene manuals, who condemned wet nursing and urged mothers to breast-feed their babies. Some mothers breast-fed their infants, whereas others preferred to hire a live-in wet nurse – affordable, however, only for the well-to-do. Conversely, employment of wet nurses increased among artisans and the urban working classes, for these working women found it increasingly difficult to reconcile their jobs with breast-feeding and infant care.[61]

Historians have estimated that the infant mortality rate in the early nineteenth century was about 190 to 200 deaths per 1,000 births in the department of the Seine. Hygienists attributed most of these deaths to bad feeding practices, lack of maternal nursing, and abuses associated with wet nursing. They argued that wet nursing, as it was practiced, presented a clear threat to the health and life of many babies and urged regulation and surveillance of urban wet-nursing agencies – municipal and private – and rural wet-nursing sites that served large cities.[62] There had been a long tradition of farming out Parisian babies and of state interest in the problem, and ordinances regulating the industry dated from the seventeenth and eighteenth centuries. In 1769 the *Bureau des nourrices*, or the municipal

61 On Paris, see Sussman, *Selling Mothers' Milk*; on Lyon, see Maurice Garden, *Lyon et les Lyonnais au XVIIIe siècle* (Paris: Flammarion, 1975), pp. 59–84; Jean-Pierre Thouvenin, *Hygiène populaire à l'usage des ouvriers des manufactures de Lille et du département du Nord* (Lille: Durieux, 1842), pp. 43, 61–4; Pierre Pierrard, *Lille et les lillois* (Paris: Bloud and Gay, 1967), pp. 140–1, 169–70; pamphlet "Breton-Biberons," in Bibliothèque nationale, T 129.30. See the frequent advertisements for the Biberon-Breton in the *Journal des Débats*, passim. See Mme. Breton [F. S. Ratier, the actual author] *Avis aux mères qui ne peuvent pas nourrir ou instruction pratique sur l'allaitement artificiel* (Paris: Baillière, 1826) in BN, T 129.30.

62 Etienne van de Walle and Samuel H. Preston, "Mortalité de l'enfance au XIXe siècle à Paris et dans le département de la Seine," *Population* 29 (1974): 101; Dr. Boys de Loury, "Mémoire sur les modifications à apporter dans le service de l'administration des nourrices," *Annales d'hygiène publique* 27 (1842): 7.

wet-nursing office, was founded. The private wet-nursing industry, which dated from the 1820s, however, drew most of the business away from the municipal office. An 1821 reform establishing a bureaucracy to stem existing abuses and provide for more regulation and surveillance of the municipal bureau, as well as on-site inspection and reporting, resulted in the rapid growth of private wet-nursing establishments. Sussman suggests that the best explanation for this rapid growth of the private wet-nursing offices is that the fifty-two *meneurs*, or rural wet-nursing recruiters, who were replaced by the new bureaucracy, went into business for themselves, taking their clientele with them. These private agencies virtually took over the wet-nursing business in Paris. Alfred Donné, a physician and reformer of the wet-nursing service, suggested another reason for the decline of the municipal wet-nursing bureau. He believed that once the *Direction générale des nourrices* was placed under the authority of the *Conseil général des hospices* (in 1801), the institution carried an image of charity, so that the public considered it to be for poor rather than middle-class families. After the middle classes stopped patronizing the municipal bureau, it was abandoned to the poor, the quality of wet nurses declined, and the bureau's business decreased drastically. Before the 1821 reforms the municipal office had placed about 5,000 to 6,000 nurses annually, but by the 1830s the number had fallen to 1,200 to 1,500.[63]

In the 1840s, hygienists, the administration of the *Conseil général des hospices*, the prefect of police, and the municipal administration began discussing public health concerns related to wet nursing and the inability of the municipal agency to compete with the private establishments. The Minister of the Interior charged Donné with inspection of all private wet-nursing agencies in Paris and the preparation of a report on their status, methods of surveillance, and a general plan to improve the service. Donné, author of a widely read manual on infant care, had a low opinion of private wet-nursing agencies, finding them dirty, unsanitary, and unregulated, with unsatisfactory nurses. Given the importance of wet nursing for public health, he urged surveillance of private agencies and medical examination of wet nurses. In the second edition of his baby care book (1846), Donné continued to lament the lack of surveillance and regu- lation of the wet-nursing industry, contending that private agencies had overwhelmed the municipal bureau, because they offered bounties to midwives and doctors. The administration, although aware of the prob- lem, was powerless to redress it. Donné accurately assessed the situation at

63 Boys de Loury, "Mémoire sur les modifications," pp. 11–22; Sussman, "Wet-Nursing Business," pp. 314–16, 326–7; Alfred Donné, *Conseils aux mères sur la manière d'élever les enfans nouveau-nés, ou l'éducation physique des enfans du premier âge* (Paris: Baillière, 1842), pp. 92–7.

midcentury, when radical reform of the wet-nursing industry was called for. Plans were discussed but no reforms were forthcoming, and the high infant mortality rate continued.[64]

Donné's reform proposals included regulation and surveillance of private agencies, examination of wet nurses, and chemical and microscopic analysis of their milk. He had a special interest in the microscopic analysis of human milk, which he hoped would be a scientific way to determine the composition and quality of a wet nurse's milk. Common sense seemed to dictate that healthy women would have higher-quality milk than unhealthy women. Impressed with Donné's 1837 work on the analysis of milk, entitled *On Milk, and in Particular That of Nurses*, a commission of the *Conseil général des hospices* chose him to be in charge of examining mother's milk at the municipal bureau and appointed a group to study Donné's research on human milk. By the early 1840s his research was being discussed in the Royal Academy of Sciences. When in 1843 the city of Bordeaux planned to establish a municipal wet-nursing bureau, it adopted Donné's reform program as the model. The main features of that program were examination of both wet nurses and babies; registration of wet nurses; certification of the age and morality of nurses; and chemical analysis of the milk of each wet nurse to ensure its quality. At one point, Donné even broadened his proposed reforms to include the inspection of the 15,000 milk cows in Paris.[65]

Jules Boys de Loury, a physician writing in the early 1840s, noted that many improvements had been made in the wet-nursing office since its administration had been placed under the *Conseil général des hospices* in 1806, and he referred specifically to the 1821 reforms. Boys de Loury

64 Donné, *Conseils aux mères*, pp. 92–108; Donné, *Conseils aux mères sur l'allaitement et sur la manière d'élever les enfants nouveau-nés*, 2nd ed. (Paris: Baillière, 1846), pp. 9–13. The book went through numerous editions and was still being published in 1905. Editions were published in 1842, 1846, 1869, 1880, 1894, and 1905. An American edition was published in 1859: *Mothers and Infants, Nurses and Nursing* (Boston: Phillips, Sampson and Co., 1859). On Donné's pediatric interests, see Ann F. La Berge, "Mothers and Infants; Nurses and Nursing: Alfred Donné and the Medicalization of Child Care in Nineteenth-Century France," *J. Hist. Med.*, 46 (1991): 20–43.

65 Donné, *Conseils aux mères* (1842), ch. 3; Alfred Donné, *Du lait et en particulier de celui des nourrices considéré sous le rapport de ses bonnes et de ses mauvaises qualités nutritives* (Paris: l'auteur, 1837). Alfred Donné, "Académie des Sciences," *Journal des Débats*, March 28, 1838, p. 2; F. S. Barrière, review of Al. Donné's "Mémoire sur le lait des nourrices," *Journal des Débats*, July 3, 1838, pp. 1–2. Members of the commission were de Gérando, Valdruche, Orfila, Moreau, Blandin, Velpeau, Baron, and Louis (chairman). Bureau central d'indication des nourrices. *Quelques préceptes sur le choix des nourrices et le régime général des enfans nouveau-nés*. Extrait de l'ouvrage du Dr. Donné, *Conseils aux mères sur la manière d'élever les enfans nouveaux-nés* (Bordeaux: Coudert, 1843), pp. 1–2. Barrière, review of Donné, "Mémoire sur le lait."

wanted to centralize all wet-nursing establishments, the municipal office, and the private agencies under the prefect of police. He suggested limiting the number of private agencies to twelve to simplify surveillance, and urged that no new agency be established without the approval of the health council and the prefectoral architects. The new program would include examination of wet nurses by a physician both at the Paris office and in the communes outside Paris. In the rural communes, physicians would visit wet nurses every eight days, or daily for sick nurses, and each wet nurse would have a *livret* (pass book) to be filled in by the doctor. Inspectors from the wet-nursing office in Paris would conduct tours throughout the countryside to check on wet nurses and babies.[66]

Hygienists writing in the 1830s and 1840s believed the wet-nursing problem could best be addressed by regulation and surveillance of individual agencies and examination of wet nurses, babies, and mothers' milk. In their proposals for reform, Boys de Loury and Donné reflected the trends common at the time in professional hygienic circles: proposals for centralization of the service, regulation and surveillance, and attempts to assess scientifically the quality of the nurses' milk. Physicians' overall goal remained the same: to reduce the rate of infant mortality and morbidity. Before effective reforms were forthcoming, however, economic and social developments from midcentury on made the wet-nursing and infant mortality situations worse than ever. George Sussman described how the wet-nursing industry was headed for a crisis by midcentury, because there were not enough good wet nurses available to meet the growing demands of the working classes at a price they could afford. Thus increasing numbers of babies were artificially fed by "dry nurses," with the result that infant mortality increased in the third quarter of the century. Hygienists achieved one of their goals with the passage in 1874 of the Roussel law, which brought all infants being cared for outside their parents' homes under the protection of the state. The law did not solve the problem of high infant mortality, however, since many infants fell outside its jurisdiction. A more effective solution became available after 1890 with the introduction of a safe milk supply subsequent to the development of pasteurization. Ultimately, the problem of infant mortality was solved not by reform measures advocated by hygienists, but by scientific advances and cultural changes that made possible the phasing out of the wet-nursing business in the early twentieth century. Cultural acceptance of artificial feeding and its safety coupled with the decreasing supply of wet nurses brought the institution to its demise after World War I.[67]

66   Boys de Loury, "Mémoire sur les modifications."
67   Sussman, "Wet-Nursing Business"; Sussman, *Selling Mothers' Milk.*

FOUNDLINGS

The foundling question – a social, moral, economic, and public health problem like prostitution – also occupied the attention of public hygienists. Hygienists investigated the foundling situation to determine why children were abandoned, how mothers could be encouraged to keep their children, what could be done about the high infant mortality rate, whether the foundling system was at fault, and if so, what reforms were necessary. The Chamber of Deputies, the scholarly societies and academies, and leading hygienists, namely, Louis F. Benoiston de Châteauneuf, Louis-René Villermé, Jean-Baptiste Monfalcon, and Jean-François Terme, debated the foundling question in the late 1830s. At stake were the lives and health of 30,000 babies abandoned each year and 120,000 babies and children being cared for annually by the state.[68]

Although the foundling service had a long history, the early-nineteenth-century service was based on an imperial decree of 1811 that provided for adoption of foundlings by the state under the aegis of the hospital administration. Each arrondissement was to have a foundling hospice and each hospice a turn box where infants could be deposited outside the building and the box then turned so that the infant could be received inside. Babies were thus received with no questions asked, and within a few days were farmed out to rural wet nurses, to be supported by the state until the age of twelve. The original purpose of the turn boxes was humanitarian – to prevent infanticides. But by the 1820s, problems with the system had developed. Not only had the number of abandoned babies vastly increased, but the system was fraught with abuses. Expenses had escalated dramatically, and the number of abandoned babies had more than tripled between the 1780s, when 40,000 were reported (1784), and the 1830s, when the estimate was 127,000. Departmental councils complained of the increasing number of abandoned infants, and by the 1820s and 1830s many councils were calling for reform of the foundling system – specifically, suppression of turn boxes. In effect, departmental councils and reformers demanded a complete revision of the 1811 foundling legislation.[69]

Departmental councils urged reform, primarily because of the expense, but hygienists wanted reform because of the high mortality rate and their

68 These figures were the ones given by Benjamin Delessert in the Chamber of Deputies debate on foundlings. See *Journal des Débats*, May 31, 1838, p. 3. For background information on foundlings, see Alan Forrest, *The French Revolution and the Poor* (New York: St. Martin's Press, 1981). For a full treatment of the foundling question, see Rachel Fuchs, *Abandoned Children: Foundlings and Child Welfare in Nineteenth-Century France* (Albany: State University of New York Press, 1984).

69 Fuchs, *Abandoned Children*; Editorial, *Journal des Débats*, March 14, 1838, pp. 1–2; *Journal des Débats*, May 31, 1838, p. 3. See Faure, *Genèse de l'hôpital moderne*.

skepticism over a system that seemed to encourage abandonment. Speaking in the Chamber of Deputies, politician Benjamin Delessert noted that the cost of the service had increased from 4 million francs in 1811 to 10 million francs in 1838, whereas the number of children supported by the state had tripled since 1784. In 1838, of the 30,000 babies abandoned each year, 33 ⅓ percent died before the age of one and 33 percent more before the age of twelve. The infant mortality rate of foundlings was twice that of other babies. Ironically, improved mortality rates since the eighteenth century had only exacerbated the problem of supporting foundlings. According to Benoiston de Châteauneuf, in the 1780s the mortality rate for foundlings was 90–91/100, which dropped to 60/100 for all of France by 1824. Villermé's figures for Paris indicated a mortality of 75/100 in 1818, decreasing to 50/100 by 1838.[70]

One abuse concerned admission procedures. Before the Revolution an official report had been required before an infant could be admitted to the foundling home. During the Revolution, however, admittance procedures became lax, and some babies were received without the official report. M.A. Valdruche, a member of the Paris hospital council, reported that the Paris foundling hospital then became a general dumping ground for many vices. The principal complaint of hygienists and administrators was the abandonment of babies out of convenience rather than necessity. Lyonnais physicians Jean-François Terme and Jean-Baptiste Monfalcon maintained that many legitimate children abandoned out of convenience consequently lost their civil status. Furthermore, some mothers tried to cheat the system, abandoning their babies only to take them back as foundlings to nurse, and thereby getting paid for their motherly duties. Some reformers argued that it would be simpler for the state to pay the mother to nurse her own baby than to make her give it up, only to take it back underhandedly. The government tried to stem such abuses by moving babies from one department to another and decreasing the number of turn boxes, and sixty-seven turn boxes in thirty departments were closed by 1838. One theory was that if parents knew they would lose all trace of their children, they would be more reluctant to abandon them, and some departments began to implement the policy of displacement as early as 1827. A national government measure of 1834 provided for sending foundlings from one department or arrondissement to a neighboring one so that mothers could

70 *Journal des Débats*, May 1838, p. 3; Louis-René Villermé, "De la mortalité des enfans-trouvés considérée dans ses rapports avec le mode d'allaitement et sur l'accroissement de leur nombre en France," *Annales d'hygiène publique* 19 (1838): 47–60. Villermé cites the data of Benoiston de Châteauneuf in this article. See also Louis F. Benoiston de Châteauneuf, *Considérations sur les enfans-trouvés dans les principaux états de l'Europe* (Paris: Martinet, 1824).

not wet-nurse their own children and therefore would, it was hoped, decide not to abandon them.[71]

Jean-François Terme was one of the leading authorities on the foundling question. As president of the Lyonnais hospital administration, he was in charge of 12,000 foundlings, having to provide for almost 2,000 babies a year left at the turn boxes. In 1837, Terme collaborated with Jean-Baptiste Monfalcon, head physician at the Charité hospital in Lyon, to produce the definitive French work on the history of foundlings. Terme and Monfalcon, like many of their contemporaries, blamed the foundling service for the high rate of abandoned babies. They called for suppression of turn boxes, registration and identification of babies before abandonment, and an end to the commerce of foundlings from neighboring departments. Abandonment of legitimate babies out of convenience also had to be stopped.[72]

Villermé and Benoiston de Châteauneuf also investigated the foundling question. In an 1829 review, Villermé compared the situation in countries with and without foundling hospitals, concluding that the existence of the hospitals encouraged infant abandonment. Villermé deplored the high mortality rates at the founding hospitals, which were much higher than those among the indigent classes, and observed that the suggested inscription on foundling homes, "Ici on fait mourir les enfans aux frais du public," was well deserved. Villermé agreed with Thomas Malthus, who had suggested that one way to limit population growth was to multiply foundling hospitals.[73]

Villermé believed that internal improvements in the foundling system, principally reforms of infant feeding methods, would increase survival rates, and opposed reformers who sought to lower mortality rates by

71 Valdruche, "Rapport fait au Conseil-général des hospices par le membre de la commission administrative chargé du service des enfans-trouvés," *Journal des Débats*, April 3, 1838, p. 2; Jean-François Terme and Jean-Baptiste Monfalcon, *Histoire statistique et morale des enfants trouvés* (Paris: Baillière, 1837); the next year, they came out with *Nouvelles considérations sur les enfants trouvés* (Lyon: Bajat, 1838); and in 1840 they published a revision of the 1837 work, *Histoire des enfants trouvés* (Paris: Paulin, 1840). For their 1837 work, they received the Montyon prize from the Académie française; *Journal des Débats*, May 31, 1838, p. 3; Villermé, "Enfans-trouvés." Several cities, such as Strasbourg, had never had any turn boxes. There were neither turn boxes nor foundlings in the department of the Haute-Saône. See the speech by Benjamin Delessert to the Chamber of Deputies in *Journal des Débats*, May 31, 1838, p. 3.

72 Jean-François Terme, *Enfants trouvés. Discours de réception à l'Académie de Lyon* (Lyon: Boitel, 1836); Terme and Monfalcon, *Histoire statistique et morale des enfants trouvés*.

73 Louis-René Villermé, review of Gouroff, *Essai sur l'histoire de enfans-trouvés, depuis les temps les plus anciens jusqu'à nos jours* in "Notices bibliographiques," *Annales d'hygiène publique* (1829); 489–95.

reducing the number of foundlings. Villermé established a definite relationship between mortality and feeding methods in an 1838 study in which he found that breast-fed foundlings had a much better chance of survival than bottle-fed foundlings. He credited Lyon with having the best foundling service in France. There, he observed, after visiting the city in 1835, all foundlings were breast-fed. This was not the case throughout France, however. Although most foundlings in Paris were breast-fed, almost all were artificially fed in Reims. There were simply not enough wet nurses for all foundlings. Some wet nurses refused to take foundlings, because they feared contracting diseases – especially venereal diseases – from them. The result was that many foundlings were fed animal milk. Although Villermé's proposed reforms in feeding methods would have reduced mortality rates, they would have done nothing to solve the larger problem of the increasing number and expense of abandoned babies. In fact, reducing the mortality rate would have exacerbated the economic problem, since more foundlings would have survived to be supported at government expense.[74]

An 1837 decree (January 25) of the *Conseil général des hospices* reformed the Parisian foundling program by requiring each foundling to have a visa from the prefect of police. According to the decree, an official report from the police commissioner of the quarter in which the baby was born would state whether the infant was exposed or abandoned. Admission to the maternity hospital was also made more difficult in an attempt to convince mothers to keep their babies. Only mothers who agreed to nurse their babies and take them home would be admitted, and impoverished women who agreed to care for their babies would receive aid. The 1837 legislation resulted in an outpouring of articles and books on foundlings, as well as debates in scholarly societies, academies, and the Chamber of Deputies. Critics assailed the legislation as inhumane and as contributing to infanticide, the crime that the turn boxes were originally instituted to prevent. Responding to such critics, one author, Bernard Remâcle, presented data demonstrating that those departments that had the greatest number of turn boxes also had the most infanticides and argued that turn boxes did not

---

74 Louis-René Villermé, "De la mortalité des enfans-trouvés"; see also Abbé Adolphe Henri Gaillard, "Résultats du défaut d'allaitement des nouveau-nés et de la suppression des tours, sur la mortalité des enfans-trouvés," *Annales d'hygiène publique* 19 (1838): 39–47. Gaillard noted that at one hospital (unnamed) in 1834, out of 127 babies only 29 were alive at the end of the year; they were artificially fed; out of 655 babies born, only 66 reached 12 years, a mortality rate of 90/100. This article was extracted from Gaillard's larger work: *Recherches administratives, statistiques et morales sur les enfans-trouvés, les enfans naturels et les orphelins en France et dans plusieurs pays de l'Europe* (Paris: Leclerc, 1837). See the review in *Annales d'hygiène publique* 19 (1838): 238–40. A. Gendron, "Note sur la création d'un dépôt d'enfans trouvés de Paris," *Annales d'hygiène publique* 6 (1831): 81–9.

serve their intended purpose. Reformers used his data as a powerful argument to support suppression of turn boxes.[75]

Reformers were pleased with the results of the 1837 decree. In the first two months after it became law (November 1837), the number of admissions to the foundling hospital decreased by 33 percent compared with the same months of the previous seven years. The number of babies given up at the maternity hospital (Maternité) decreased by 20 percent, an improvement reformers attributed to the new requirement that mothers nurse their babies during the first forty-eight hours after birth and also to the aid given those who kept their babies. Presumably, the more babies who were reared by their own mothers, the lower the infant mortality rate would be. Prefect of Police Delessert reported a much improved foundling situation in Paris after enforcement of the decree began. The formalities for admission of a baby were simple. First, police officers determined if the woman depositing the baby was actually the mother; then, aid in the form of money and/or a layette was offered to mothers who would keep their babies. Delessert denied critics' charges that the required measures were equivalent to suppression of turn boxes and had increased infanticides, citing Remâcle's data. The turn box was still there; only its use was modified, he argued.[76]

The foundling problem was only partially solved before 1850 because, like other social and public health problems, it was a complex issue that defied easy and quick answers. In their investigation of wet nursing and foundlings, the early nineteenth-century hygienists foreshadowed the major infant welfare concerns of reformers and hygienists in the second half of the century.[77]

75 "Mesures de police prises à Paris, à l'égard des enfans trouvés," *Annales d'hygiène publique* 19 (1938): 65–75. On the history of foundlings in Paris, see Albert Dupoux, *Sur les pas de Monsieur Vincent: Trois cent ans d'histoire parisienne de l'enfance abandonnée* (Paris: Revue de l'Assistance publique à Paris, 1958). See, for example, Alphonse de Lamartine's eloquent plea for the maintenance of the 1811 legislation and the foundling service in the Chamber of Deputies in *Journal des Débats*, May 31, 1838, p. 3. For a defense of the foundling institutions as they were, see also Gaillard, *Recherches administratives, statistiques et morales sur les enfans-trouvés*; Bernard-Benoît Remâcle's work, *Des hospices d'enfans-trouvés en Europe* (Paris: Treuttel et Wurtz, 1838), is discussed in an editorial in the *Journal des Débats*, March 14, 1838, pp. 1–2.

76 "Rapport du préfet de police au ministre de l'intérieur," *Journal des Débats*, April 3, 1838, pp. 1–2; Valdruche, "Rapport fait au Conseil général des hospices." Valdruche had gathered data to show that the mortality of those infants kept by their mothers was 1/14 but in the foundling hospitals it was 1/3. The figure 1/14 seems highly suspect, although Valdruche admitted that his sample was quite small.

77 On the late-nineteenth-century infant hygiene movement, see Jane Ellen Crisler, "Saving the Seed: The Scientific Preservation of Children in France during the Third Republic" (Ph.D. dissertation, University of Wisconsin, 1984), and La Berge, "Mothers and Infants."

A regulatory, statist approach dominated the discussion of public health and social welfare. Moralization did not figure prominently in the case of wet nursing, foundlings, or prostitution. Rather, hygienists accepted reality as they found it. This was in sharp contrast to their attitudes toward workers. In the case of foundlings, there was some attempt to change behavior, or what today would be called *social engineering*, with regulations being changed and made with an end to modifying mothers' behavior. Wet nursing and prostitution were considered both social evils and businesses. There was little notion of changing the behavior of mothers, wet nurses, prostitutes, or the men who patronized prostitutes. Regulation was employed to reduce the negative social and public health effects of the two industries. There was little attempt at moral reform, since neither was considered by public hygienists to be a predominantly moral problem. It was not immorality that led to the abuses of wet nursing; it was the demands of parents' work, on the one hand, and the insouciant attitude of some wet nurses, on the other. Wet nursing, like prostitution, was an accepted, if unfortunate, fact of life in the hygienic literature. Like any other industry, wet nursing and prostitution had to be regulated to protect clients, their families, and the public health. This lack of moral indignation on the part of public hygienists suggests a sophisticated understanding of the socioeconomic situation and cultural traditions that allowed both industries to flourish in nineteenth-century France.

CONCLUSION

Public health concerns in early-nineteenth-century Paris illustrate the wide range of urban health problems that confronted hygienists. As part of their mission, urban hygienists sought to investigate all possible causes of disease and death and to make recommendations for their solution. The domain of the hygienist included not only sanitary reform, but pure food and drink and more complicated social welfare problems such as prostitution, wet nursing, and foundlings. Their approach to social welfare problems varied: All hygienists urged regulation, inspection, and legislation to improve public health. A few advocated more thorough social and cultural reform to modify or eliminate the problem itself; yet no public hygienist really thought complex social problems – prostitution, for example – could be eliminated. Some hygienists believed the wet-nursing industry was capable of radical modification: A change in infant hygiene – a major shift to maternal breast-feeding – would result, they thought, in substantial alteration of the industry and its resulting public health problems. Some hygienists advocated major reform of the foundling policy as well, arguing that if infant abandonment could not be eliminated entirely, at least it could be significantly reduced.

Although inspection, regulation, and legislation helped solve some urban health problems, such as the provision of pure food and drink and the salubrity of public establishments, they did not solve the more complicated problems associated with unhealthy dwellings. Like social welfare problems, unhealthy dwellings could not be managed by superficial remedies. Although building codes and regulations could provide a palliative, and ultimately might improve public health, hygienists realized that all public health problems were concentrated in the dwellings of the poor. Unsanitary living conditions were nearly always accompanied by profound poverty and overcrowded conditions. Some hygienists were optimistic, looking to industrialization eventually to improve the standard of living for all. But in the meantime, while recognizing the complexity of the problems with which they dealt, hygienists had to content themselves with superficial measures that they hoped in the long run – when accompanied by an improved standard of living – would have profound public health ramifications.

One way to assess the public health improvements made in Paris during the Restoration and the July Monarchy is to look at Paris after Haussman and consider the major changes made in the city under Napoleon III, when Paris was transformed, it has been suggested, from a medieval to a modern city. This approach can make reforms made before 1850 seem almost inconsequential. Starting with Haussman's Paris and looking back, the accomplishments of public hygienists and municipal authorities seem like simple stopgap measures, and from this vantage point the reforms of Chabrol, Rambuteau, Delessert, and the public hygienists can be dismissed as inadequate.

A second way, however, is to adopt the method of the early-nineteenth-century hygienists and compare Paris of the 1840s with pre-1800 Paris. If one does this, the achievements are noteworthy, although they were still stopgap measures, as many hygienists realized. Practical reforms included tripling the mileage of sewers in Paris and improving their construction; increasing the water supply; increasing the number of fountains for personal use and street cleaning; suppression of the city dump and modernization of the horsebutchering industry; increased sanitary surveillance of prostitutes; improved sanitary conditions in prisons and hospitals; moving dangerous and unhealthy industries outside the city center; and greater surveillance and regulation of food and drink. These improvements were due to increased awareness of public health problems among public hygienists and administrators, resulting in part from the detailed investigations by hygienists and from chemical and technological advances.

The major public health problems confronting Paris had still not been solved by 1848, however. The rapidly increasing population of the city had made many unsanitary conditions worse, and hygienists and reformers called for major reform of municipal institutions and systems. The sewerage system was still grossly inadequate, the water supply was still insufficient, and the distribution system was so poor that much of the available water could not be used. The housing situation was critical, with much of the lower class living in unsanitary conditions. The problem of garbage disposal had not been solved, and the streets were still dirty, in spite of major street-cleaning efforts.

In the final analysis, the principal contribution of urban hygienists was their recognition, identification, and scientific investigation of the major urban health problems. They proposed reforms, and in some cases they succeeded in effecting them. Public hygienists brought before their professional colleagues, the municipal authorities, and the informed public the most pressing urban health problems, and by their detailed investigations laid the foundation for the major public health reforms that would come in the second half of the century.[78]

78 On public health in Paris during the Second Empire, see David Pinkney, *Napoleon III and the Rebuilding of Paris* (Princeton, NJ: Princeton University Press, 1958); on public health and the public health movement in late-nineteenth-century France, see Martha Hildreth, *Doctors, Bureaucrats, and Public Health in France, 1888–1902* (New York: Garland, 1987); Shapiro, *Housing the Poor of Paris*; Claire Salomon-Bayet, *Pasteur et la révolution pastorienne* (Paris: Payot, 1986); Bruno Latour, *The Pasteurization of France* (Cambridge, MA: Harvard University Press, 1987); Goubert, *Conquest of Water*.

III

Public health before Pasteur

8

Public health and public health movements: Comparison and assessment

The early-nineteenth-century public health movement that ultimately spread to many areas of Western Europe and the United States had its origins in eighteenth-century France. The French were the leaders in public health theory and reform up to the 1830s, when the French public health movement reached its culmination. During the 1820s and 1830s there was considerable cross-fertilization of ideas between public health advocates in Britain and France, and British public health leaders such as Edwin Chadwick, Southwood Smith, and William Farr were influenced by French developments. The beginnings of the British public health movement dated from 1837–8, and by the 1840s, the British were enjoying some legislative and administrative success. By the 1850s, the French acknowledged British superiority in practical public health matters, such as sewerage and water supply, and leadership passed from the French to the British. Although Chadwick was familiar with the works of the French hygienists, frequently citing them in his 1842 *Sanitary Report*, by 1854 Ambroise Tardieu, one of the leading French hygienists and legal medicine specialists, included in his *Dictionnaire d'hygiène publique* the British parliamentary inquiries of the late 1830s and 1840s into public health conditions as some of the most important public health works the French hygienist should consult. Although the French were the early leaders in public health, the French and British movements developed simultaneously for a while and hence invite comparison. The public health movement in the United States, by contrast, more properly belongs to the second half of the nineteenth century, so that comparisons made between public health theory and practice in France and the United States before 1850 refer to the origins of the American public health movement rather than to the movement itself.

PUBLIC HEALTH IN THE EARLY NINETEENTH CENTURY

Urban health problems caused by the immigration of poor, often diseased people into cities ill-equipped to handle them in terms of housing, water supplies, and sewerage systems created the nineteenth-century public health crises in France, Britain, and the United States. By the 1830s and 1840s, statistical data showed that disease and death rates were increasing in some cities and were higher in cities than in the countryside. Recurring epidemics of cholera, typhus, and, in the United States, yellow fever illustrated the deteriorating urban sanitary situation, according to contemporary observers. Social problems related to disease and death also motivated reformers and municipal authorities: Crime, immorality, and poverty could all be shown to be related to an increasing incidence of disease and death.

The most troublesome epidemic diseases – for endemic diseases such as consumption aroused little fear and were an accepted part of life – in the United States before 1850 were yellow fever and cholera, and it was primarily these two diseases that motivated municipal authorities to action and acted as a stimulus to public health reformers.[1] Fevers, mainly typhus and typhoid, were the immediate instigation of the British public health movement, with the 1832 cholera epidemic being a motivating factor as well. Unlike the British and American movements, the French public health movement did not develop in response to any particular disease or epidemic. Although the cholera epidemic served as a further impetus to reform, the French public health movement was well underway by 1832, its basic theories having already been enunciated and institutionalized by the 1820s.

Similar theories of disease causation were articulated in France, Britain, and the United States. Most physicians and hygienists attributed disease to either environmental or social causes, often both. Those, like Chadwick, who emphasized environmental causes, primarily filth and bad odors, urged sanitary reform. Hygienists such as Villermé who emphasized social and moral causes, especially poverty, with its attendant unsanitary living conditions, urged social and individual moral reform. Many hygienists advanced moral causes of disease. A common popular belief, also held by hygienists, was that sickness, disease, and poverty resulted from immorality, and that conversely, health, wealth, and happiness were proof of adherence to moral laws. Although some hygienists agreed that disease was the result of immorality, a more prevalent attitude, especially among French hygienists but also common in Britain and the United States, was that bad morals were a *result*, not a cause, of disease and substandard living

---

1 John Duffy, *The Healers: The Rise of the Medical Establishment* (New York: McGraw-Hill, 1976), p. 195; Charles Rosenberg, *The Cholera Years* (Chicago: University of Chicago Press, 1962). On yellow fever, see John Harvey Powell, *Bring Out Your Dead: The Great Plague of Yellow Fever in Philadelphia in 1793* (New York: Arno Press, 1970; originally published 1949); and John Duffy, *Sword of Pestilence: The New Orleans Yellow Fever Epidemic of 1853* (Baton Rouge: Louisiana State University Press, 1966). Before the nineteenth century, smallpox and yellow fever caused the greatest fear.

conditions, and that public health reforms would result in improved morality.[2] A specific example of how public health reform might improve morals was the widespread belief that cleanliness predisposed people to good morals. Isaac Parrish, a Philadelphia physician, expressed the idea succinctly: "By facilitating the means of frequent bathing in families – particularly the poor and labouring classes – the effect would soon be apparent, by removing a prominent cause of disease, and contribute to the moral and physical improvement of the lower classes of society."[3] The Paris health council held a similar point of view, noting that uncleanliness was degrading, accustoming people to filth and making them incapable of "ideas of order and lofty sentiments." "How many people," the health council asked, "live in debauchery who would change their habits if they had those [habits] of frequent ablutions?"[4]

With few exceptions, nearly all hygienists believed that filth and bad odors were a principal cause of disease. But not all could agree on the role poverty played in disease causation. Although Villermé, Virchow, and other social epidemiologists asserted that poverty was the primary determinant of high mortality rates, other hygienists, notably Chadwick himself, turned the same argument on its head. Josiah Curtis of Massachusetts, echoing the Chadwickian philosophy, but also that of some of the French hygienists, asserted that disease and untimely death were a cause of pauperism, rather than vice versa, and that bad health led to bad morals. Public health reform, according to Curtis and other hygienists, could solve some of the socioeconomic problems associated with poverty and immorality.[5]

A public health theory shared by hygienists in France, Britain, and the United States was that public health improvements were concomitant with the advance of civilization, and statisticians presented data to support this belief. Chadwick shared the optimistic viewpoint of most French hygienists with regard to the concomitance of civilization and public health. Like the French hygienists, Chadwick was familiar with and influenced by the work of the Swiss statisticians Marc d'Espine, Edouard Mallet, and Francis d'Ivernois. Using their data, Chadwick concluded that public health improvements could hasten the progress of civilization by favorably affecting birth rates, death rates, and the age distribution of the population.[6]

Other hygienists took the opposing point of view – that civilization

---

2 Duffy, *The Healers*, pp. 189–205. See also the recent work by Duffy, *The Sanitarians* (Chicago: University of Illinois Press, 1990).

3 Isaac Parrish, *Report on the Sanitary Condition of Philadelphia* in *The First American Medical Association Reports on Public Hygiene in American Cities* (New York: Arno Press, 1977, reprint; originally published in 1849), p. 479.

4 A.N., F^{8}77, [Paris] health council report on public baths, February 4, 1818.

5 Josiah Curtis, *Public Hygiene of Massachusetts* in *First AMA Reports*, p. 523. Curtis was familiar with the work of Villermé. See p. 518.

6 Edwin Chadwick, *Report on the Sanitary Condition of the Labouring Population of Great Britain, 1842*, ed. Michael W. Flinn (Edinburgh: Edinburgh University Press, 1965), pp. 238–50.

created as many or more health problems than it solved. This attitude seemed justified by the 1830s, when statistical data showed that in Paris and New York mortality rates had increased. An American public health reformer, physician John Griscom of New York City, was an exponent of this outlook. Sounding like a disciple of Rousseau, he put forward the "noble savage" argument: The American Indian was naturally healthy, since health was the natural state of humans, and the American Indian lived in a natural state. Civilization, Griscom asserted, had a generally corrupting influence on health. But he was not completely pessimistic, noting that civilization was not necessarily provocative of disease. Public health measures could overcome the unhealthy influences of civilization, and even civilized city dwellers might remain healthy, Griscom maintained.[7]

Hygienists in France, Britain, and the United States put forward a similar case for public health reform. In the 1840s, Griscom presented the typical arguments. Chadwick's influence is obvious, but his ideas might well have come from the French hygienists. Echoing one of the major points made by French hygienists since the late eighteenth century, Griscom contended that health was one of the natural rights to which citizens were entitled; then, espousing a concept that dated back at least to Johann Peter Frank, and also to Frank's French contemporaries, he insisted that public health was the duty of the state. Griscom also urged public health reform for economic reasons. His assertions that health equals wealth and that a healthy nation is a wealthy nation were reminiscent of the mercantilist philosophy and the early-nineteenth-century French point of view. Even more to the point was the "sanitary economics" argument, advanced so persuasively by Chadwick and enthusiastically adopted by American hygienists, that a sick population is more costly than a healthy one; that it is cheaper to prevent sickness and death by public health reform than to pay for the results with socioeconomic dislocation. Griscom also maintained that disease led to immorality and that therefore moral benefits would result from public health reform. A final argument in favor of public health reform was the statistically proven fact that there was more sickness and death in large cities that in the countryside. Using Chadwick's figures (noting that no American figures were available), Griscom advanced the Villermé hypothesis that poverty leads to disease and premature death. The solution, Griscom suggested, was public health reform, which was to be carried out by a professional public health administration.[8]

7 John Griscom, *Anniversary Discourse Before the New York Academy of Medicine* (New York, 1855), reprinted in *Origins of Public Health in America: Selected Essays, 1820–1855* (New York: Arno Press, 1972), pp. 46–8. Griscom had been city inspector of New York City.
8 John H. Griscom, *The Sanitary Condition of the Laboring Class of New York* (New York: Arno Press, 1970; reprint of the 1845 edition published in New York by Harper and Bros.), pp. 20–3; The term *sanitary economics* was used by Josiah Curtis of Massachusetts. See Curtis, *Public Hygiene of Massachusetts*, p. 534.

Griscom's arguments illustrate the early-nineteenth-century hygienic viewpoint and indicate the influence of French and British hygienic thought on American public health reformers. Although the primary influence on Griscom appears to have been Chadwick, he was also familiar with the work of Parent-Duchâtelet. But like many American public hygienists, his knowledge of the work of the French hygienists was through Chadwick, whose *Sanitary Report* propagated French public health ideas to the American hygienists at a time when the deteriorating sanitary state of American cities was making them receptive to public health theories.

The sanitary survey, of which Griscom's *The Sanitary Condition of the Laboring Class of New York* is a good example, was a principal source of hygienic investigation in the early nineteenth century. The medical topography, the classical hygienic treatise, much used by French public health reformers in the eighteenth and nineteenth centuries, had its theoretical basis in the environmental theory of disease causation. With a tradition going back to Hippocrates, the medical topography emphasized geography, climate, and other environmental conditions to determine the salubrity of an area. Attention was also given to the population and habits of the inhabitants. The medical topography continued to be a popular form for hygienic treatises in early-nineteenth-century France. A typical M.D. thesis was a local medical topography of the candidate's home town or district. One of the best of the classical medical topographies published in France was Lachaise's *Topographie médicale de Paris* (1822).

The emphasis on climatic and general environmental factors in disease causation and hence the traditional medical topography began to undergo modification in France in the 1820s. Once again, the work of Villermé was central, for in his studies of varying mortality in Paris he demonstrated that the traditional climatic and geographical conditions used to explain disease and mortality did not correlate statistically with the rates of disease and mortality in the twelve arrondissements of Paris. From the 1820s, hygienists began to pay more attention to the social causes of disease and increasingly relied on social statistical data. In the 1830s and 1840s in France, Britain, and the United States, the medical topography emerged in its more modern form, the sanitary survey or sanitary inquiry. These surveys became the typical form used to describe public health conditions. Because of the interrelationship of industrialization, working-class problems, and public health, much information on public health conditions was published in working-class inquiries. Classic examples were James Phillips Kay's study of the working class of Manchester and Villermé's study of French textile workers. Both Chadwick and Griscom's classic studies concerned the "laboring population" as well.

A new feature of many early-nineteenth-century public health investigations that distinguished them from traditional medical topographies was the inclusion of statistical data, which gave them a scientific basis. Although many reform proposals were not new – nor were many of the problems – the inclusion of this scientific proof, usually comparative disease and death rates, made reformers' arguments more compelling and convincing. Statistical data became scientific rhetoric that hygienists used to their own advantage. Hygienists got their figures from a variety of sources: actuarial tables, army recruitment figures, hospital records, official statistical collections such as the *Recherches statistiques sur la ville de Paris*, and finally, dating from the late 1830s, British civil registration figures. Arming themselves with quantitative evidence, reformers demonstrated through their inquiries, surveys, investigations, and reports the urgency and economy of public health reform.

The typical nineteenth-century public health institution was the health council, or board of health. As the scope of public health changed in response to new problems and shifting theories of disease causation, health councils underwent important modifications. Before 1850 in the United States, Britain, and France, during times of medical emergency temporary health boards were established, for example, during the 1793 yellow fever epidemic in Philadelphia or the 1832 cholera epidemic in Britain. After the danger had passed, these boards were either disbanded or simply ceased to function. In some cities, volunteer citizens' commissions took charge of public health and welfare during an epidemic. Examples are the Howard Association in New Orleans, active during the 1853 yellow fever epidemic, and the leading citizens' commissions (*commission des notables-commissaires*) in Lyon before the 1832 cholera epidemic. Most public health institutions in the United States before midcentury were quarantine agencies. This was true of the health committees and boards of health in New York City and the first state board of health in Louisiana, founded in 1855.[9] The situation was different in France, where a separate agency, the sanitary intendancy, was in charge of quarantines. Although some French health councils functioned as temporary boards to deal with medical emergencies, the Paris health council was exceptional in that it was established in 1802 as a permanent public health institution. In theory, all the French provincial health councils established before 1850 were intended to be permanent institutions modeled after the Paris council. In practice, some of them were, such as the health council of the Nord at Lille, and some were not, such as the councils in Rouen and Troyes.

French hygienists defined public health broadly. The domain of public health was everywhere; its scope was all-encompassing. The French health councils embodied this broad interpretation of public health. But in the

9 Duffy, *The Healers*. pp. 197–201; Frederick F. Cartwright, *A Social History of Medicine* (London and New York: Longman, 1977), pp. 100–1; Duffy, *Sword of Pestilence*, pp. 31–2, 54–5, 125–8, 145.

United States before 1850, public health was still traditionally conceived of as quarantine and nuisance removal. A shift to a more all-encompassing view was perceptible by the 1840s in the work of Griscom and in the physicians' reports prepared for the Committee of Hygiene of the recently founded American Medical Association in 1848. But not until the second half of the century did American boards of health include the many duties of the French health councils. (The New York City Board of Health created in 1866 was the first permanent effective board of health in the United States.)[10]

Hygienists in Britain, France, and the United States debated the most effective kind of public health administration. In France, the health councils had served a useful function, and French hygienists defended their utility. But they complained that these institutions lacked power and initiative, and urged independent health councils with power to execute and enforce decisions. Parent-Duchâtelet did not believe that physicians were the most competent professionals to be in charge of public health unless they were specialists in public hygiene. Instead, he emphasized the importance of a variety of technical experts serving on the health councils, and by the 1830s their composition reflected his suggestions. Chadwick was skeptical of boards of health, finding them ineffective. Instead, he advocated one district medical officer of health, a physician, to oversee public health reforms. Chadwick postulated that in this district medical officer could be centralized the myriad duties that various physicians performed in an official capacity.[11]

Like many of the French hygienists, Griscom stressed the importance of physicians in public health administration and in positions of authority. Like the French hygienists – Parent-Duchâtelet excepted – Griscom believed that physicians were the best qualified to deal with sanitary matters. Reminiscent of the French Enlightenment viewpoint out of which grew the dual mission of the epidemic physicians, Griscom considered his proposed sanitary police health missionaries, teaching middle-class values of personal hygiene and household cleanliness in addition to performing official functions.[12] Hygienists in all three countries agreed that public health should be in the hands of technical and professional experts – engineers, architects, pharmacist-chemists, physician-hygienists – not in citizens' councils, the elected representatives of the people, or appointed administrators like prefects.

10 Griscom, *Sanitary Condition*. See the reports in *First AMA Reports*; Duffy, *The Healers*, pp. 308, 315.
11 Alexandre Parent-Duchâtelet, "Quelques considérations sur le Conseil de salubrité de Paris," *Hygiène publique*, 2 vols. (Paris: Baillière, 1836), 1: 1–11; also see "Des obstacles que les préjugés médicaux apportent," *Hygiène publique*, 1: 12–58; Chadwick, *Sanitary Report*, pp. 397, 408–10.
12 Griscom, *Sanitary Condition*, pp. 41–55.

Although one cannot speak of a public health movement in the United States before 1850, its public health problems, theories, and institutions in many ways paralleled those in Britain and France. The work of the Committee of Public Hygiene of the American Medical Association (AMA) provides a convenient way to compare the public health situation in the United States with those of Britain and France. Given the popularity of the sanitary survey by the 1840s, it is not surprising that the new AMA's Committee of Public Hygiene undertook as its first order of business the preparation of sanitary surveys of towns and cities. In these reports, written by leading local physicians, such as John Griscom of New York City and Josiah Curtis of Boston, there are many similarities with the French public health situation.[13] American hygienists complained about inhabitants' noncompliance with public health ordinances, the perpetual lament of French hygienists. Waste disposal was particularly troublesome in both French and American towns, and it was made worse because citizens continued to throw their wastes into the street, in spite of all prohibitions and threats. Echoing Chadwick and Parent-Duchâtelet, the committee recommended a copious water supply accompanied by an underground sewer system. The committee affirmed the relationship of poverty and disease, recognizing that much disease was a result of poverty. On this issue, the physicians on the committee resembled the French social epidemiologists much more than Chadwick, who had maintained that disease caused poverty, and not vice versa. Believing that the poor would use water if it were readily available, the committee suggested that plentiful water would relieve much poverty-related disease. This point of view was shared by many British and French hygienists, although a substantial number of French hygienists, recognizing the cultural tradition of uncleanliness in France, questioned whether habits would change even if adequate water was available.

The physicians who served on the AMA's Committee of Public Hygiene were knowledgeable about the French and British public health movements, especially the British. They believed that although their own problems were urgent, the United States was better off than Europe in terms of public health, owing to the newness of the cities and the fact that mistakes made in Europe might still be prevented in the United States by a good sanitary police. For example, before it was too late, the construction of buildings could be regulated. The reports, taken individually, are interesting in terms of the scope of public health in the United States by midcentury compared with that in Britain and France. With a few exceptions, the reports demonstrate that American physician-hygienists were interested in enlarging the domain of public health to include more

13   AMA commission reports in *The First AMA Reports*, pp. 431–40.

than quarantines and nuisance removal, traditional areas of public health concern and activity in the New World.[14] By the 1840s, American hygienists were thinking along the same lines as their British and French counterparts.

For public health movements before 1850, we must look to Britain and France. In Britain, as in France, there had been a long history of public health interest when Edwin Chadwick took over in the late 1830s as the self-appointed leader of the public health movement. As in France, since the late eighteenth century, hygienic treatises, primarily in the form of medical topographies, had been published, mainly by physicians, dealing with the correlation of poverty, filth, and disease. In Britain, physicians led the public health movement; the best known of them are James Phillips Kay (later Kay-Shuttleworth), Neil Arnott, Southwood Smith, and William Farr. The notable exception, was, of course, Chadwick himself, a lawyer by training, a civil servant by profession.[15]

There is no consensus on when Chadwick became interested in public health or the beginning of the British public health movement. Although he had been interested in public health, medicine, and administrative reform since the late 1820s, Chadwick himself dated the beginning of general interest in public health reform from 1832, the year of the initiation of the Poor Law Inquiry and the first cholera epidemic. Michael W. Flinn, the modern editor of the *Sanitary Report*, takes the years 1837 and 1838, respectively, as the major turning points in the history of public health in Britain and the beginning of the public health movement: 1837 saw the establishment of the General Register Office and the introduction of civil registration; and 1838 the publication of the reports of Smith, Kay, and Arnott on fever in London, which instigated Chadwick's investigation of the sanitary condition of the British laboring population. In any case, until Chadwick entered the picture (having been occupied with Poor Law Reform and administration up to 1838), there was no public health movement, even though ideas of public health reform had been circulating for decades. Until 1837-8, the French were the acknowledged leaders in public health. But in these pivotal years the British movement came into existence and quickly took on a momentum, organization, and leadership that the French movement lacked.[16]

Because the French were the leaders in public health in the 1820s and

14 Ibid.; see the reports on various cities, pp. 445–634 in *First AMA Reports*.
15 Flinn, "Introduction" to Edwin Chadwick, *Sanitary Report*, pp. 1–73.
16 Flinn, "Introduction," pp. 2–3, 27–9, 35–45.

1830s, it is not surprising that British public health reformers were familiar with and influenced by medical and public health developments in France. William Farr was a medical student in Paris from 1829 to 1831 and undoubtedly became acquainted with French hygienic and statistical work, especially that of Pierre Louis and his "numerical method."[17] Smith and Chadwick were also intellectually indebted to French hygienic ideas, especially the work of Villermé and Parent-Duchâtelet. In his two-volume *Philosophy of Health*, published in the late 1830s, Smith drew heavily on Villermé's research for his chapter on mortality statistics.[18] Most important, Chadwick's *Sanitary Report* contains numerous references to the work of Villermé and Parent-Duchâtelet and to the reports of the Paris health council and the Royal Academy of Medicine. But long before he began the *Sanitary Report*, Chadwick had incorporated French hygienic ideas into his own research.

In his introduction to Chadwick's *Sanitary Report* (1965), Flinn paid considerable attention to Chadwick's use of French and other continental sources, noting that Chadwick read widely, calling upon a variety of European sources to strengthen his arguments. Flinn commented on French leadership in public health, acknowledging the vitality and contributions of the French hygienists. Early French influences on Chadwick are readily apparent in his 1828 article on life insurance, "Life Assurances." Chadwick relied on Villermé's data and on French statistical collections, the *Annuaire* of the Bureau of Longitude and the *Recherches statistiques sur la ville de Paris*, to show that the value of life had increased with the progress of civilization. Unable to obtain a statistical comparison of the mean duration of life among the differing classes from British data, Chadwick turned to Villermé's research on varying mortality in Paris. Stating, "It is only in Paris that the collection of any satisfactory information of this kind has been attempted," Chadwick discussed Villermé's research on the morbidity and mortality of the affluent and poor classes in Paris, which showed that mortality among the poor was almost twice that among the affluent. Adopting the Villermé hypothesis, Chadwick stated that the gradations of wealth or the means of providing comforts may almost be taken as the scale of mortality, and asserted that "poverty and bad diet, which weakens the general constitution, must be always taken into account as one of the predisposing causes of mortality."[19] Later in the *Sanitary Report*, however,

17 David E. Lilienfeld and Abraham M. Lilienfeld, "The French Influence on the Development of Epidemiology," in *Times, Places and Persons*, ed. Abraham M. Lilienfeld (Baltimore: Johns Hopkins University Press, 1980), pp. 28–38.
18 Southwood Smith, *The Philosophy of Health*, 2 vols. (London: Charles Knight and Co., 1837–8), v. 1, ch. 4. This chapter was translated into French and published in the *Annales d'hygiène publique* 15 (1836): 87–114.
19 Edwin Chadwick, "Life Assurances," *Westminster Review* 9 (1827–8): 384–421. Quotes, p. 413.

Chadwick greatly modified his position on the relation of poverty to disease and mortality.

Villermé's research on the causes of differing mortality rates contributed to Chadwick's early formulation of what his biographers have called the *sanitary idea*, that is, the Chadwickian principle that the length and healthiness of life are determined by the circumstances in which it is lived. According to Benjamin W. Richardson, Chadwick's contemporary, biographer, and compiler of his work, Chadwick told him that he began thinking about the sanitary idea while working on the question of the probability of mortality and sickness in the life assurances article. If the gradations of wealth or the means of providing comforts could be taken as the scale of mortality, as Villermé had asserted, then this led Chadwick to consider the revolutionary idea that it was not sickness, but conditions independent of sickness, that governed mortality. If this was the case, then by altering these conditions, one could modify mortality rates. Richardson suggested that this revolutionary sanitary idea was the key to three-fourths of Chadwick's work and supplied for the first time the notion that mortality might be separated from disease and treated preventively.[20]

Although Chadwick formulated his sanitary idea in 1828, it did not dominate his thinking until a decade later. Most of Chadwick's attention in these intervening years was occupied by his job as assistant poor law commissioner, wherein he engineered the Poor Law Reform Act of 1834 and became subsequently Secretary of the Poor Law Commission.[21] By the late 1830s, the sanitary idea had become the motivating principle behind the work of Chadwick and Smith, the chief theorists of the public health movement. The sanitary idea was quite simply that mortality was determined by the physical conditions in which one lived, by which Chadwick and Smith meant primarily the environment, or the sanitary condition, rather than the level of poverty.

In the *Sanitary Report* Chadwick made extensive use of French sources to illustrate his major points. He continued to rely heavily on Villermé: to demonstrate the advantages of draining marshes for the reduction of fevers (161); to show the difference in disease and mortality in different districts in the same city (236–7); to show how improvements in public health had

20 Richard A. Lewis, *Edwin Chadwick and the Public Health Movement, 1832–1854* (London: Longman, Green, 1952), pp. 29–59; Benjamin Ward Richardson, *The Health of Nations: A Review of the Works of Edwin Chadwick*, 2 vols. (London: Dawsons of Pall Mall, 1965; first published 1887), 1: 33–4. For a more detailed analysis of French influences on Chadwick, see Ann F. La Berge, "Edwin Chadwick and the French Connection," *Bull. Hist. Med.* 62 (1988): 23–41.

21 Flinn, "Introduction," p. 35; Margaret Pelling, in *Cholera, Fever and English Medicine: 1825–1865* (Oxford: Oxford University Press, 1978), pp. 11–13, takes exception to this interpretation, citing Chadwick's enthusiasm for medical aspects of the "condition of the people" question shown by the *Examiner* under Chadwick's subeditorship.

followed structural improvements in Paris (238); to show the correlation of adult physical strength to increased duration of life and the improved sanitary condition of an individual (250–1); and to show how sanitary improvements in prisons had resulted in greatly decreased mortality (232).

But if Chadwick's major theoretical contribution, the sanitary idea, had been arrived at in part owing to his reading of Villermé, his principal practical contribution to sanitary reform, his notion that the key to public health reform lay in the major overhaul of water services and sewer systems, was reminiscent of Parent-Duchâtelet.[22] Whether Chadwick's ideas on sewage disposal were actually influenced by Parent-Duchâtelet is unclear, but the two men shared similar ideas. Both were concerned with the dual problem of how to dispose of sewage in a healthful manner while conserving valuable wastes. Parent-Duchâtelet had suggested that liquid wastes attenuated in enough water could be disposed of through sewers, with no attendant problems. Chadwick was even more radical, proposing that, with ample water, solid wastes could also be sent through sewers, out into the surrounding countryside to irrigate and fertilize agricultural lands. Parent-Duchâtelet adhered to the more traditional method of collecting solid wastes in closed barrels and then transporting them outside the city for fertilizer. Chadwick respected Parent-Duchâtelet's work, calling him "the most industrious and able of modern investigators into questions of public health" (149). He cited Parent-Duchâtelet in the Sanitary Report to demonstrate that poor-quality water was a cause of sickness (149); to show the great advantages of public sewers for the health of towns (161); to explain the insufficiency of the Parisian water supply (162); for a discussion of drainage (161–2); to discuss the effects of bad ventilation (173); in his discussion of the influence of occupations and working conditions on health (183–4); and to demonstrate the futility of leaving preventive measures up to individual workers (320–1).

Chadwick also used the studies of other French hygienists, the reports of the Paris health council and the Royal Academy of Medicine, to strengthen his arguments. He discussed the debunking controversy of Parent-Duchâtelet and Joseph d'Arcet, that is, the influence of occupation and working conditions on health, inserting in his Appendix a long section from their work and providing in the text a lengthy discussion of the traditional viewpoint discussed by Patissier (183–7 and Sanitary Report), Appendix 17, 424–6). To support preventive health measures and state regulation of public health, Chadwick turned to a French example, citing a report of the epidemic commission of the Royal Academy of Medicine for 1838–40 (217–18);[23] to demonstrate the effects of bad ventilation on cattle,

22 Ann F. La Berge, "A. J. B. Parent-Duchâtelet, Hygienist of Paris, 1821–1836," Clio Medica 12 (1977): 279–301.
23 Isidore Bricheteau, "Rapport de la Commission des épidémies, 1839–40," Mémoires de l'Académie Royale de Médecine 9 (1841): 31–64.

Chadwick quoted from a report done by the Paris health council (172–3); and to broaden the Villermé hypothesis and buttress his own point of view, he cited evidence from a Paris health council report that attributed the varying mortality in Paris not just to misery, but more specifically to the insalubrity of private dwellings (218). Although he recognized the contributions of the Paris health council, Chadwick also saw its shortcomings:

In Paris a Board of Health has been in operation during several years, but if their operations, as displayed in their reports, be considered, it will be evident that, although they have examined many important questions and have made representations, recommending for practical application some of the principles developed in the course of the inquiry; still as they had no executive power, their representations have produced no effect, and the labouring population of Paris is shown to be, with all the advantages of climate, in a sanitary condition even worse than the labouring population of London. (397)

Impressed with the work of the health council in spite of its shortcomings, in his Appendix, Chadwick included a translation of a report that described the council's work (App. 14, 409–23). In another section, discussing the influence of working conditions on health, Chadwick relied on preventive rules outlined by the Paris health council (319). True, Chadwick recognized the main weakness of the Paris council: that it was advisory only, possessing no initiative and no power. But in his discussion of boards of health, Chadwick chose the Paris health council for his prime example, because it was the most successful council and the only permanent one. Although boards of health had been established in Britain before and during the cholera epidemic, these institutions were not useful for Chadwick's discussion because of their singular purpose and temporary nature.[24] Chadwick did not regard boards of health as the most effective public health organization, but his choice of the Paris council for discussion suggests that it was the preeminent health council.

Chadwick was well informed about public health in France. Adopting Parent-Duchâtelet's explanation, he attributed the filthy state of Paris to powerful interest groups who profited from the status quo (163–4).[25] Citing Villermé's statistical data, Chadwick noted that public health had improved following structural reforms in Paris but that these changes had been unequal, some districts benefiting more than others (238–9). Chadwick acknowledged French leadership in occupational hygiene, commenting on the particular attention given by French hygienists, especially Parent-Duchâtelet, to the diseases of the working class (320–1).

Although the influence of Villermé on Chadwick is apparent, in the end

24 Cartwright, *Social History*, p. 101. At the end of the 1832 epidemic, over 1,200 local boards of health had been set up: 822 in England and Wales, 400 in Scotland.
25 See the original article by Parent-Duchâtelet: "Rapport sur les améliorations à introduire dans les fosses d'aisance," *Hygiène publique*, 2: 350–407.

Chadwick turned the Villermé hypothesis on its head. In the *Sanitary Report* Chadwick consistently maintained that indigence or destitution was not the primary cause of disease and high mortality among the laboring classes.[26] Rather, Chadwick had found that "the attacks of disease are upon those in full employment, the attack of fever precedes the destitution, not the destitution the disease"(210). By their fundamental disagreement on the cause of disease, Chadwick emerged as the principal advocate of sanitary reform, whereas Villermé remained one of the leading spokesmen for a social theory of epidemiology. How Chadwick arrived at this complete reversal of the original Villermé hypothesis, which had had such a formative influence on his thought, requires some discussion, for this above all was the key to Chadwick's emphasis on sanitary reform.

The idea that poverty caused disease had been a recurring theme of British and French medical writers since the eighteenth century, and Villermé had argued that poverty was the principal underlying cause of disease and premature death. By the 1830s the Paris health council, the *Annales d'hygiène publique*, and the Royal Academy of Medicine had adopted his hypothesis. Villermé's ideas were influential outside France as well. In addition to Chadwick, Rudolf Virchow was intellectually indebted to him and other French hygienists, emerging by 1848 as a leading social epidemiologist and advocate of social medicine. Acceptance of the Villermé hypothesis of the role of poverty in disease causation did not necessarily mean rejection of the traditional miasmatic theory, even though hygienists usually emphasized one over the other. But the leading French hygienists did not deny poverty as a cause of disease, as Chadwick did. Although many hygienists subscribed to the miasmatic theory of disease causation and recommended sanitary reform, most acknowledged poverty or misery as a major predisposing cause of the greater incidence of disease and death among the poor and laboring classes compared with the comfortable classes. However, some French hygienists questioned the miasmatic theory and the utility of sanitary reform alone in combatting disease. Most prominent was Parent-Duchâtelet, who showed in his study of the Bièvre River and the horsebutcher yards of Paris that bad odors did not always correlate with disease and death.[27]

In the *Sanitary Report* Chadwick challenged the Villermé hypothesis. An explanation may be found in the background for the inquiry. The immediate question instigating the inquiry was whether Poor Law Administration funds could be spent for sanitary reform. More broadly put, could sanitary

---

26 Chadwick, *Sanitary Report*, p. 210.
27 Erwin Ackerknecht, *Rudolf Virchow: Doctor, Statesman, Anthropologist* (Madison: University of Wisconsin Press, 1953), pp. 46, 128–38; Benoiston de Châteauneuf et al., *Rapport sur la marche et les effets du choléra-morbus dans Paris* (Paris: Baillière, 1834). Parent-Duchâtelet was a member of the commission.

reform lead to a decrease in poverty, and were insanitary conditions, therefore, a cause of poverty?[28] Given this background and Chadwick's role in Poor Law reform, one can argue that Chadwick was predisposed to find unsanitary conditions a cause of disease, and disease, in turn, a cause of poverty. Chadwick emphasized the economic consequences of lack of public health to show that Poor Law funds could justifiably be spent for sanitary reforms. Inadequate public health measures led to sickness, death, discomfort, and misery, and the expenditure of additional funds for poor relief.

Second, in the *Sanitary Report*, although concerned about disease in general, Chadwick addressed himself specifically to typhus and typhoid fever, as had Kay, Smith, and Arnott in their earlier inquiries. Typhus was on the upsurge in Europe and was occurring in epidemic proportions in some areas of Britain. Chadwick's observations and those of most medical writers before him attributed fevers to unsanitary conditions. Although acknowledging the correlation between class, profession, state in society, and mortality, Chadwick still asserted that, since many of the laboring classes received a sufficient income to keep them adequately fed, their greater mortality must be determined not by their level of poverty or comfort, but by the physical, or sanitary, condition in which they lived. Chadwick had found that improved material conditions had not exempted the laboring classes from fevers. Thus both Chadwick and Smith maintained that fever was not necessarily the result of poverty, but of unsanitary conditions, which might or might not be the result of poverty. Therefore, Chadwick and Smith asserted that it was more likely that poverty was the result of fever than the reverse. Cleanliness, or sanitary reform, would eliminate the cause of fever, which was filth. Thus, Chadwick espoused an environmental theory of fever causation and rejected the social theory.[29]

Another reason Chadwick was reluctant to attribute to poverty a primary role in fever causation was that he himself had engineered the reform of the British Poor Law, which had supposedly solved the problem of poverty. Yet the incidence of disease, or rather fever, was on the

28 Flinn, "Introduction," pp. 37–43.
29 Ibid., pp. 8–9; Chadwick, *Sanitary Report*, pp. 210, 422; Flinn, "Introduction," p. 4. Chadwick and Smith were referring to one class of disease, the fevers, typhus and typhoid. In the 1830s in Britain, *fever* was a catchall term, which could and often did include cholera, plague, and yellow fever, in addition to typhus and typhoid. In fact, for Southwood Smith, the term *fever* was synonymous with epidemic. As Smith explained it," The term epidemic, considered etymologically, merely signifies *generally prevailing*, but in medicine, it is universally appropriated to designate a certain class of fever." Southwood Smith, "Contagion and Sanitary Laws," *Westminster Review* 3 (1825): 141. Now the French hygienists talked about disease in general, not just one class of disease; hence, the focus of Chadwick and his colleagues was narrower than that of the French hygienists.

increase. Poor Law reform had already occurred, and the reform now urgently needed was sanitary reform. Thus, reasoning like a Poor Law reformer, Chadwick turned the whole poverty–disease argument on its head. Chadwick emphasized disease as a cause of poverty, which was increasing the amount of poor relief the state was required to provide. Sanitary reform was the answer, for by reducing disease, it would reduce poverty. Furthermore, sanitary reform would have a beneficial effect on society, resulting in more happiness and less misery.[30]

Not all British health reformers agreed with Chadwick and Smith's emphasis on sanitary reform or with Chadwick's contention that poverty was not a cause of fevers. A leading critic was physician William Alison of Edinburgh. Like the French hygienists, Alison did not believe that sanitary measures alone would go far to reduce disease, for he contended as did Parent-Duchâtelet, that bad smells and unsanitary conditions did not necessarily cause disease. Like Villermé, Alison suggested that poverty could predispose a person to fever. If destitution was not the actual cause of fever, Alison maintained that it was the cause of its rapid spread. To reduce the incidence of fever, Alison proposed Poor Law reform. This is not surprising, considering that at the time Alison was working for reform of the Scottish poor law. Thus, Alison had every practical reason to stress the relationship of poverty and disease, just as Chadwick had every reason to argue against it.[31] In the end, critics like Alison were silenced, and sanitary reform emerged as the main focus of the British public health movement.

Chadwick's indebtedness to the French hygienists is clear; they, in turn, made considerable use of foreign sources. Villermé was familiar with and used many foreign sources, especially statistical collections, and his life-long professional relationship with Quetelet is well known. In addition, he turned to Britain to investigate the public health ramifications of industrialization and relied on British sources to test general public health hypotheses. He urged the French to emulate the British by enacting a civil registration act.[32]

There was considerable cross-fertilization of ideas between French and British public health circles, an exchange facilitated in France by the *Annales d'hygiène publique* and elsewhere by medical journals and general journals that reported on public health developments abroad. Although

30 Flinn, "Introduction," pp. 65–6.
31 Ibid., pp. 63–4. In his formal rebuttal to Alison, Arnott claimed that as a result of the New Poor Law there was no destitution in England.
32 Erwin Ackerknecht, "Villermé and Quetelet," *Bull. Hist. Med.* 26 (1952): 317–29. One example was his theory that mortality rates were higher in marshy areas. See L. R. Villermé, "Influence des marais sur la vie des enfans," *Annales d'hygiène publique* 12 (1834): 31–7.

transmission of ideas between British and French hygienists is easily established, the United States is more problematic. Many American physicians studied in Paris in the 1820s and 1830s, but they went to work with leading clinicians, not to investigate public health. There appears to have been little or no influence of the French public hygienists on the Americans. By the time the American public health movement began to emerge in the 1840s, the British example was more compelling than the French. One exception was Lemuel Shattuck, who in his sanitary report on Massachusetts displayed familiarity with Paris health council reports, with the *Annales d'hygiène publique*, and with several French public health treatises such as Monfalcon and Polinière's comprehensive *Traité de la salubrité dans les grandes villes*. There was virtually no American influence on the French at this time. Nor was there any reporting in France of the public health situation in the United States, with the possible exception of the controversy over the contagion or noncontagion of yellow fever.[33]

The British public health movement emerged as a full-fledged movement by the 1840s, its goal being sanitary reform by administrative and legislative means. Traditionally, historians have looked to the British public health movement as the model, the prototype. In light of the present investigation, this interpretation should be reconsidered. The two movements invite comparison and assessment. Not only has the British movement been the prototype, Chadwick has been the model reformer, to the exclusion of leading continental hygienists and other British reformers. One of the reasons is the availability of two good biographical studies of Chadwick and Flinn's modern edition of the *Sanitary Report*.[34] A strong case can be made that Chadwick *was* the most influential of the early-nineteenth-century reformers in terms of the British experience and influence on the English-speaking world. Chadwick was the reformer who most influenced American public hygienists, making it reasonable for American historians to have concentrated on him. The emphasis that has been placed on Chadwick invites a comparison of him with his French counterparts.

33 George Rosen, "An American Doctor in Paris in 1828," *J. Hist. Med.* 6 (1951): 64–116; Russell M. Jones, *The Parisian Education of an American Surgeon: Letters of Jonathan Mason Warren (1832–1835)* (Philadelphia: American Philosophical Society, 1978); Lemuel Shattuck et al., *Report of the Sanitary Commission of Massachusetts 1850*, foreward by C.-E.-A. Winslow (Cambridge, MA: Harvard University Press, 1948), pp. 16–24, 87, 106, 113–114; see also the original work, Lemuel Shattuck, et al., *Report of a General Plan for the Promotion of Public and Personal Health* (Boston: Dutton and Wentworth, 1850), p. 539, in which he discusses French publications to be included in a hygienist's library.
34 Lewis, *Edwin Chadwick*; Samuel E. Finer, *The Life and Times of Sir Edwin Chadwick* (London: Methuen, 1952).

PHYSICIANS, THE MEDICAL PROFESSION,
AND PUBLIC HEALTH

The important role of physicians in the British, French, and American
public health movements should be highlighted. Physicians were prominent as social investigators. In local medical topographies, sanitary
surveys, and official reports they investigated disease patterns and health
conditions and recommended reforms. Although one cannot really speak
of a public health movement in Britain until Chadwick, Smith, Kay,
Arnott, and Farr came on the scene in the late 1830s, or in France until the
hygienists founded the *Annales d'hygiène publique* in 1829, it is clear that
these dates represent the culmination of a general trend that had been
developing in each country for about fifty years – sanitary investigations
carried out by physicians, accompanied by recommendations for reform.
With the exception of Chadwick in Britain and Shattuck in the United
States, nearly all the major British and American hygienists were
physicians.

Physicians were also at the forefront of the French public health movement, but a significant proportion of French hygienists were pharmacist-
chemists and other specialists in related scientific and professional fields.
The primary occupation of some of the leading physician-hygienists was
not the teaching or practice of medicine. The examples of Farr, Kay,
Villermé, and Parent-Duchâtelet immediately come to mind. Although
trained as a physician, very early in his career Farr became interested in
population statistics and public health, accepting the position of compiler
of abstracts at the newly established General Register Office in 1837 and
achieving prominence as the founder of vital statistics and an avid
promoter of public health reform.[35] Kay, trained as a physician, became
interested in social questions, occupying himself with public health and
working-class reform until 1839, then devoting himself to educational
reform. Villermé, although achieving considerable recognition in medical
circles in the early years of his career, by the 1820s turned first to prison

35 Flinn is the primary source for these general comments about the British public
    health movement. See also the works of Chadwick, Kay, and Smith. On Farr, see
    Noel Humphrey's introduction to *Vital Statistics: A Memorial Volume of Selections
    from the Reports and Writings of William Farr* (London: The Sanitary Institute, 1885),
    pp. vii–xxiv; Lilienfeld and Lilienfeld, "The French Influence"; and John M. Eyler,
    "The Conceptual Origins of William Farr's Epidemiology: Numerical Methods
    and Social Thought in the 1830s," in *Times, Places, and Persons*, pp. 1–21; John M.
    Eyler, *Victorian Social Medicine: The Ideas and Methods of William Farr* (Baltimore:
    Johns Hopkins University Press, 1979). A good general treatment is Anthony
    Wohl, *Endangered Lives: Public Health in Victorian Britain* (Cambridge, MA:
    Harvard University Press, 1983).

reform, then to statistics and public health reform, and finally, in the 1830s and 1840s, to working-class reform, while continuing his interest in public health and statistics. His profession, rather than the practice or teaching of medicine, was that of researcher, writer, editor, sociologist, and academician. Parent-Duchâtelet gave up his private practice of medicine in the early 1820s to become a full-time public hygienist, on the advice of his mentor, Jean-Noël Hallé. Although he held a hospital post at the Pitié, his primary occupation from 1825 until his death in 1836 was as an urban and occupational hygienist. Of course, many physician-hygienists practiced or taught medicine, in addition to their public health interests. Southwood Smith, for example, was physician to the London Fever Hospital for over forty years. Neil Arnott was Chadwick's personal physician, and Charles Marc was personal physician to King Louis-Philippe.

The principal contribution of the medical profession to public health reform was that by their investigations and publications, physicians stimulated the growth of awareness of public health problems, which led to administrative and legislative reform. In the case of Britain, Flinn emphasized the medical profession's "contribution to a growing awareness of the correlation between dirt and disease." In France also, this period witnessed the increasing involvement of medical men in social questions. Of the British physicians Flinn has this to say, but his comment would apply equally well to France and the United States: "More than any other social group, the doctors of the nineteenth century were responsible for stirring the social conscience." Flinn's assessment of the contributions of the medical profession to the British public health movement was that the doctors generated the movement by their supply of persuasive statistical and descriptive material. In short, in Britain the contribution of the medical profession to the public health movement was substantial.[36]

One historian of the American public health movement, John Duffy, makes a similar assessment of the role of the medical profession in the American public health movement, asserting that "the public health movement in America was led by physicians and was strongly supported by medical associations at all levels until World War I." Throughout the nineteenth century, public health leadership in the United States was supplied by physicians. The early presidents of the American Public Health Association were all prominent physicians, and the membership of municipal and state boards of health consisted primarily of outstanding physicians and surgeons. Indicative of the early aims of the AMA was that one of its first actions was to instigate sanitary surveys of major American cities. In the nineteenth century the American medical profession was the vanguard of

36 Flinn, "Introduction," pp. 21–6. Quotes, p. 21.

public health reform. The situation would change, however, in the twentieth century.[37]

In France, involvement of the medical profession in public health
matters dated from the eighteenth century and the Royal Society of Medicine. The goals of the Society were public health related, and the epidemic
physicians and provincial correspondents appointed by the Society formed
an elite with public health interests. In the early nineteenth century, before
the creation of health councils, local medical societies served as public
health advisory boards. The Royal Academy of Medicine was founded
with public health goals and served as the national public health advisory
board. Leading French physician-hygienist were respected members of the
medical profession at both the national and local levels, participating as
permanent and corresponding members of the Royal Academy of Medicine, holding positions at the Faculties of Medicine and in the secondary
schools of medicine, and serving as members of local and national medical
and public health establishments such as departmental medical juries,
health councils, vaccine committees, and sanitary intendancies.

Although physicians were at the forefront of the French public health
movement, the French case differs from the British and American. For
with the exception of Chadwick and Shattuck, in Britain and the United
States nearly all the leading public health reformers were trained as
physicians or were practicing physicians, whereas in France many leading
hygienists, such as Adolphe Trébuchet, Alphonse Chevallier, and Joseph
d'Arcet, were scientists or administrators. Trébuchet, like Chadwick, was
trained as a lawyer and worked as an administrator. Chevallier was a
pharmacist-chemist and d'Arcet an industrial chemist. If one looks at the
memberships of the Paris health council, the provincial health councils,
and the editorial staff of the *Annales d'hygiène publique*, it is clear that
although most hygienists were physicians, a sizable minority were
pharmacist-chemists, veterinarians, architects, engineers, and administrators. So French hygienists were a more diversified group than their
British and American colleagues.

THE BRITISH AND FRENCH MOVEMENTS COMPARED
AND ASSESSED

The early-nineteenth-century British and French public health movements
were similar in many ways. Both were urban movements, the primary
concern of hygienists being reform in cities and manufacturing towns.
Both were professional movements, with physicians being the single most

---

37 Quote in Duffy, *The Healers*, p. 313; *First AMA Reports.* On public health in the
United States, see Paul Starr, *The Social Transformation of American Medicine* (New
York: Basic Books, 1982), ch. 4.

important professional group. Unlike the French movement, however, the British movement had its popular or voluntary side, with reformers attempting to sway public opinion through public meetings and publications such as parliamentary inquiries, the most important of which was Chadwick's *Sanitary Report*. But the impetus for reform was professional, not popular. Both in France and in Britain, humanitarians, philanthropists, and socialists who supported other types of social reform were not necessarily attracted to the public health movements. Rather, the leading public health reformers in both countries were members of the Establishment, respected physicians, scientists, and administrators, most of whom held official positions at the national or local level.

The British public health movement was an official movement led by professional administrators and instigated by an arm of the national administration, the Poor Law Commission. The sanitary reports and inquiries done from 1838 to 1848 were official in origin, the investigators either commissioners themselves or appointed by commissioners. But if the Public Health Act of 1848 was the culmination of ten years of an active, official, professional public health movement, the movement itself, like the French movement, was also the culmination of fifty or more years of unofficial but professional interest and activity on the part of physicians.

Although the French movement was quasi-official rather than official, there were many similarities with the British movement. French hygienists did not hold national administrative positions, as Chadwick did, nor did they serve on comparable parliamentary investigative commissions, like the leading British reformers; nevertheless, much of their investigation and reporting was done in an official capacity. For example, Paris health council memberships were appointive, salaried positions; although members devoted varying amounts of time to health council activities, evidence suggests that Parent-Duchâtelet spent much of his time on health council investigations and reports. Health council reports were official reports, undertaken on the recommendation of the prefect of police. Other major hygienic investigations were done by official commissions appointed by the municipal council or one of the two prefects. The leading hygienists served on these commissions. The investigation of the horsebutcher yards was one example; the report prepared following the cholera epidemic was another.[38]

Many major public health investigations were done by the Royal Acad-

38 Some leading French public health reformers did hold important administrative positions, such as Adolphe Trébuchet, head of the sanitary office at the prefecture of police, and Jean-François Terme, mayor of Lyon from 1840 to 1847. Parent-Duchâtelet, chairman, "Recherches et considérations sur la nécessité d'établir à Paris un clos central d'écarrissage" (Paris: Baillière, 1827); Benoiston de Châteauneuf et al., *Rapport sur le choléra*.

emy of Medicine at the request of the Minister of the Interior or the Minister of Commerce and Public Works. Thus, these reports had an official origin. A good example was the report of the Royal Academy of Medicine commission on the establishment of departmental health councils.[39] The permanent vaccine and epidemic commissions of the Royal Academy of Medicine published annual or periodic reports. Leading hygienists served on both permanent and temporary Royal Academy of Medicine commissions. Another landmark report with an official origin was the inquiry of Villermé and Benoiston de Châteauneuf on the state of French textile workers, prepared for the Academy of Political and Moral Sciences.

Now if the main vehicles in Britain for influencing official and public opinion were the inquiries undertaken by the Poor Law Commission and by both Houses of Parliament, the main source for influencing official and professional opinion in France was the *Annales d'hygiène publique*, wherein the numerous official investigations and reports were published, either in their entirety or as extracts or reviews. There was no British equivalent of this journal, although there were publications, such as *Lancet*, that reviewed French works and reported on French public health activities.[40] French hygienists made little or no effort to influence public opinion, and popular agitation had nothing to do with the success or failure of the French movement. Given the nature of the French government, the hygienists' emphasis on reform from the top was reasonable. The French parliament was in no way popularly elected; and the suffrage was much narrower than in Britain, where by this time the bulk of the middle classes had been given the vote. In France, the encouragement of popular participation, given the rather paranoid nature of the July Monarchy, might have seriously harmed the movement, had it associated with elements that the government regarded as subversive. It was important to the success of the French movement that it remain professional, with the most active hygienists recognized as members of the Establishment. But in Britain, with the organization of the Health of Towns Association in 1844 and the Metropolitan Working Classes Association for the Improvement of the Public Health, Chadwick, Smith, and others attempted to sway public opinion through public meetings and publications. The instigation was,

39 Charles C. H. Marc, chairman, "Rapport d'une commission de l'Académie royale de Médecine à M. le Ministre du Commerce et des Travaux Publics sur l'establissement de conseils de salubrité départementaux," *Annales d'hygiène publique* 18 (1837): 5–36.
40 *The Journal of Public Health and Monthly Record of Sanitary Improvement*, issued under the auspices of the Metropolitan Health of Towns commission, was published from 1847 to 1849. One student of the subject suggested that publication ceased in 1849, because the Health of Towns commission believed its work had been completed. See Robert G. Paterson, "The Health of Towns Association in Great Britain, 1844–1849," *Bull. Hist. Med.* 22 (1948): 381, 397.

however, official, administrative, and professional. Thus, in spite of this "voluntary" side, which much impressed contemporary French observers such as Antoine Ostrowski and Ambroise Tardieu, the British movement, like the French, was essentially professional and administrative.[41]

Discussing the British public health movement, Flinn emphasized that, although there was a long tradition of interest in public health questions in Britain, before Chadwick came on the scene in 1838 the movement was unorganized, aimless, and leaderless. Without organization, leadership, and specific goals, he argued, there was no public health movement. Although spearheaded by the administrative energies of Chadwick, the movement was also ably led by Smith, with major contributions by Kay, Arnott, and Farr. An army of Poor Law medical officers contributed a vast amount of data that Chadwick was able to use in compiling and writing the *Sanitary Report*. Nevertheless, in its early phase, the movement did have one leader, Chadwick, and several right-hand men. By contrast, there was no one leader of the French movement. Instead, leadership was invested in the society of the *Annales d'hygiène publique* and the Paris health council, whose membership was overlapping. The leaders of the French public health movement were Villermé and Parent-Duchâtelet, but their leadership was not comparable to Chadwick's. Nor did either of them ever consider himself the leader of the public health movement, as Chadwick did. No one emerged as the leader of the French movement. Although hygienists and their contemporaries considered their collective actions as a movement, and could identify its goals, no one ever claimed to lead it. Rather, leadership was always attributed to groups: to the Paris health council, to the society of the *Annales d'hygiène publique*, and to leading spokesmen within the various academies.

Flinn asserted that before the British public health movement had specific legislative goals it was aimless, suggesting that legislative goals are a necessary precondition for a movement. Now the specific legislative goal of the British reformers was the passage of a national law acknowledging that public health was the duty of the state, accompanied by a centralized national public health administration. French hygienists had similar goals, but the more advanced state of the French public health movement accounts for the fact that the goals were less specific and more diffused. For one thing, the idea that public health was the duty of the state had been commonplace in France since the late eighteenth century. Left unresolved was which areas of public health were appropriate for the national government and which ones were better handled at the local level. Also, the

---

41 Antoine Ostrowski, "Etudes d'hygiène publique sur l'Angleterre," *Annales d'hygiène publique* 37 (1847): 5–43; Ambroise Tardieu, "Introduction" to the second edition of *Dictionnaire d'hygiène publique et de salubrité*, 4 vols. (Paris: Baillière, 1862), 1: viii–x.

French already had the centralized organization and administration that Chadwick admired and Britain lacked.[42] The machinery for an effective national public health program already existed in France: Thus, French hygienists gave priority to defining appropriate areas of involvement and getting the power of enforcement into the hands of professional hygienists instead of elected or appointed representatives. Although Chadwick thought boards of health were inefficient, one of the oft-cited achievements of the British movement was the establishment in 1848 of a (albeit short-lived) National Board of Health. In France, the health councils dated from 1802, and by the 1830s many major cities had such councils. France also had (since 1822) a national board of health, the *Conseil supérieur de santé*, although its duties were very circumscribed. Part of the 1848 reform in France comparable to the British movement was the abolition of the by then defunct *Conseil supérieur de santé* and the establishment of a new national institution, the *Comité consultatif d'hygiène publique*, which was intended to reflect the changes that had occurred in public hygiene since the early 1820s. Since the health councils already existed in France, the goal of the public health movement was to make the institution nationwide and empower the councils. Thus, whereas one of Chadwick's primary goals was to establish a national centralized public health administration in Britain comparable to the Poor Law Administration on the French model, in France such an administration – although not precisely comparable – was already in place.

Thus, two of Chadwick's primary goals, a national public health law acknowledging the responsibility of the state in public health matters and the establishment of a nationwide public health administration, to some extent already existed in France. The goals of the French hygienists, then, were to encourage the government to define more precisely its area of public health activity, to increase its public health involvement in response to the enlarged scope of public health, and to expand and make more effective the existing health council organization.

Another difference in the goals of the French and British movements was that the British movement aimed almost exclusively at practical sanitary rather than social reform. In France, social aspects were also important. Part of the explanation for the difference in approaches was that France had not experienced factory reform comparable to that in Britain, and in France, working-class and factory reforms were considered the realm of the public hygienist. Thus contemporaries considered the 1841 child labor law a major piece of public health and social legislation. In

---

42 [Edwin Chadwick] unsigned, "Centralization. Public Charities in France," *London Review* 2 (1829): 536–65.

France throughout the 1840s, ideas of social hygiene, social medicine, and schemes for social reform abounded. Most French hygienists agreed that sanitary living conditions provided by adequate salaries and accompanied by decent working conditions were as important to public health as clean, abundant water and good sewage disposal. Although the idea of *assainissement*, which meant primarily keeping the streets clean, was a central focus of French hygienists, most never believed that sanitary reform alone would reduce disease and death rates or solve the public health problems confronting the nation.

A final area of comparison and assessment of the two movements is the events of 1848. In both Britain and France, 1848 was the culmination of the early nineteenth-century public health movements. In Britain, the principal goal of reformers was achieved in 1848 with the passage of the national public health law, which formally declared the responsibility of the state in public health matters. The law established local boards of health and a national board of health. The French legislation of 1848 also achieved one of the principal aims of reformers: The health councils became a nationwide institution, with every department and arrondissement having its own council. Like the British law, it set up a national health council composed of leading hygienists to act as a national public health advisory board. There was one big difference: The British boards were to have their own power, whereas the French remained advisory only. In each case, however, the 1848 legislation missed the mark: Chadwick had not advocated boards of health as the best means for administering public health, for he found them inefficient; in France the health councils remained advisory, so that they still lacked the power of initiative and enforcement that French hygienists believed essential to an effective public health institution. And in both cases, the immediate results of the legislation were not so gratifying as reformers had hoped. The National Board of Health in Britain was short-lived, ceasing to exist in 1854, and in France by the late 1850s, most of the councils were either defunct or ineffective.

Finally, in Britain, the 1848 law initiated a program of practical public health reform, with the emphasis on sanitary reform, which continued throughout the century. The French law did not initiate the same practical reforms that the British did. Instead it was the rather unsatisfactory culmination of an era of much public health activity. Many practical sanitary reforms resulted from the urban transformations of the Second Empire. But French contributions to public health took a different turn with the advent of the era of bacteriology, the emphasis shifting from street-cleaning activities to the laboratory and to social problems related to depopulation such as infant mortality, venereal diseases, tuberculosis, and alcoholism.

THE FRENCH MOVEMENT ASSESSED

The French public health movement was characterized by its breadth of research. French hygienists published numerous articles and books on virtually every aspect of public health. Exchange of ideas was greatly facilitated by the existence of the *Annales d'hygiène publique et de médecine légale,* to which there was nothing comparable elsewhere.[43] It was the first journal in the West devoted exclusively to public health and legal medicine, and provided a focal point for the community of hygienists. The journal published or reviewed most of the major French hygienic works and served as an international forum on public health matters, devoting considerable attention to foreign developments and publications.

Another distinguishing feature of the French movement was the long hygienic tradition dating from the eighteenth century and its legacy of public health institutions: the health councils, the vaccine administration, the epidemic physicians, and the Royal Academy of Medicine. The vaccine administration and the network of epidemic physicians demonstrated the national government's involvement in public health, and the health councils and the Royal Academy of Medicine offered forums for research and debate, gave hygienists a shared sense of identity, and provided public health advice to the government.

Another characteristic of the French movement, which set it apart from the British and American movements, was the centralized and bureaucratic nature of the French government. Although Raspail complained that in France everything ended up in bureaucracy, reformers such as Chadwick attributed French leadership in medicine and public health to its centralized administration.[44] The French military experience in the Revolutionary and Napoleonic wars also contributed to French leadership in public health. One of the lessons learned from the military experience of physicians who later had important roles in the public health movement was the effectiveness of preventive medicine.[45]

43 Evidence that this was the first public health journal in the West is in *Annales d'hygiène publique* 48 (1852): 235. See also Charles C. H. Marc, "Introduction," *Annales d'hygiène publique* 1 (1829): ix–xxxix. Marc did mention several short-lived eighteenth-century German public health journals. A journal of public health and legal medicine was not founded in Prussia until 1852, by Johann Ludwig Casper, a physician and statistician who had been a contributor to the *Annales d'hygiène publique*. A review of the new journal, *Vierteljahrsschrift für Gerichtliche und Oeffentliche Medicin*, appeared in *Annales d'hygiène publique* 48 (1852): 235.

44 This is what François Raspail said of France in general and of reform in particular, "Tout se termine ainsi en bureaucratie..." in Raspail, *Réforme pénitentiaire. Lettres sur les prisons de Paris*, 2 vols. (Paris: Tamisey and Champion, 1839), 2: XLIIIe lettre, p. 259; [Chadwick] unsigned, "Centralization."

45 Erwin Ackerknecht, *Medicine at the Paris Hospital, 1794–1848* (Baltimore: Johns Hopkins University Press, 1967), p. 149; David M Vess, *Medical Revolution in France, 1789–1796* (Gainesville: University Presses of Florida, 1975).

The prestige and international position of the Royal Academy of Medicine were attributable to France's leadership in both clinical medicine and public health. Many hygienists were members of the Academy, which was the scene of major debates and commission reports on public health questions; indeed, its four permanent commissions were public health related. Working through the Royal Academy of Medicine, physician-hygienists reformed the French sanitary administration, subsequent to the French medical profession's acceptance of an environmental theory of disease causation. Reform of the quarantine system was begun in 1828, and by the 1840s substantial modifications of the sanitary administration opened the way for other preventive measures against epidemic diseases, primarily sanitary reform.

Hygienists' investigations of working-class conditions contributed to the passage of a child labor law in 1841. A notable achievement of the public health movement, the 1841 child labor law was in part attributable to the publicity efforts of Villermé. The only major piece of social legislation passed before 1850, the law was unenforceable and therefore in practice had little effect. Nevertheless, its passage was a tangible achievement of the public health movement. At the very least, the problem of child labor had been recognized and addressed.

Hygienists were also successful in getting other public health legislation passed. In 1848 hygienists called for a national public health law, and the Medical Society of Strasbourg even went so far as to ask for the creation of a separate Ministry of Public Health. No ministry was established, but two laws were passed reforming the health councils and instituting a national health committee to replace the Superior Health Council.[46] A law of December 18, 1848, set up health councils throughout France at the departmental and arrondissement levels and provided for the establishment of health commissions at the cantonal level. Organized on the Paris model, the councils were strictly advisory, acquiring no separate and distinct power. The passage of this law was the culmination of efforts that had been made since the 1830s by Ministers of Commerce, the Royal Academy of Medicine, and public hygienists to establish a nationwide system of health councils. Another law set up a national public health committee to be in charge of the institution and organization of the health councils. Appointed to the new Consultative Committee on Public Health (*Comité consultatif d'hygiène publique*) were physicians François Magendie, Louis Aubert-Roche, Hippolyte Royer-Collard, François Mélier, and Villermé.[47]

---

46 Information about 1848 comes from Pierre Astruc, "1848 et la médecine," *Le Progrès médical*, no. 12 (June 24, 1946), pp. 269–82 and no. 13 (July 10, 1946), pp. 297–302.

47 *Recueil des textes officiels concernant la protection de la santé publique 1790–1935*, 9 vols. (Paris: Ministère de la Santé Publique, 1957), 2: 230. A specific function of the

This new committee replaced the old and defunct Superior Health Council, which had been instituted in conjunction with the 1822 sanitary law. The creation of a new public health institution and the suppression of the Superior Health Council (*Conseil supérieur de santé*) signaled the formal end of the old French quarantine system. In the new institution, the older and more general term *santé* was replaced in the title of the new committee by the newer and now generally accepted term *hygiène publique*, meaning, of course, public health or public hygiene but also referring specifically to the scientific discipline developed by the public hygienists. By the end of the century the Committee replaced the Paris health council as the most important public health authority in France. It was not until 1902 that a national public health law such as the one advocated by the early-nineteenth-century hygienists was finally passed, and a Ministry of Health was created only in 1919.

The year 1848 was the culmination, if only symbolic, of the goals, attitudes, successes, and failures of the public health movement. Many ideas and programs advanced by hygienists came to a head that year. One program advocated by some hygienists and physicians was social medicine or social hygiene. These hygienists had stressed the social nature of both medicine and public health and had emphasized the interrelatedness of medicine, public health, and social reform. In keeping with Revolutionary and socialist aspirations, *social medicine* was a term much discussed in 1848. Two examples illustrate what hygienists meant by it. Michel Lévy, author of a widely used hygiene manual, editor of the *Annales d'hygiène publique*, and director of the Val-de-Grâce hospital, commented: "A government which lives by universal suffrage is forced to ask our profession to do all the good it can; history shows us the social value of medicine increasing with the price of human life, and this price is very simply the measure of civilization."[48] Jules Guérin, physician and editor of the *Gazette médicale de Paris* since 1830, also came forward as an advocate of *social medicine*, defined by him as medicine in the service of society and including sanitary police, public health, and legal medicine. Advocacy of social medicine by Lévy and Guérin illustrates the continuing dialectic between social and liberal medicine that prevailed in hygienic circles and within the larger French medical profession throughout the century.

French hygienists made major contributions to urban hygiene, investigating and reporting on most urban health problems. Partly as a result of their recommendations, important sanitary reforms were made in Paris. In

new committee was to indicate to the Minister of Agriculture and Commerce (to whom the committee was responsible) questions to be submitted for consideration to the National Academy of Medicine (in 1848 the Royal Academy of Medicine became the National Academy of Medicine).

48   Quote from Pierre Astruc, "1848 et la médecine," no. 12 (June 24, 1946), p. 275.

some instances, even though actual reforms postdated 1848, hygienists and administrators had already outlined and prepared plans for reform. Public health reforms in Paris included a fivefold increase in the Paris water supply accompanied by improved distribution via fountains and underground pipes; an increase in public bathing facilities, with the number of public bathtubs multiplying from 500 in 1816 to 3,760 in 1832; tripling the underground sewer mileage; improvements in the horsebutchering industry and suppression of the city dump; the introduction of better ventilation and drainage systems and an increased water supply in prisons, hospitals, and other public and industrial establishments; regulation of dangerous and unhealthy industries, which improved urban sanitary conditions and working conditions in some workshops and factories; and the establishment of a sanitary program to regulate prostitution. Although some reforms were stopgap measures, Paris was far ahead of other French cities in public health and compared favorably with other European and American cities. Indeed, Paris served as a public health model for other departments and cities.[49]

French hygienists carried out important research in occupational hygiene, investigating most dangerous and unhealthy industries and analyzing the impact of industrialization on health. In the 1820s, Parent-Duchâtelet began a project to investigate all Parisian trades and industries, and his reports on the horsebutchering industry, the dock workers of Paris, sewer workers, tobacco workers, and hemp retting became the definitive works on these trades. Alphonse Chevallier, Joseph D'Arcet, Louis Tanquerel des Planches, and Théophile Roussel also made important contributions in occupational hygiene. The industrial investigations done by the health councils included most of the dangerous and unhealthy urban trades, and on a broader level, sociomedical investigations provided penetrating analyses of the impact of industrialization on workers' health.

French hygienists achieved partial success in epidemic prevention and control. Smallpox was the only disease for which a specific preventive was available, and hygienists encouraged vaccination by publicizing its benefits and participating in municipal and departmental vaccine commissions. Supported by hygienists and operating through vaccine commissions, the government distributed vaccine throughout the nation. Since vaccination was not compulsory, local initiative, the educational level of the inhabitants, and resistance to interference in their private lives explain the varying results of the program.

49 The city of St. Louis, for example, tried to put the Paris sanitary program for prostitutes into effect. It was advocated for New York City as well. See John C. Burnham, "Medical Inspection of Prostitution in America in the Nineteenth Century: The St. Louis Experiment and Its Sequel," *Bull. Hist. Med.* 45 (1971): 203–18. See Jill Harsin, *Policing Prostitution in Nineteenth-Century Paris* (Princeton NJ: Princeton University Press, 1985).

Public hygienists had some success with cholera. Their role was three-fold: first, investigation of the disease so that effective preventive measures might be taken; second, publication of instructions on preventive measures and actual implementation of such measures; and third, development of a system to care for the sick if prevention failed. Hygienists participated in government commissions sent throughout Europe to determine the etiology of the disease, observe its course, and make recommendations for administrative procedures. Physicians and health councils publicized instructions, conducted clean-up campaigns, and set up the administrative machinery and facilities to handle the sick in case prevention failed. The Paris health council developed a cholera plan for the city, but its success was only partial, since cholera invaded Paris in spite of all precautions. The cholera programs initiated in Paris and other French cities illustrate the shift in emphasis on disease prevention since the yellow fever scare of the early 1820s. At that time the defense had been the traditional quarantine system and the use of the *cordon sanitaire*. But the experience of other countries showed that cholera was not deterred by quarantine, so by the early 1830s the principal French defense was sanitary reform and, if that failed, backup measures to care for the sick.

Another contribution of the public hygienists was their early use of statistics as a tool for public health investigation and analysis. During the 1820s and 1830s, French hygienists used statistical analysis to study public health theories and problems. Their task was made easier by the publication of official statistical collections, the most useful being the *Recherches statistiques sur la ville de Paris*. Villermé, for example, used statistical data to test public health theories, to measure the level of health and the incidence of disease and death of varying classes and groups of the population. With statistical data, proofs and comparisons were possible, and hygienists could make public health arguments more compelling.

French hygienists transformed public hygiene into a professional scientific discipline based on firsthand observation, interviews, statistical data, and experiments. Central to the development of public hygiene was the *Annales d'hygiène publique*, which served as the rallying point for the specialty. In their selection of material, the founders and editors of the journal defined the limits of the discipline. Illustrative of the development of public hygiene were the hygienists' attempts to define its terminology more precisely. By midcentury old terms such as *police médical, police sanitaire, salubrité, and santé*, all of which had been used at one time or another to mean "public health," had acquired more precise meanings and were being replaced in professional works by the term *hygiène publique*, meaning "public health" but also referring specifically to the scientific discipline of public hygiene. Exemplary of the contributions of the public hygienists by midcentury were the monumental works of Monfalcon and

Polinière, *Traité de la salubrité dans les grandes ville* (1846), and Ambroise Tardieu's *Dictionnaire de l'hygiène publique* (1854), which attempted to bring together all aspects of the discipline and define its boundaries.

Hygienists failed, however, to achieve their aims in several important areas. First, they did not convince the monied classes, who controlled both the national and municipal governments, of the importance of public health, with the result that many of their recommended reforms were never tried for lack of money. Although public health measures were intended to benefit the whole community, reforms were aimed principally at the poor and working classes. Given the attitudes of many of the bourgeoisie toward poverty and the working classes, it is not surprising that many comfortable and wealthy people had little or no interest in public health reform. They did not perceive reforms, such as industrial restrictions to protect public health or regulations requiring landlords to maintain rental properties, to be in their self-interest. The middle and upper classes were deeply suspicious of the intrusion of the government into their private lives and private property in the name of the public health and therefore resisted reform. This attitude would change later in the century, when public health became a central feature of the national agenda.

Municipal authorities were often reluctant to undertake public health reforms. In addition to dominant liberal economic and political beliefs that upheld individual rights, the sanctity of private property, and the privacy of the individual, there was the more practical reason that those in power believed their own interests and those of their constituents threatened by reform. Another compelling reason for opposition to public health reform was the expense entailed. Money had to be found, interest groups appeased, and the rights of individuals reconciled with the claims of hygienists. In Paris reforms to improve the garbage collection and sewerage systems were never implemented because of inadequate funds and opposition from powerful interest groups like ragpickers and proprietors, who profited from the status quo. Unable to resolve these problems, municipal councils remained conservative and tight-fisted.

Another area of failure for hygienists was lack of enforcement of public health ordinances and laws. Public health regulations were only sporadically enforced and, in the case of the 1841 national child labor law, unenforceable, so hygienists' success in getting such measures passed was in a sense a hollow victory. This situation points up the primary weakness of the public health movement: Hygienists were powerless to enforce decisions. Although they could exert a certain amount of pressure through the Royal Academy of Medicine and the health councils, and although the government was often willing to take their recommendations, health councils had no separate and distinct power, and hygienists could not see their programs through by enforcing public health regulations.

One disappointment of the French hygienists was their inability to get a national public health law passed before or during 1848. The 1822 sanitary law dealt only with contagious disease, and many hygienists opposed it on principle. Hygienists wanted the national government to reaffirm health, along with liberty and property, as a natural right of French citizens. In addition to a national public health law, some hygienists urged the establishment of a Ministry of Public Health. In both cases, hygienists' goals were not realized before the twentieth century.

A final area of failure concerns the stopgap nature of many of the public health programs and reforms. Yet given available funds and the various interest groups whose demands had to be met, it is hard to imagine how major overhauls of sewer or water systems could have been achieved. Accustomed to dealing with pennypinching administrators, most hygienists – Parent-Duchâtelet excepted – did not have the vision to advocate major urban reform programs. It is difficult to see how the reforms of Haussmann could have been accomplished under Louis Philippe and the Paris municipal council. As David Pinkney suggested, only a despotic government such as that of Napoleon III was in a position to undertake a major rebuilding of Paris, which in the final analysis was the most efficient way to accomplish the major sanitary reforms advocated by hygienists. Even then, the public health problems confronting the city were still not solved, although the sanitary condition of the city improved greatly. But without the vast urban transformations of the Second Empire, had only the programs of the early-nineteenth-century hygienists continued to be implemented – stopgap measures and piecemeal reforms – it is probable that the sanitary state of Paris and other French cities would not have improved significantly for decades and might even have deteriorated.

French public hygienists exerted much influence on public health reform and reforming administrators both in France and abroad. But they made their greatest impact by their scientific investigations of public health problems. Napoleon III and Baron Haussmann, for example, were influenced by the research of the leading public hygienists. The rebuilding of Paris was in part a response to hygienists' publicity of health conditions in Paris. By 1848, hygienists, urban planners, and administrators were aware of the public health problems facing the city, recognizing the inadequacy of attempted solutions. The questions raised by the hygienists, the problems investigated, and the solutions proposed helped pave the way for the transformation of some French cities after 1850. The rebuilding of Paris under Haussmann, with its accompanying public health reforms, was an expanded version of a reform program already outlined by Prefect of the Seine Rambuteau, urban planners, and public hygienists. A similar situation prevailed in Lyon, where Jean-François Terme, mayor from 1840 to 1847, had proposed far-reaching reforms, which were finally effected only during the Second Empire.

In the final analysis, the achievements of the French hygienists attest to the vitality of the public health movement. A group of devoted professionals produced a prodigious amount of research on all the major public health problems of the age and, by publicity of their investigations, influenced policy at the professional level both in France and abroad. In terms of actual public health reform, limited but significant accomplishments were tempered with many frustrations.

Thus between 1820 and 1840, fifty years of interest in public health coalesced into an active public health movement. The French were the leaders in public health until the late 1830s, when French leadership was challenged by the British. During the 1840s, the British public health movement gathered momentum, whereas the French movement, weakened by the loss of Parent-Duchâtelet, consolidated the discipline of public hygiene and continued along the same general lines as in the earlier decades, but without the legislative achievements made by the British. France was the undisputed and acknowledged public health leader before the 1840s. The extent and type of hygienic literature, the activities of the public hygienists, the public health institutions, the scholarly journal of the movement, and the influence of French hygienists on foreign public health reformers all support such a thesis.

9

Before Pasteur: Hygienism and the French model of public health

The overarching mission of the French public health reformers was hygienism, a belief that all areas of life should be medicalized and moralized to prevent disease and promote public health in the interest of social order and national security. Hygienism was developed within a statist context. French society was to be medicalized and moralized by state agencies and institutions, with professional hygienists serving the state as advisors and hygienic missionaries. This did not necessarily imply the bureaucratization of medicine, however, although some favored this approach, since physicians in private practice might also carry out these goals. The notion of hygienism was derived in part from prevailing theories of disease causation, which attributed most diseases to environmental and social causes. Since almost anything might potentially cause disease, hygienism had to be all-encompassing. The experts, the professional hygienists who were to act as advisors and help determine policy, had to achieve authority and legitimacy by cloaking their work with the mantle of science. The increasing scientism of French society required that if a particular approach or discipline was to be taken seriously, it had to be scientific. Hygienism thus incorporated a community of practitioners, professional hygienists who applied scientific methods to the study of public health problems and sought to transform public hygiene into a scientific discipline. The method was an important part of the mission.

Hygienism outlived Pasteur. Indeed, Pasteur's discovery that micro-organisms caused some diseases provided further scientific justification for the program of the hygienists. Pasteur's germ theory and the ensuing bacteriological revolution did not immediately alter French public health. Indeed, hygienism, the legacy of the early-nineteenth-century public health movement, became even more pronounced as a key item on the national agenda, emerging as the secular religion of the Third Republic. After the French defeat in the Franco-Prussian War, politicians and reformers invoked medical reasons to account for the perceived weakening of moral fiber and national strength, characterized by depopulation and physical degeneracy. Some reformers and social observers contended that French society was fundamentally disease-ridden and advocated hygienism to address the sociomedical problems that they thought to be the cause of military, economic, and moral deterioration. Public health reform became a key item on the national agenda of the Third Republic long before the pasteurization of France occurred.[1]

The legacy of the early-nineteenth-century public health movement included not only the ideology of hygienism, but also a model of public health that determined the course of French public health for the rest of the century. The French model, which emerged in clear form by the 1830s, consisted of a particular theoretical approach to public health that was embodied in French public health institutions. The French model incorporated a new definition of and approach to public health; the concept of public hygiene as a social and administrative science; the establishment of advisory boards of health composed of technical experts from a variety of specialties as the institutional embodiment of the scientific discipline of public hygiene; the articulation and exemplification of these concepts of public health and public hygiene by a group of physicians, scientists, and administrators who formed a public health movement; and a centralized national bureaucracy through which public health could be administered.

Characteristic of the French model of public health was the new approach to and definition of public health, institutionalized in the Paris health council and the Royal Academy of Medicine. Public health was broadly interpreted to include everything that was in any way related to health. Until the 1830s, this new approach coexisted with the traditional notion of public health exemplified by the Restoration government's sanitary policy. The new approach to public health became dominant in the 1830s as a result of a shift in national public health policy and the emergence of the public health movement. The new public health emphasized administrative and legislative reform, to be undertaken by the state, as well as individual moral reform, and its proponents saw public health as an integral part of a more general reform of society upon the basis of scientific principles.

> 1   On public health in the Third Republic and the transmission and acceptance of Pasteurian ideas and techniques, see Martha Hildreth, *Doctors, Bureaucrats, and Public Health in France, 1888–1902* (New York: Garland, 1987); Ann-Louise Shapiro, *Housing the Poor of Paris, 1852–1902* (Madison: University of Wisconsin Press, 1985); and Bruno Latour, *The Pasteurization of France* (Cambridge, MA: Harvard University Press, 1987). Latour argues that French physicians were not pasteurized before about 1895, when they realized that the use of diphtheria serotherapy, developed by the Pasteurians, could have an impact on their private practices. Hildreth emphasizes the tension between the Parisian public health leaders, who promoted public health and the bureaucratization of medicine, and the provincial practitioners, who resisted both the Parisian physicians and Pasteurism. On the invocation of medical explanations to account for national decline, see Robert Nye, *Crime, Madness, and Politics in Modern France: The Medical Concept of National Decline* (Princeton, NJ: Princeton University Press, 1984).

In the development of the French model of public health, the idea of science, particularly social science, which the nineteenth-century hygienists incorporated into their notion of public hygiene, was especially important. For the hygienists, the word *scientific*, as it applied to public hygiene and to the health council, had two meanings, both grounded in an Enlightenment approach to science and society: First, it meant the application of the scientific or empirical method to the study of public health problems; second, it meant the transformation of a mass of hygienic information into a coherent administrative science, a codification. With the French hygienists, public hygiene became a social and administrative science with practical applicability to the public health reform of society.[2]

The health council was a central feature of the French model of public health. As a permanent board, the health council exemplified the dominant French approach to public health. It was the place where scientific hygiene was learned and practiced, the training ground of the professional public hygienist. A key component of the French model of public health was a vocal, articulate community of hygienists that functioned through existing public health institutions and through its own journal, the *Annales d'hygiène publique*. This group of hygienists defined, exemplified, and publicized the new approach to public health and the scientific discipline of public hygiene. The journal they founded demonstrated their ideas of disciplinary development and professionalization. They wanted to separate public hygiene from medicine, to make it something more than a medical specialty – a collaborative effort of specialists from a variety of scientific backgrounds. Although ostensibly retaining the traditional relationship between public health and legal medicine, hygienists asserted and demonstrated in the organization and publication of the journal the separateness and distinctiveness of public hygiene.

The ideological and institutional framework within which the French model was conceived and exported was a centralized, national bureaucracy through which public health could be administered. Given this statist approach to public health, the French model could be most appropriately applied on the continent, where similar bureaucratic organizations existed. This aspect of the French model was a powerful attraction to reformers like Chadwick, who sought to create a centralized bureaucracy through which to administer both Poor Law and public health reforms. However, because such structures did not traditionally exist, the French model proved to be not especially well suited to the Anglo-American situation.

In conclusion, the most important contributions of the French hygienists were theoretical and institutional. From 1770 to 1840 a community of

2 Keith Baker, *Condorcet: From Natural Philosophy to Social Mathematics* (Chicago: University of Chicago Press, 1975).

hygienists including physicians, scientists, and administrators articulated the public health idea that grew into the ideology of hygienism, developed the scientific discipline of public hygiene, and institutionalized these notions nationally in the Royal Society of Medicine and its successor, the Royal Academy of Medicine, and locally in the health councils, especially the Paris health council. Viewed against the backdrop of broader intellectual and social currents in the late eighteenth and early nineteenth centuries, the French public health movement is representative of the reform movements that characterized the period. Hygienism, the new approach to public health, and the scientific discipline of public hygiene were a direct outgrowth of Enlightenment and Revolutionary ideas and programs about natural rights, the role of government in preserving these rights, and the role of science in society. Although there were many points of view represented by individual hygienists, the dominant ideology of the public health movement seems to have been, first, that any area of investigation could and should be made scientific – hence, scientific hygiene – and, second, that society could and should be reformed upon the basis of scientific principles and administered accordingly.[3]

3   Much of this conclusion has appeared in Ann F. La Berge, "The Early Nineteenth-Century French Public Health Movement: The Disciplinary Development and Institutionalization of *hygiène publique*," *Bull. Hist. Med.* 58 (1984): 363–79.

EPILOGUE

Hygienists writing in the 1850s considered the science of public hygiene mature. In the decades after 1848 public hygiene came of age both as a scientific discipline and in terms of practical results. According to Adolphe Trébuchet, the Paris health council and the society of the *Annales d'hygiène publique et de médecine légale* established the science of public hygiene on a firm basis and made possible its propagation both in France and abroad.[1] In terms of practical results, reforms that were advocated in the first half of the century were effected in some cities with the urban transformations of the Second Empire. Paris and Lyon, where water supplies and sewerage systems were enlarged and improved, are obvious examples. After 1850 some of the problems that had preoccupied early-nineteenth-century hygienists were solved by industrial improvements and chemical discoveries. But new ones appeared, such as health concerns related to railway hygiene.[2] Subsequent to the public health law of 1848, health councils proliferated throughout the nation. And in 1854, the editors of the *Annales d'hygiène publique* commenced the second series of the journal, with a commitment to continue to publicize all aspects of public health and legal medicine, as they had done in the first series (1829–54).[3]

The work of the leading hygienists, such as Jean-Baptiste Monfalcon and A. P. Isidore de Polinière, Alexandre Parent-Duchâtelet, Alphonse Chevallier, Michel Lévy, and Louis-René Villermé, continued to be widely cited and in most cases remained the definitive studies on the subjects they had treated.[4] Many of the leading hygienists, such as Villermé, Chevallier, and Trébuchet, continued to serve on the Paris

1 Adolphe Trébuchet, review of Ambroise Tardieu's *Dictionnaire d'hygiène publique et de salubrité* in *Annales d'hygiène publique* 2e série, 2 (1854): 222.
2 Maxime Vernois, *Traité pratique d'hygiène industrielle et administrative*, 2 vols. (Paris: Baillière, 1860), 1: xxix–xxx. See, for example, Prosper Pietra Santa, *Chemins de fer et santé publique ou hygiène des voyageurs et des employés* (Paris: Hachette, 1861).
3 *Annales d'hygiène publique* 2e série, 1 (1854): 1–4.
4 For example, a third and enlarged edition of Parent-Duchâtelet's *De la prostitution dans la ville de Paris* was published, edited and completed by A. Trébuchet and Poirat-Duval, 2 vols. (Paris: Baillière, 1857). The edition included a *Précis sur la prostitution dans les principales villes de l'Europe*.

health council and/or as editors of the *Annales d'hygiène publique*, but some of the most influential hygienists had died: Parent-Duchâtelet, Fodéré, and Marc, just to mention a few.[5]

Whereas in the first half of the century the principal repositories of hygienic knowledge were the annual reports of the Paris health council, the *Annales d'hygiène publique*, Monfalcon and Polinière's treatise on urban hygiene, and the collected writings of Parent-Duchâtelet, in the 1850s hygienists like Ambroise Tardieu and Maxime Vernois attempted to systematize the body of doctrine of public hygiene.[6] The most important such work was Tardieu's three-volume *Dictionnaire de l'hygiène publique*, first published in 1854, with a second edition appearing in 1862. Vernois's work on industrial hygiene, *Traité pratique de l'hygiène industrielle et administrative*, published in 1860, brought together the work of the health councils and industrial legislation in an organized fashion. Meanwhile, the Paris health council continued to publish its reports, as did many provincial health councils.[7]

By the 1850s, hygienists were writing the history of public health in France, dating the beginnings of the public health movement from the late eighteenth century and the Royal Society of Medicine. There was a consensus that France was the leader in public health before the 1840s, by comparison with other European countries.[8] Writers in the 1850s were already looking at some of Parent-Duchâtelet's studies as history, and when one reads through the *Annales d'hygiène publique* or looks at the work of the health councils in the 1850s, the sense of continuity is striking: the same problems, the same solutions, and many of the same names. For example, Villermé continued to be actively involved with public health and social questions throughout the 1850s. He maintained his earlier concern for the condition of the working class with his interest in mutual aid societies and working-class housing projects, or *cités ouvrières*. He

5 See Appendixes 8 and 11 for a list of members of the Paris health council in 1852 and editors of the *Annales d'hygiène publique* in 1854, respectively.

6 *Traité de la salubrité dans les grandes villes* (Paris: Baillière, 1846); *Hygiène publique*, 2 vols. (Paris: Baillière, 1836).

7 Ambroise Tardieu, *Dictionnaire d'hygiène publique et de salubrité ou Répertoire de toutes les questions relatives à la santé publique*, 3 vols. (Paris: Baillière, 1862). For a review of the first edition, see Trébuchet's review in *Annales d'hygiène publique* 2e série, 2 (1854): 221–39; Maxime Vernois, *Traité pratique de l'hygiène industrielle et administrative*, 2 vols. (Paris: Baillière, 1860). For a review of Vernois's work, see *Annales d'hygiène publique* 2e série, 9 (1858): 216–31. Signed B.; probably Boudin. Adolphe Trébuchet, ed., *Rapport général sur les travaux du Conseil d'hygiène publique et de salubrité du département de la Seine depuis 1849 jusqu'à 1858 inclusivement* (Paris: Imprimerie municipale, 1861); Maxime Vernois, "Des rapports généraux des Conseils d'hygiène de l'Empire," *Annales d'hygiène publique* 2e série, 15 (1861): 453–69.

8 See, for example, Trébuchet's review of Tardieu's *Dictionnaire* in *Annales d'hygiène publique* 2e série, 2 (1854): 221–2.

continued to investigate epidemics, with a study on the 1853 typhoid fever epidemic in Paris. His long-lived interest in statistics continued, as did his support for and encouragement of the work of Adolphe Quetelet. A new area of investigation after 1848, the therapeutic uses of mineral water and mineral water treatment as an aspect of public assistance, also attracted Villermé's attention.[9]

The health council idea of the 1830s came to fruition in 1848, when a national law established councils throughout the nation at the departmental and arrondissement levels. The results were not so gratifying as hygienists had hoped. By 1858, few councils were sending their annual reports to the Minister of Commerce, as required by law. In fact, only the council of the Meurthe had regularly sent in its report since 1850. The problem was typically lack of funds, many departmental general councils being reluctant to vote the funds necessary for printing and distribution of annual reports. In 1858 only six departments had allocated enough money, and thirty-three departments had provided no funds. Hygienist Maxime Vernois, a member of the Paris health council and an industrial hygienist, concluded that practical and administrative hygiene in France were still – even in 1861 – at the early stages of their development.[10]

The general concerns of the Paris health council in the 1850s illustrated both new and traditional areas of interest. New areas included increased attention to working-class housing, day-care centers, and the medical service for theaters and swimming pools. Traditional areas included the

9 Pierre Astruc, "Louis-René Villermé, médecin-sociologue (1782–1863)," *Le Progrès médical* (1932) supplément illustré, 1 Oct., p. 53; L. R. Villermé, "Sur les cités ouvrières," *Annales d'hygiène publique* 43, (1850): 241–61; L. R. Villermé, "De l'épidémie typhoïde qui a frappé la ville de Paris pendant les cinq premiers mois de 1853," *Annales d'hygiène publique* 2e série, 2 (1854): 83–95; L. R. Villermé, "Considérations sur les tables de mortalité, à l'occasion d'un travail de M. Quetelet sur le même sujet," *Annales d'hygiène publique* 2e série, 1 (1854): 7–31. This work was presented to the Academy of Political and Moral Sciences, in which Villermé continued his active involvement. See also L. R. Villermé, "De l'application de la méthode statistique aux opérations de recrutement," *Annales d'hygiène publique* 2e série, 8 (1857): 5–13; L. R. Villermé, "Des eaux minérales dans leurs rapports avec l'assistance publique," *Annales d'hygiène publique* 42 (1849): 241–53. On mineral water, see George Weisz, "Water Cures and Science: The French Academy of Medicine and Mineral Water in the Nineteenth Century," *Bull. Hist. Med.* 64 (1990): 393–416.

10 See the important article by Vernois, "Des rapports généraux des Conseils d'hygiène de l'Empire," esp. p. 468. This article is of the utmost importance for health council history, for Vernois gives a list of all the published works of all the health councils from 1802 to 1860, as well as an analysis of the most interesting reports and works published by the various health councils. The Paris health council was an exception. By a law of 1851, the Paris health council's organization was left unchanged. On this see A. Trébuchet, "Note sur l'organisation du Conseil d'hygiène publique et de salubrité du département de la Seine," *Annales d'hygiène publique* 47 (1852): 286–314. Trébuchet's article gives a good general history of the Paris health council, with special emphasis on the various organizational changes.

salubrity of private dwellings and public establishments, public baths, garbage collection and street cleaning, occupational hygiene, pure food and drink, first aid, epidemics, and dangerous and unhealthy establishments. Hygienists were finally successful in their attempts to secure passage of laws and ordinances to clean up unhealthy dwellings. A police ordinance of November 20, 1848 (reissued in 1853), regulated unhealthy dwellings in Paris, and in 1850 (April 13) a national law on the same issue was passed. The two measures differed in that the Paris ordinance aimed at the elimination of exterior causes of insalubrity, whereas the 1850 law dealt with interior problems. With their increased interest in workers' dwellings, hygienists also favored the construction of special housing projects for workers, called *cités ouvrières*. The Paris health council, for example, approved an experiment to build a model project for 4,000 workers. Hygienists generally opposed barrackslike structures and favored individual or duplex cottages.[11]

The Melun law of 1850 on unhealthy dwellings reflected the goals of hygienists and led to the creation of Unhealthy Dwellings Commissions that functioned like health councils, conducting investigations and making recommendations. These commissions met a fate similar to that of the provincial health councils. Just as by the 1860s many of these councils had ceased to function, by the 1870s in major cities like Marseilles, Lyon, Bordeaux, Nantes, and Rouen, the commissions no longer existed or met only sporadically. Only in Paris and Lille did the Unhealthy Dwellings Commissions continue to function, but with restricted powers. The inspection of private dwellings versus the public health raised the question of individual rights and private property versus the right of the state to interfere in the name of public health. This problem of conflicting interests between private property and public health continued unresolved throughout the nineteenth century, exemplifying the tension between liberalism and statism.[12]

Increased attention to the health and condition of the working classes

---

11 The *service médical des théâtres*, created in 1852, provided for a physician to be on duty at each theatrical performance to give first aid. At each theater a stall for medicine and first aid was made available. The Paris health council also wanted a physician attached to each swimming school (*école de natation*). Information on the Paris health council in the 1850s is taken from Alphonse Guérard, review of Adolphe Trébuchet, ed., *Rapport général sur les travaux du Conseil d'hygiène publique et de salubrité du département de la Seine, depuis 1849 jusqu'à 1858 inclusivement* in *Annales d'hygiène publique* 2e série, 16 (1861): 446–77. See also Villermé, "Cités ouvrières." Villermé opposed the idea of constructing one large building to house many workers and families, favoring instead building small individual or duplex cottages to allow more privacy. He also wanted to exclude single males from the *cités ouvrières* for fear that they would lower moral standards.

12 Ann-Louise Shapiro, *Housing the Poor of Paris, 1850–1902* (Madison: University of Wisconsin Press, 1985).

was also shown by hygienists' interest in day-care centers for the children of workers and in the mineral water question. In 1853 the Paris health council conducted a special study on *crèches*, or infant day-care centers. The primary interest of the members included the salubrity of the locale, the influence of the crowding together of small children on their health, dangers posed by changes of temperature from home to *crèche*, the incidence of contagious infections, the number of cradles and the number of babies, hygienic measures to be taken, relative mortality figures, and general improvements needed.[13]

The hygienists' concern about mineral water was to make possible its therapeutic use by the indigent, since they assumed that mineral water was a valid form of treatment and an aspect of public assistance. Use of mineral waters had increased greatly in the first half of the century as their therapeutic value for certain diseases became accepted, and hygienists and physicians addressed the public health issues associated with mineral waters in the years after 1848. In 1848, mineral water sources were declared to be of national utility. After 1848, the idea that "taking the waters," like medical care in general, was an aspect of public assistance, the right of all in a democratic society, became generally accepted among public hygienists. Some hygienists felt that everyone was entitled to mineral water therapy and that provisions for sick indigents had to be made available at sources. Many indigents were already receiving free treatments. Reporting to the mineral water commission of the National Academy of Medicine in 1848, mineral water specialist Philippe Patissier noted that at Eaux-Chaudes, a source in the Basses-Pyrénées, in 1827, 2,040 indigents had received free baths. At about the same time Jules François, a mining engineer in charge of the mineral water service (engineer of medical hydrology), published a work on the relationship of mineral waters and public assistance. François asserted the therapeutic value of mineral water and urged the government to accept the responsibility of ensuring that even the poor would have access to mineral water for medical treatment.[14]

13 Guérard, review of Trébuchet, ed., *Rapport général*. On the crèches, see Ann F. La Berge, "Medicalization and Moralization: The Crèches of Nineteenth-Century Paris," *J. Soc. Hist.*, 25 (1991): 66–87.
14 By a decree of March 8, 1848, the French government declared mineral water of public utility. See Villermé, "Eaux minérales," p. 248. For legislation pertaining to mineral waters, see Maxime Durand-Fardel et al., *Dictionnaire général des eaux minérales et d'hydrologie médicale...* 2 vols. (Paris: Baillière, 1860). See the review of the work by Maxime Vernois in *Annales d'hygiène publique* 2e série, 14 (1860): 473–8. Mineral water was not a major concern of the public hygienists in the first half of the nineteenth century. For example, before 1848 no article on mineral water appeared in the *Annales d'hygiène publique*. See, for example, Villermé, "Eaux minérales," and Philippe Patissier, "Des eaux minérales considérées au point de vue de l'assistance publique," *Annales d'hygiène publique* 43 (1850): 189–94. Jules

In the late nineteenth century the ideas and all-encompassing scope of the early-nineteenth-century public health movement, with its emphasis on both sanitary and social reform, gave way to a narrower interpretation. Late-nineteenth-century hygienists concentrated their efforts on sanitary engineering and control of contagious diseases, their general goal being comprehensive public health legislation, finally enacted only in 1902. The mission of the early-nineteenth-century public health movement had been sanitary, social, and moral reform, but little social and moral reform had been forthcoming. Sanitary reform had occurred but had not succeeded in eliminating epidemic and contagious diseases. By the end of the century, the acceptance and promotion by hygienists of the germ theory of disease shifted the emphasis of sanitary reform from general street-cleaning activities to more specific measures of vaccination, disinfection, and inspection of individual dwellings. The dwellings of the poor continued to be considered breeding places of disease, but now because they harbored "microbe factories" instead of filth and bad smells.[15]

One of the main stumbling blocks to effective public health reform remained the lack of enforcement of public health legislation. Health councils had no power of enforcement, and mayors, although charged with protection of the public health, in fact often did not have the means to enforce public health measures either, because their municipal councils would not allocate money or because the appropriate sanitary and public health administrations and institutions did not have the power to enforce their measures. Like their early-nineteenth-century counterparts, late-nineteenth-century hygienists sought to transfer power on health issues from political bodies such as municipal councils to competent professional bodies with advisory functions such as health councils.

Resistance to public health measures came from many quarters. Popular resistance to vaccination, for example, continued throughout the century. Many practicing physicians joined with the general population and landlords in resisting hygienic measures that seemed annoying, expensive, an invasion of privacy, and a challenge to the sanctity of private property and private practice. Since the early nineteenth century, hygienists had succeeded in establishing their profession independently of the medical profession in general. Although many hygienists were physicians, not all physicians were hygienists or were especially interested in public health reform. Leading Parisian bureaucratic physicians, the "princes of

François, *Des eaux minérales dans leur rapports avec l'assistance publique* (Bagnères-de-Bigorre: Dossun, 1849), reviewed in Villermé, "Des eaux minérales," pp. 241–53. François's treatise was a twenty-seven-page pamphlet. See also Weisz, "Water Cures and Science."

15 Martha Hildreth, *Doctors, Bureaucrats, and Public Health in France, 1850–1902* (New York: Garland Press, 1987). Shapiro, *Housing the Poor of Paris*.

medicine," those who sat on the *Comité consultatif d'hygiène publique*, the principal public health institution of the late nineteenth century, pushed vigorously for public health reform and the bureaucratization of public health. Their efforts were staunchly resisted, however, by average practitioners in the provinces who were active in the medical syndicates and who saw public health and bureaucratization as a threat to their private practices.[16]

By the late nineteenth century, French preoccupation with declining military strength and a falling rate of population growth increased the urgency of public health reform. By the 1880s, the health of the nation had been identified with national security, and the national government seemed ready to take a larger role in public health matters. Much of the motivation came from the French defeat in the Franco-Prussian War and what this seemed to indicate about French society. The campaign to reduce infant mortality by applying scientific principles to infant care was an important part of this effort. By the end of the century, a group of professional hygienists mounted an intense lobbying effort to enlarge the jurisdiction of public health professionals and to produce effective guidelines, codes, and procedures relating to sanitary matters. The goals of this late-nineteenth-century movement were similar to the principal goals of the early-nineteenth-century reformers. The immediate practical result of the efforts of the late-nineteenth-century public health movement was the public health law of 1902, which invites comparison with the public health laws of 1848, the political culmination of the efforts of the early-nineteenth-century movement. The 1902 law embodied some, but not all, of the goals of the public hygienists. Smallpox vaccination was made mandatory a little more than 100 years after its introduction into France. The 1902 law also closed some of the loopholes of the Melun law, thereby increasing its effectiveness. Minor improvements in the organization of health services and in enforcement of sanitary standards resulted, but final authority and enforcement in health matters still rested with elected local officials instead of professional hygienists. As in the first half of the century, legislators were reluctant to interfere too much in private lives and private property in the name of public health.[17]

---

16 Hildreth, *Doctors, Bureaucrats, and Public Health.*
17 Robert Nye, *Crime, Madness, and Politics in Modern France: The Medical Concept of National Decline* (Princeton, NJ: Princeton University Press, 1984); Jane Crisler, "Saving the Seed: the Scientific Preservation of Children in the Third Republic" (Ph.D. dissertation, University of Wisconsin, 1984); Ann F. La Berge, "Mothers and Infants, Nurses and Nursing: Alfred Donné and the Medicalization of Child Care in Nineteenth-Century France," *J. Hist. Med.*, 46 (1991): 20–43. See also Claire Salomon-Bayet, *Pasteur et la révolution pastorienne* (Paris: Payot, 1986), and Bruno Latour, *The Pasteurization of France* (Cambridge, MA: Harvard University Press, 1987).

In 1827 the Paris health council suggested that one of the ways to measure industrialization was by counting the number of steam engines in use and their rate of proliferation (*R. G....1827*, 7). According to Roger Price in the *French Second Republic: A Social History* (Ithaca, NY: Cornell University Press, 1972), p. 16, in 1832 there were 525 steam engines in all of France; by 1847 the number had risen to 4,853, an increase of more than 900 percent. By 1870 the number of steam engines was 27,958, an increase since 1847 of 575 percent. Thus the proliferation of steam engines was more rapid between 1832 and 1847 than between 1847 and 1870.

In 1835 the *Géographie industrielle et commerciale de la France* [cited in Dr. Thouvenin, "De l'influence que l'industrie exerce sur la santé des populations dans les grands centres manufacturiers," *Annales d'hygiène publique* 36 (1846): 20] stated that in all France there were 1,448 steam engines. Of these, 1,105 were concentrated in ten departments:

Nord	297	Aisne	49
Seine	197	Haut-Rhin	48
Loire	175	Saône et Loire	45
Seine-Inférieure	160	Marne	34
Rhône	60	Gard	25

The Paris health council supplied some interesting information on the increase in requests for authorization of steam engines in Paris in this same period (*R. G....1837*, 54; *1838*, 200; *1839*, 244).

1835	33
1836	39
1837	49
1838	66
1839	82

Information on the French working-class population is furnished by Thouvenin ("l'influence de l'industrie, p. 20). He put the French working-class population in 1846 at 11 million, or roughly one-third of the total population, but this figure included agricultural laborers. He estimated the number of industrial workers (including those in the handcraft and domestic industries) at 5 million. Out of this 5 million, about 1 million were employed in the cotton industry, 500,000 in the wool industry, 300,000 in the silk industry, and 25,000 to 30,000 in the linen industry. This means that out of 5 million industrial workers, approximately 1,925,000 were employed in the textile industry. Thouvenin estimated that out of this number of textile workers, 400,000 were weavers (Thouvenin, "l'influence de l'industrie," pp. 20, 25, 29, 35–6, 38, 43–5, 283).

Examples of the rapid growth of some industrial towns in the period were Roubaix, whose population increased from 8,000 at the turn of the century to 25,000 by 1846, and Mulhouse, whose population more than doubled from 1832 to 1840 ["Rapport de M. Villermé sur l'ouvrage intitulé 'Recherches statistiques sur Mulhouse par M. Achille Penot (1843),' in *Séances et trav. de l'Acad. des Sci. Mor. et Pol.* 4 (1843): 116]. In Mulhouse, a textile center, this rapid population growth is explained by an increase in the number of spindles from 500,000 in 1828 to 1,150,000 in 1847, or one-third of all the spindles in France [J. H. Clapham, *The Economic Development of France and Germany, 1815–1914,* 4th ed. (Cambridge: Cambridge University Press, 1968), p. 53].

Cities with large working-class populations were Paris and Lyon. Paris, for example, had a working-class population of more than 400,000 [Paul Gagnon, *France Since 1789* (New York: Harper and Row, 1964), p. 134]. Other cities with sizable working-class populations were Ste.-Marie-aux-Mines in Alsace, with 20,000 workers; Rouen, with 23,000; Amiens, with 40,000; and Lille, with 50,000, or about one-half the total population of the city (Thouvenin, "l'influence de l'industrie," pp. 278, 285–90; L. R. Villermé, *Tableau de l'état physique et moral des ouvriers,* 2 vols. (Paris: Renouard, 1840, 1: 283).

APPENDIX 2: COMMISSION CENTRALE SANITAIRE AND CONSEIL SUPÉRIEUR DE SANTÉ

Members of the *Commission centrale sanitaire* of 1820
  Councilors of state:
    Gérando
    Hély d'Oissel
    Forestier
  Physicians:
    Desgenettes
    Kéraudren
    Duméril
    Pariset
    Bally
    Devèze
  Intendants of the Marseilles health intendancy:
    Majestre
    Rostan
  Moreau de Jonnès, a naval officer
  Laffon de Ladébat, head of the *Administration des hospices* of the Ministry
    of the Interior
  Two Parisian businessmen and two legal scholars.[1]

Members of the *Conseil supérieur de santé, 1822*
  Councilors of State:
    Baron Capelle
    Gérando
    Hély d'Oissel
    Saint-Cricq

---

1 This list is in George Sussman, "From Yellow Fever to Cholera: A Study of French Government Policy, Medical Professionalism and Popular Movements in the Epidemic Crisis of the Restoration and the July Monarchy" (Ph.D. dissertation, Yale University, 1971), n. 36, p. 403. The existence of the commission is mentioned in Alexandre Moreau de Jonnès, *Rapport au Conseil supérieur de santé sur le choléra-morbus pestilentiel* (Paris: Cosson, 1831), p. 157, but no list of members is given. The creation of the commission was not reported in the *Moniteur*.

Physicians:
  Bally
  Kéraudren
  Pariset
André, a banker
Moreau de Jonnès, a former military officer.[2]

Members of the *Conseil supérieur de santé, 1835*
  Gérando
  André
  Bally[3]
  Kéraudren[3]
  Moreau de Jonnès
  Pariset[3]
  B. de Montfort
  Odier
  Fleuriau de Bellevue
  David
  Dubois[3]
  Lefebvre
  Vernos
  Pellet-Will
  Pouyer
  Jacqueminot
  Marc[3]
  Gay-Lussac
  Virey[3]
  Ferrus[3]
  Sollicoffre
  Désurgiess
  Reynard

Comité consultatif d'hygiène publique, 1848
  Louis Aubert-Roche
  François Magendie
  François Mélier
  Hippolyte Royer-Collard
  Louis-René Villermé

2 *Moniteur universel*, September 3, 1822, pp. 1829 and 1894.
3 Physicians. This information in *Almanach Royal*, 1835. By 1835 the superior health
  council was under the *Service sanitaire*, attached to the Ministry of Commerce.

APPENDIX 3: MEMBERS OF THE MEDICAL SECTION OF THE ROYAL ACADEMY OF MEDICINE IN 1828

Titular Members
Adelon[1,2]
Alibert[5]
Bally[3,4]
Broussais
Coutanceau
Desgenettes
Double
Esquirol[1,2]
Girard[1]
Huzard[1]
Kéraudren[2,3]
Leroux
Lucas
Magendie[5]
Marc[1–3]
Moreau de la Sarthe
Orfila[1,2]
Pariset[1,3,4]
Portal

Free Associates (Associés libres). From related sciences and living in Paris, 1828
Chabrol de Volvic, Prefect of the Seine
Chaptal
D'Arcet[1,2]
Gay-Lussac

[1] Member of the Paris health council.
[2] Editor of the *Annales d'hygiène publique et de médecine légale.*
[3] Member of the *Conseil supérieur de santé.*
[4] Participant in government commissions sent to observe yellow fever.
[5] Participant in 1831 government commissions sent to observe cholera.

There were eighty ordinary associates, twenty of whom were from Paris; they were well-known doctors, pharmacists, and surgeons. There was also an undetermined number of adjunct members – people who had sent observations and essays to the Academy. Some of the hygienists and well-known doctors who were adjunct members in 1828 were:

Andral fils[1,2]
Bourdon
Bricheteau
Londe[5]
Louis
Olliviers d'Angers[1,2]
Parent-Duchâtelet[1,2]
Patissier
Piorry
Roche
Rochoux
Rostan
Villermé[1,2]

1845 Members of Section No. 8, Public Health, Legal Medicine, and Medical Police, Mémoires, 11 (1845).

Adelon[1,2]
Chevallier[1,2]
Eméry[1]
Forestier
Gérardin[5]
Kéraudren[2]
Labarraque[1]
Lecanu[1]
Londe[5]
Nacquart
Renauldin
Royer-Collard[1]
Villermé[1,2]

1 Member of the Paris health council.
2 Editor of the *Annales d'hygiène publique et de médecine légale*.
3 Member of the *Conseil supérieur de santé*.
4 Participant in government commissions sent to observe yellow fever.
5 Participant in 1831 government commissions sent to observe cholera.

APPENDIX 4: PREFECTS OF POLICE, 1815–1848[1]

Julien Anglès	September 1816–December 1821
Guy Delaveau	December 1821–January 1828
Louis Debelleyme	January 1828–August 1829
Jean Mangin	August 1829–1830
Jacques Bavoux	July 1830
Louis Girod de l'Ain	August 1830–November 1830
Achille Treilhard	November 1830–December 1830
Jean Baude	December 1830–February 1831
Alexandre Vivien	February 1831–September 1831
Sébastien Saulnier	September 1831–October 1831
Henri Gisquet	October 1831–September 1836
Gabriel Delessert	September 1836–February 1848

1 John Phillip Stead, *The Police of Paris* (London: Staples Press, 1957), p. 210.

APPENDIX 5: ORGANIZATION OF THE PREFECTURE OF POLICE: THE ADMINISTRATION OF PUBLIC HEALTH, 1846[1]

First Division:	Police of order and public safety, judicial affairs, prisons and hospices
Second Bureau:	Interrogations, dispensary
Second Section:	Prostitution and the dispensary
Third Bureau:	Prisons
Fifth Bureau:	Hospices, foundlings, the insane
Second Division:	Administrative police, provisions, commerce, navigation, public works, health
First Bureau:	Provisions, navigation, commerce
First Section:	Police of markets and food establishments
Second Section:	Upkeep and cleaning of rivers, first aid to the drowning, morgue, destruction of falsified drinks
Second Bureau:	Public works (*petite voirie*), railroads
First Section:	Dwellings, hindrances to circulation, surveillance of public buildings, water supply, construction of sewers, sidewalks, cleaning of cesspits, city dump, movable cesspits, public urinals
Third Bureau:	Vehicles, fires, cleaning and watering down of streets, public lighting
First Section:	Water carriers, fountains
Second Section:	Street cleaning and lighting, sewers, aqueducts, wells, reservoirs
Fourth Bureau:	Unhealthy establishments, sanitary police
First Section:	Dangerous, unhealthy, incommodious establishments; flaying and cutting up of horses, epizootics, fireworks, falsified foods, all related to the public health; health council, laws regulating medicine and pharmacy, secret remedies, dissection rooms, inspection of mineral waters, epidemics, vaccine, cemeteries, mortality statistics
Second Section:	Execution of law relative to child labor

1 APP, D²79, Budget des dépenses de la Préfecture de police pour l'exercice 1846.

APPENDIX 6: COMPARISON OF BUDGETS OF THE PREFECTURE OF POLICE FOR THE YEARS 1831 AND 1847, AND MONEY SPENT FOR VARIOUS ASPECTS OF PUBLIC HEALTH ADMINISTRATION[1]

1831		*1847*
7,240,646	Total budget	10,720,072
118,750	Directors' salaries for street cleaning and inspection for lighting	122,400
885,665	Public lighting	1,622,220
1,080,003	Street cleaning	1,086,750
3,000	Morgue	5,345
75,934	Dispensary	35,627

1 APP, D²69, Personnel. Budget de 1831. APP, D²79, Ville de Paris. Compte, au 16 mai 1848, des Dépenses de la Prefecture de police pour l'exercice 1847. Certain expenditures cannot be easily compared, as the offices were organized differently in 1831 and 1847, and in some cases expenditures were classified differently.

APPENDIX 7: PUBLIC HEALTH TERMINOLOGY

At the beginning of the nineteenth century a number of terms were used, often interchangeably, to refer to public health: *santé publique, salubrité, police médicale, police sanitaire, hygiène publique*. But by the 1850s, when the scientific discipline of public hygiene was firmly established, the term most widely used for public health was *hygiène publique*. *Santé publique* was the more general term used to refer to *the* public health, but *santé* was less used by nineteenth- than eighteenth-century hygienists. In the eighteenth century, there had been *intendants de santé* and local *bureaux de santé*. In the early nineteenth century these were transformed into *intendants sanitaires* and *commissions sanitaires*, or *conseils de salubrité*. *Police médicale* was an eighteenth-century term connoting public health administration, which continued to be widely used into the nineteenth century. The term *salubrité* was often used interchangeably with *hygiène publique* in the Revolutionary and Napoleonic periods and throughout the first half of the century.[1] The boards of health founded in the first half of the century were called *conseils de salubrité*. After 1848, they became *Conseils d'hygiène publique et de salubrité*. By the 1840s and 1850s, many terms used to refer to public health had acquired more precise definitions.

Three examples of the use of public health terminology from the early part of the century are those of Hallé, Prunelle, and Sainte-Marie. In his 1818 entry "Hygiène" in the *Dictionnaire des sciences médicales*, Hallé distinguished between private and public hygiene and used the term *hygiène publique* to mean the knowledge of laws, customs, and the administration of peoples relative to hygiene.[2] That same year Gabriel Prunelle, professor at the medical faculty of Montpellier, was still using the

1 For a good treatment of public health terminology, see Dora Weiner, "Public Health Under Napoleon: The Conseil de salubrité de Paris, 1802–1815," *Clio Medica* 9 (1974): 271–84.

2 J. N. Hallé and P. S. Nysten, "Hygiène," in *Dictionnaire des sciences médicales*, 60 vols. (Paris: Panckoucke, 1812–22), 22 (1818): 510. On Hallé, see William Coleman, "Health and Hygiene in the *Encyclopédie*: A Medical Doctrine for the Bourgeoisie," *J. Hist. Med.* 29 (1974): 413–14. See also Weiner, "Public Health," p. 272.

eighteenth-century term *police médicale* to describe public health. He taught a course in *police médicale*, which he defined as the application of medicine to public administration, including the administration of public health. In speaking of public health matters, Prunelle also employed the terms *médecine politique* and *médecine du corps social*, which he distinguished from clinical or private medicine.[3] In 1824, Etienne Sainte-Marie, a physician and member of the Rhône health council, was still thinking in terms of *police médicale*, which he defined as the science of legislation and regulations to preserve public health. One aspect of *police médicale* was *hygiène publique*, along with *médecine publique* and *police de la médecine*. *Police médicale* and *médecine legale* formed the two branches of the general area of medical administration called by Sainte-Marie *médecine politique*.[4]

By 1829, when a group of public hygienists founded the *Annales d'hygiène publique et de médecine légale*, they articulated more precisely the definition of public hygiene and the goals of the discipline. In the introduction to the first volume, Charles Marc defined public hygiene as a scientific, professional, administrative discipline, completely distinct from legal medicine, encompassing more than *police médicale* or *police sanitaire*. Marc emphasized that public hygiene was more than an administrative discipline, however. It was also a body of doctrine, a scientific discipline.[5] From 1829 on, the term *hygiène publique* was most commonly used by hygienists to refer to public health, and *police médicale* was rarely used. It is indicative of this shift that when Marc translated the title of Frank's influential work into French, it became *Traité complet d'hygiène publique*, the term *medicinische Polizey* being translated as *hygiène publique* instead of *police médicale*.[6] The decade of the 1830s was the period of most intense public health activity in France. By the 1840s and the 1850s, the discipline of public hygiene had matured and definitions were more precise. Still, however, the terms *hygiène publique* and *salubrité* were being used almost interchangeably, although some authors made a distinction. Writing in 1844, Michel Lévy defined public hygiene simply as the extension of individual hygiene, differing only by the scale of its application. But he went on to call it a new science with its foundation in medical statistics. Lévy differentiated between *hygiène publique* and *hygiène sociale*, the latter term, which he considered even broader, encompassing a class of men, a population, a nation, all of humanity.[7]

3 Gabriel Prunelle, "De l'action de la médecine sur la population des états," *Revue médicale historique et philosophique* I (1820): ix–xiii.

4 Etienne Sainte-Marie, *Précis élémentaire de police médicale* (Paris: Baillière, 1824), pp. 1–6.

5 Charles C. H. Marc "Introduction," *Annales d'hygiène publique* I (1829): ix–xx.

6 Ibid., p. xix.

7 Michel Lévy, *Traité d'hygiène publique et privée*, 2 vols. (Paris: Baillière, 1844), I: 50.

In their work on urban hygiene, *Traité de la salubrité dans les grandes villes*, published in 1846, Monfalcon and Polinière used both terms, *hygiène publique* and *salubrité*, to refer to public health. *Hygiène* included anything that in any way could modify the organism, whereas *salubrité* was the practical application of hygiene, the goal of hygiene. *Salubrité* was defined as a medico-administrative science, the concern of physicians and administrators. However, when the authors defined *hygiène publique*, the distinction between it and *salubrité* was none too clear. *Hygiène publique* was defined as a new science, based on observation, not theoretical illusions, whose primary interest was in practical applications. For these hygienists, the highest expression of the new science was the health councils, still called *Conseils de salubrité*.[8]

When the *Conseils de salubrité* were established on a nationwide basis in 1848, they were renamed *Conseils d'hygiène publique et de salubrité*, reflecting that *hygiène publique* had become the generally accepted term for public health. When Ambroise Tardieu published his public health dictionary in 1854, its title included both terms: *Dictionnaire d'hygiène publique et de salubrité*. Adolphe Trébuchet, who reviewed Tardieu's dictionary for the *Annales d'hygiène publique*, admitted it was difficult to make a distinction between *hygiène publique* and *salubritè*. *Hygiène*, Trébuchet said, was more general in its application, whereas *salubrité* was one of its consequences.[9] Tardieu's definition of *hygiène publique* was a catalog list of all that the discipline encompassed. Indeed, the domain of public health was everywhere. Here is his definition:

The general administration of cities, that is to say, concerns of cleanliness, lighting, the surveillance of markets, the sale of foodstuffs, the adulteration of food and drink, burials, the construction of streets, squares, dwellings, sewers, canals; public establishments, prisons, hospitals, hospices, asylums, welfare, workhouses, prostitution; educational institutions, schools for the deaf, dumb and blind, etc.; all that is in the domain of public hygiene. There was more. Public hygiene also encompassed *la police sanitaire*, or the prevention and control of contagious and epidemic diseases. This area which had been the primary aspect of public health until late in the eighteenth century was now only one of the concerns of the new scientific discipline of *hygiène publique*.[10]

---

8   Jean-Baptiste Monfalcon and A. P. Isidore de Polinière, *Traité de la salubrité dans les grandes villes* (Paris: Baillière, 1846), pp. 9–11, 25.

9   Adolphe Trébuchet, review of Ambroise Tardieu's *Dictionnaire d'hygiène publique et de salubrité* in *Annales d'hygiène publique* 2e série, 2 (1854): 232–4.

10 Ambroise Tardieu, *Dictionnaire d'hygiène publique et de salubrité ou répertoire de toutes les questions relatives à la santé publique* 2e édition, 2 vols. (Paris: Baillière, 1862), 1: xi–xii. Actually, Tardieu's definition is even longer and more detailed than this. See the work itself.

APPENDIX 8: MEMBERS OF THE PARIS HEALTH COUNCIL 1852[1]

Titular members:

Juge	M.D.
Huzard	Member of the Royal Academy of Medicine
Chevallier	Professor at the School of Pharmacy
Lecanu	Professor at the School of Pharmacy
Beaude	M.D.
Bussy	Member of the Institute, director of the School of Pharmacy
Emery	Member of the Royal Academy of Medicine
Guérard	Hospital physician
Boutron	Member of the Royal Academy of Medicine
Cadet-Gassicourt	Pharmacist
Devergie	Hospital physician
Payen	Member of the Institute
Boussingault	Member of the Institute
Flandrin	M.D.
Lélut	Member of the Institute

Adjunct members:

Soubeiran	Director of the Central Pharmacy
Combes	Member of the Institute
Trélat	Physician at Salpêtrière
Vernois	Hospital physician
Boudet	Doctor of Sciences
Bouchardat	Chief pharmacist at Hôtel-Dieu

Members because of their positions:

The secretary-general of the prefecture of police (unnamed)

P. Dubois	Dean of the Faculty of Medicine
Adelon	Professor of legal medicine at the Faculty of Medicine

1 This information exactly as found in A. Trébuchet, "Note sur l'organisation du Conseil d'hygiène publique et de salubrité du département de la Seine," *Annales d'hygiène publique* 47 (1852): 313–14.

Bégin	President of the army health council
De Sermet	Chief engineer of bridges and highways for the department of the Seine
Dupuit	Chief engineer of the municipal service of Paris
Fournel	Chief engineer of mines
Dubois	Head of the second division at the prefecture of police
Bruzard	Architect-commissioner of small public works
Trébuchet	Head of the sanitary office at the prefecture of police

APPENDIX 9: FIGURES ON BATHING

Bathtubs

1780	250
1789	300
1816	500
1818	998
1832	2,374 (fixes)
	3,760 (all bathtubs)
1835	3,768 (fixes)
	3,778 (all bathtubs) (notice discrepancy)

Bathing establishments

1817	30
1818	37
1831	74
1835	75 (78 according to Parent-Duchâtelet)
	58 establishments provided *bains à domicile* with 1,059 portable tubs

Baths taken annually

1817	270,000
1818	400,000 for an estimated 30–50,000 bathers
1849	2,000,000 or 21/4 baths per capita

Cost of baths

1818	Simple bath: 1.25–1.50 francs plus linen at 1.25 francs
	Barèges bath: 3–3.50 francs
	Oleogelatinous bath: 4 francs
	Shower: 3–8 francs
1835	Simple bath: 75 centimes

See Appendix 10 for a detailed price list for the Néothermes establishment.

Bathhouses by arrondissement according to a health council report of 1818 (list incomplete)

1er	7
2^e	8
3^e	6
4^e	2
5^e	3
6^e	1
7^e	2
8^e	0
9^e	1
10^e	6
11^e	1
12^e	0
	37 total

Sources:

P. S. Girard, "Recherches sur les établissements de bains publiques à Paris depuis le IVe siècle jusqu'à present," *Annales d'hygiène publique* 7 (1832): 44–8.

L. F. Benoiston de Châteauneuf, *Recherches sur les consommations de tout genre de la ville de Paris en 1817*, 2nd part. Consommation industrielle (Paris: Cosson, 1821), p. 141.

Elouin, Trébuchet, and Labat, *Nouveau dictionnaire de police*, 2 vols. (Paris: Béchet jeune, 1835), p. 92.

A.N., F^{8}77, Paris health council report on public baths, February 4, 1818.

Parent-Duchâtelet, "Bains" (Hygiène) in *Dictionnaire de l'industrie manufacturière*, ed. A. Baudrimont et al., 10 vols. (Paris: Baillière, 1833–41), 2: 24–9. Parent-Duchâtelet cites Girard as his source for statistics.

"Revue administrative," *Annales d'hygiène publique* 46 (1851): 457–62.

APPENDIX 10: ETABLISSEMENT HYGIÉNIQUE DES NÉOTHERMES PRIX DES BAINS ET DOUCHES

	Bain et douche f. c.		Abonnem^t de six f. c.		Abonnem^t de douze f. c.		Service et linge f. c.	
Hydroconion, ou Bain de pluie	6		5		4		1	
Bain de Sable	10		5		4		1	
Bain de Vapeur émolliente, aromatique ou sédative	5		4		3	50	1	
Bain de Vapeur sèche mercurielle, de succin, etc.	6		5	50	5		1	
Bain de Vapeur sulfureuse	5		4		3	50	1	
Bain Hydrosulfure	6		5	50	5		1	
Bain de Vapeur sèche aromatique	5		4		3	50	1	
Bain de Vapeur alcoolique aromatisée	5		4		3		1	
Bain partiel de Vapeur émolliente ou aromatique	5		4		3	50	1	
Bain partiel de Vapeur sèche de camphre, baies de genièvre, assafoetida, absinthe, armoise, belladonna, etc.	5		4	50	4		1	
Bain partiel de musc, opium, castoréum. (Le prix variera suivant la prescription des médecins)	5		4		4		1	
Bain d'eau de Savon parfumé	5		4	50	4		1	
Bain de Vapeur cosmétique odoriférante	5		4	50	4		1	
Bain d'Eau cosmétique odoriférante	4		3	50	3		1	
Bain de Lait. (Le prix variera suivant la composition)	4		3		3		1	
Bain Égyptien avec massage, friction, etc.	12		10		9		2	
Bain Russe avec immersion d'eau froide	5		10		9		1	
Bain Gélatineux de force ordinaire	5		10		9		1	

	Bain et douche		Abonnem^t de six		Abonnem^t de douze		Service et linge	
	f.	c.	f.	c.	f.	c.	f.	c.
Bain Liquide de plantes émollientes ou aromatiques	5		4	50	4		1	
Bain d'Eau de son	4	50	4		3	50	1	
Bain d'Eau minérale (Barèges et autres)	5		4	50	4		1	
Bain d'Eau de mer	5		4	50	4		1	
Bain d'Iode. (Le prix variera suivant la dose)	5		4		4		1	
Bain de Siège composé	2		4		4		1	50
Bain de Siège d'eau minérale	2	50	4		4		1	50
Bain d'Ondée	2		4		4		1	
Douche de Vapeur émolliente, aromatique ou sédative	4		3	50	3		1	
Douche de Vapeur cosmétique odoriférante	4		3	50	3		1	
Douche de Vapeur hydrosulfurée	6		5	50	5		1	
Douche générale d'une heure, ou bain de vapeur par aspersion	6		5	50	5		1	
Douche d'Eau de savon parfumé	5		4	50	4		1	
Douche Gélatineuse de force ordinaire	6		4		4		1	
Douche Ascendante d'eau minérale ou naturelle	3		2	50	2		1	
Douche d'Eau de mer	3		2	50	2		1	
Douche d'Eau de mer avec bain	7		5	50	5		1	
Douche d'Eau minérale avec bain	6		5	50	5		1	
Douche Injectante pour les maladies de la vessie	6		5	50	5			50
Massage et Friction pratiquées pendant les douches	2		5		5			
Lit de repos après le bain ou la douche	1	50	1	25	1			

Nota: Les douches de vapeur, prises concurremment avec le bain, augmenteront de 2 fr. le prix de ce dernier.
Source: A.N. F⁸150 Prospectus. Etablissement hygiénique des Néothermes.

APPENDIX 11: EDITORS OF THE *ANNALES D'HYGIÈNE PUBLIQUE*

1829

Founding editors:
Nicolas Adelon
Gabriel Andral
Jean-Pierre Barruel
Jean-Pierre Joseph D'Arcet
Alphonse Devergie
Etienne Esquirol
Pierre Kéraudren
François Leuret
Charles C. H. Marc
Matthew Orfila
Alexandre Jean-Baptiste Parent-Duchâtelet
Louis-René Villermé

1841

Nicolas Adelon
Gabriel Andral
J. B. Alphonse Chevallier
Jean-Pierre Joseph D'Arcet
Alphonse Devergie
Henri Gaultier de Claubry
Alphonse Guérard
Pierre Kéraudren
François Leuret
Charles Olliviers d'Angers
Matthew Orfila
Adolphe Trébuchet
Louis-René Villermé

1854, second series

Nicolas Adelon
Gabriel Andral
Alexandre Brierre de Boismont
Jean Boudin
J. B. Alphonse Chevallier
Alphonse Devergie
Henri Gaultier de Claubry
Alphonse Guérard
Pierre Kéraudren
Ambroise Tardieu
Adolphe Trébuchet
Louis-René Villermé

APPENDIX 12: PHYSICIAN-HYGIENISTS OF LYON: BIOGRAPHICAL SKETCHES

Jean-Baptiste Monfalcon received his M.D. in Paris in 1818. He subsequently became physician at the Hôtel-Dieu in Lyon, prison physician, a member of the Rhône health council, and chief physician at Charité. He contributed to the *Dictionnaire des sciences médicales* and was coauthor (with Polinière) of several of the major public health treatises published in France during the first half of the nineteenth century. Aside from his medical and hygienic activities in the 1830s, he was editor of the conservative newspaper *Courrier de Lyon*; in the 1840s became a librarian; continued to be principal librarian and then historian of the city into the 1860s; and was the author of one of the most comprehensive histories of Lyon. See "Notice sur la vie et les ouvrages de J.-B. Monfalcon," extrait de la *Nouvelle biographie générale* (Paris: Didot, 1861), 35: 970, in Monfalcon, *Histoire monumentale de la ville de Lyon*, 9 vols. (Lyon: Bibliothèque de la ville de Lyon, 1866), 1: i–iv. On Monfalcon as editor and librarian, see Robert Bezucha, *The Lyon Uprising of 1834* (Cambridge, MA: Harvard University Press, 1974), pp. 185–6. See also J. B. Monfalcon, *Souvenirs d'un bibliothécaire* (Lyon: Nigor, 1853).

A. P. Isidore de Polinière was a military surgeon during the Napoleonic wars, received his M. D. in Paris in 1815, and subsequently came to Lyon to practice medicine. From the beginning, he was especially interested in hospital hygiene. He became chief physician at the Hôtel-Dieu and in 1832 was a member of the commission that went to Paris to study cholera. He was a member of the Rhône health council and president of the Society of Medicine of Lyon; coauthored with Monfalcon two of the major public health treatises of the era; and in the 1840s and 1850s became a member of the hospital administration and head physician at Charité, and was responsible for many of the reforms that took place there. In 1851 he was made director of Charité and administrative director of the Hôtel-Dieu. See Paul Diday, *Vie du Dr. Polinière* (Paris: Baillière and V. Masson, 1857), and Monfalcon, *Histoire monumentale*, 4: 107–9.

Jean-François Terme received his M. D. in Paris and was one of the founders of the Lyon Dispensary in 1818. Though trained as a physician, he was primarily an administrator. A leading Lyonnais liberal, he was chosen assistant mayor under Prunelle (1830) and, according to Monfalcon, virtually ran the city in Prunelle's absence. In 1832 he became president of the hospital administration and was responsible for many of the reforms that took place at the Hôtel-Dieu after 1832. He was keenly interested in hospital hygiene and in the foundling question, coauthoring with Monfalcon several major treatises on foundlings. From 1840 to 1847 (d.) he was mayor of Lyon and initiated many of the public health reforms during this time. He pushed for reform of the water supply and sewer systems, but unfortunately did not succeed. He was also a member of the general council of the department and was elected a deputy from the arrondissement of Villefranche in 1842. See Monfalcon, *Histoire monumentale*, 3: 353–7.

Ariste Potton was a physician at the Antiquaille hospice, where he worked primarily with venereal disease patients. He was author of a major work on prostitution in Lyon, as well as of several other public health–related works.

Jacques-Pierre Pointe was a physician at the Collège royale de Lyon, professor of *clinique interne* at the *clinique médicale* at the Hôtel-Dieu, and for seven years was the physician attached to the Lyon tobacco factory. He was the author of several important hygienic treatises on topics ranging from tobacco workers to school hygiene to hospital hygiene. See Monfalcon, *Histoire monumentale*, 4: 119–20. See also J. P. Bourland-Lusterbourg, *Notice biographique sur Jacques-Pierre Pointe* (Lyon: Vingtrinier, 1861).

Alexandre Bottex was a physician at the Antiquaille hospice, specializing in the mentally ill. He was also inspector for establishments for the mentally ill for the department of the Rhône. He wrote several treatises on various aspects of public health, and was a member of the Rhône health council and a member of the commission sent to Paris to observe the cholera. See A. P. I. de Polinière, *Eloge de M. le Dr. Alexandre Bottex* (Lyon: Perrin, 1850).

Gabriel Prunelle received his M.D. at Montpellier, where he studied under Chaptal. He was a professor at the Medical Faculty of Montpellier, where he held the chair of history of medicine and legal medicine (1807–19). He gave what was probably the first regular course in *police médicale* at Montpellier in 1812 and was known for the opening speeches he gave annually for his course. The most famous of these was the speech given at the opening of his 1818 course, "De l'action de la médecine sur la population des états," *Revue médicale historique et philosophique* 1 (1820): ix–ixiv. This article includes an outline of his course. See also the article on this speech in *Journal des Débats*, June 26, 1818. He was fired in 1819, probably for political reasons, and went to Lyon to practice medicine. A liberal under the Restoration, he became mayor of Lyon in 1830 after the July

Revolution and was also elected deputy from the Isère. He took an active interest in public health reform during his four years as mayor, but unfortunately was in Paris much of the time. He resigned in 1834 and became inspector of mineral water at Vichy. See A. F. Potton, *Le Docteur Prunelle. Sa vie et ses travaux* (Lyon: Savy, 1855); Monfalcon, *Histoire monumentale*, 4: 102–6; Etienne Sainte-Marie, *Précis élémentaire de police médicale* (Paris: Baillière, 1824), pp. 29–30.

Other physician-hygienists who made important contributions were Etienne Martin, Etienne Sainte-Marie, and Alphonse Dupasquier (Physician and chemist). For a listing of all physicians and their titles, see M. G., *Tableau indicateur de MM. les médecins, chirurgiens, officiers de santé...de Lyon et de ses faubourgs* (Lyon: Deleuze, 1842).

BIBLIOGRAPHICAL NOTE

The most important sources for the study of the French public health movement are printed sources. The first is the journal of the movement, the *Annales d'hygiène publique et de médecine légale* (1829–), in which most of the articles of Parent-Duchâtelet, Villermé, and the other leading hygienists were published. Twenty-nine articles by Parent-Duchâtelet were also assembled and published as a collection, *Hygiène publique*, 2 vols. (Paris: Baillière, 1836). Also essential are the two major sociomedical studies by Villermé, *Tableau de l'état physique et moral des ouvriers employés dans les manufactures de coton, de laine, et de soie*, 2 vols. (Paris: Renouard, 1840), and Parent-Duchâtelet, *De la prostitution dans la ville de Paris*, 2 vols. (Paris: Baillière, 1836). The other major sources for a study of the French public health movement are the reports of the Paris health council and the provincial health councils, published at varying intervals from the 1820s on and cited in full in Chapter 4. Other important sources addressing the public health movement in general include the *Bulletin* (1836–) and *Mémoires* (1828–) of the Royal Academy of Medicine; the *Mémoires* (1837–) and *Séances et travaux* (1842–) of the Académie des Sciences Morales et Politiques; the landmark sociomedical report on cholera in Paris, Louis-François Benoiston de Châteauneuf et al…, *Rapport sur la marche et les effets du choléra-morbus dans Paris* (Paris: Imprimerie royale, 1834) and its English translation, *Report on the Cholera in Paris* (New York: Francis Wood, 1834); and the works on urban hygiene by Jean-Baptiste Monfalcon and A. P. Isidore de Polinière, *Traité de la salubrité dans les grandes villes* (Paris: Baillière, 1846) and *Hygiène de Lyon* (Paris: Baillière, 1846). For newspaper coverage of the public health movement, the official newspaper, the *Moniteur universel*, should be consulted, as well as the Establishment newspaper, the *Journal des Débats*. The most important statistical collection for hygienists was the *Recherches statistiques sur la ville de Paris et le département de la Seine*, 5 vols. (Paris: Imprimerie municipale, 1821–9, 1844). For public health legislation, the best source is *Recueil des textes officiels concernant la protection de la santé publique (1790–1935)*, 9 vols. (Paris: Ministère de la santé publique, 1957).

Archival sources, although not as rich as printed sources, are nevertheless important. At the National Archives, the F^8 series deals with public health (*police sanitaire*). Dossiers that contain information useful for this study include 77 (prefecture of police correspondence regarding public health), 22–37 (material on sanitary intendancies during the Napoleonic and Restoration eras), 150 (Parisian bathing establishments), 171–2 (*Conseils et commissions de salubrité, département de la Seine*), departmental dossiers on vaccine: 102 (Aube), 103 (Bouches-du-Rhône), 110 (Gironde), 113 (Loire-Inférieure), 118 (Nord), 120 (Bas-Rhin), 121 (Rhône), and 124 (Paris). Important manuscript and printed materials on provincial health councils are found in departmental archives: A.D. Loire-Atlantique, 1M1373 and 1M6753; A.D. Nord, M256/1, 256/4, 257/8, and 261/4; A.D., Bas-Rhin, 5M1; A.D. Seine-Maritime, 5MP2236 and, 5MP2237; A.D. Aube, M1615. Information on the health council of the Rhône and the municipal health council of Lyons is in Archives municipales de Lyon, $I^5$2; dossiers $I^5$1, 8, 9, and 10 also deal with public health and social welfare. At the Archives of the Prefecture of Police, information pertaining to budgets is in Da 69 and Da 79; on prostitution, Da 122 can be consulted. The manuscript reports of the Paris health council from 1802 to 1825 are also available. At the Archives de la Seine, V $I^5$3 contains useful information from the 1870s on water, sewers, and cesspools.

Sources not available that would have added an important dimension to the story are personal papers of leading hygienists and the reports of the Paris municipal council. The latter were apparently burned when the Hôtel de Ville was set on fire during the uprising of the Paris Commune. No personal papers of Parent-Duchâtelet have been located. The Villermé–Quetelet correspondence is available in Brussels: Bibliothèque Royale. Académie Royale des Sciences, des Lettres et des Beaux Arts de Belgique. Centre national d'histoire des Sciences. Correspondence Villermé–Quetelet. Cat. 2560 (1826–35) and 2561 (1839–63).

A variety of secondary sources is available on various aspects of early-nineteenth-century French public health. The starting points are the works of Erwin Ackerknecht and George Rosen. The pioneer work in the field was Ackerknecht's "Hygiene in France, 1815–1848," *Bull. Hist. Med.* 22 (1948): 117–55. That same year he also published the important interpretive article "Anticontagionism between 1821 and 1867," *Bull. Hist. Med.* 22 (1948): 562–93. Ackerknecht attempted to fit the public health movement into the broader context of Paris medicine in his book *Medicine at the Paris Hospital, 1794–1848* (Baltimore: Johns Hopkins University Press, 1967), with a chapter devoted to hygiene. Most of the material in that chapter had already been published in the 1948 article, however. George Rosen's general work *A History of Public Health* (New York: MD Publications, 1958) is essential background reading, and his articles

"Mercantilism and Health Policy in Eighteenth-Century French Thought," in his volume of collected essays *From Social Police to Social Medicine* (New York: Science History Publications, 1974), pp. 201–19, and, in the same volume, "Cameralism and the Concept of the Medical Police," pp. 120–41. "The Fate of the Concept of the Medical Police, 1780–1890," pp. 142–58, and "Hospitals, Medical Care and Social Policy in the French Revolution," pp. 220–45, are important for situating the public health movement in its historical context. Central for understanding social disease and public health in Paris is Louis Chevalier, *Classes laborieuses et classes dangereuses à Paris pendant la première moitié du 19e siècle* (Paris: Plon, 1958). Recent general works on the public health movement include William Coleman, *Death Is a Social Disease: Public Health and Political Economy in Early Industrial France* (Madison: University of Wisconsin Press, 1982), which emphasizes Villermé's contributions; Ann F. La Berge, "The Early Nineteenth-Century French Public Health Movement: The Disciplinary Development and Institutionalization of *hygiène publique*," *Bull. Hist. Med.* 58 (1984): 363–79, which summarizes the principal contributions of the public health movement; and, most recently, a good summary by Bernard Lécuyer, "L'hygiène en France avant Pasteur," in Claire Salomon-Bayet, ed., *Pasteur et la révolution pastorienne*" (Paris: Payot, 1986), pp. 67–139. An important work that provides the general medical and political contexts in which the public health movement developed is Jacques Léonard, *La médecine entre les pouvoirs et les savoirs* (Paris: Aubier Montaigne, 1981). For a thorough treatment of professional and popular medicine in the late eighteenth and early nineteenth centuries, see Matthew Ramsey, *Professional and Popular Medicine in France, 1770–1830: The Social World of Medical Practice* (New York: Cambridge University Press, 1988). A related work dealing with the medical milieu of nineteenth-century France and focusing on the developing specialty of psychiatry is Jan Goldstein, *Console and Classify: The French Psychiatric Profession in the Nineteenth Century* (New York: Cambridge University Press, 1987).

The literature on the eighteenth-century background to the public health movement is prodigious. The few most important works for this study, however, are Caroline Hannaway, "Medicine, Public Welfare, and the State in Eighteenth-Century France: The Société Royale de Médecine of Paris (1776–1793)" (Ph.D. dissertation, Johns Hopkins University, 1974), and her article "The Société Royale de Médecine and Epidemics in the Ancien Régime," *Bull. Hist. Med.* 46 (1972): 257–73; Jean-Paul Desaive, Jean-Pierre Goubert, et al., *Médecins, climat et épidémies à la fin du XVIIIe siècle* (Paris: Mouton, 1972); Charles C. Gillispie, *Science and Polity in France at the end of the Old Régime* (Princeton, NJ: Princeton University Press, 1980); Keith Baker, *Condorcet: From Natural Philosophy to Social Mathematics* (Chicago: University of Chicago Press, 1975); and Martin

Staum, *Cabanis: Enlightenment and Medical Philosophy in the French Revolution* (Princeton NJ: Princeton University Press, 1980). A good general overview of eighteenth-century public health is James Riley, *The Eighteenth-Century Campaign to Avoid Disease* (New York: St. Martin's 1987). For Revolutionary contributions to public health the classic article is Dora B. Weiner, "Le Droit de l'Homme à la Santé–une Belle Idée devant l'Assemblée Constituante: 1790–1791," *Clio Medica* 5 (1970): 209–23.

A virtual industry in the history of statistics has developed in the last few years, and a spate of monographs has appeared. The most important works for understanding statistics and the French public health movement are Coleman, *Death Is a Social Disease*; Theodore Porter, *The Rise of Statistical Thinking* (Princeton, NJ: Princeton University Press, 1986); Bernard Lécuyer, "Démographie, statistique et hygiène publique sous la monarchie censitaire," *Annales de démographie historique* (1977): 215–45; the works of Villermé, many of which were published in the *Annales d'hygiène publique*, including the *Tableau de l'état physique et moral des ouvriers*, and his numerous articles addressing statistical questions; Benoiston de Châteauneuf, *Rapport sur la marche et les effets du choléra-morbus dans Paris*; and the main statistical collection utilized by the hygienists, the *Recherches statistiques sur la ville de Paris*.

Historians have taken a keen interest in the Royal Academy of Medicine, theories of disease causation, and vaccination. George Weisz is working on a major study on the Royal Academy of Medicine and has published several important articles on the institution: "The Medical Elite in France in the Early Nineteenth Century,' *Minerva* 25 (1987): 150–70; "The Self-Made Mandarin: The Eloges of the French Academy of Medicine, 1824–47," *History of Science* 26 (1988): 13–39, and on mineral waters and the Royal Academy of Medicine: "Water Cures and Science: The French Academy of Medicine and Mineral Water in the Nineteenth Century," *Bull. Hist. Med.* 64 (1990): 393–416. Another recent article on experimental science at the Academy of Medicine is John Lesch, "The Paris Academy of Medicine and Experimental Science," in *The Investigative Tradition: Experimental Physiology in Nineteenth-Century Medicine*, ed. William Coleman and Frederic L. Holmes (Los Angeles: University of California Press, 1988). Two recent books on vaccination are Yves-Marie Bercé, *Le chaudron et la lancette: Croyances populaires et médecine préventive (1790–1830)* (Paris: Presses de la Renaissance, 1984), and Pierre Darmon, *La Longue traque de la variole: Les pionniers de la médecine préventive* (Paris: Perrin, 1986). On theories of disease causation, specifically anticontagionism, the starting point is the classic article by Ackerknecht, "Anticontagionism"; also essential is Margaret Pelling, who takes exception to Ackerknecht's interpretation in *Cholera, Fever and English Medicine: 1825–1865* (Oxford: Oxford University Press, 1978); and, most recently, there is the provocative article by Roger Cooter, "Anticontagionism and History's Medical Record," in *The Problem of Medical Knowledge*, ed. P. Wright and A. Treacher (Edinburgh: Edinburgh University Press, 1983), pp. 87–108, which attempts to show how physicians used atmospheric causes of disease to bolster their professional expertise and increase their authority. All these works on theories of disease causation are discussed in William Coleman, *Yellow Fever in the North: The Methods of Early Epidemiology* (Madison: University of Wisconsin Press, 1987). On cholera, the contemporary source is Benoiston de Châteauneuf, *Rapport sur la marche et les effets du choléra-morbus*, already cited. The best treatment of cholera and yellow fever remains George Sussman, "From Yellow Fever to Cholera: A Study of French Government Policy, Medical Professionalism and Popular Movements in the Epidemic Crises of the Restoration and July Monarchy" (Ph.D. dissertation, Yale University, 1972). Two recent books on cholera are François Delaporte, *Disease and Civilization: The Cholera in Paris, 1832* (Cambridge, MA: MIT Press, 1986), and Patrice Bourdelais and Jean-Yves Raulot, *Une peur bleue: Histoire du choléra en France, 1832–1854* (Paris: Payot, 1987). The best book on yellow fever is Coleman, *Yellow Fever in the North*.

On the health councils, the sources are both printed and manuscript. Manuscript sources in the National Archives, in departmental archives, and at the Prefecture of Police have been discussed. Printed reports are available for the Paris health council, the Nantes health council (Loire-Inférieure), the Nord (Lille), Lyon, Troyes (Aube), the Bouches-du-Rhône (Marseilles), the Gironde (Bordeaux), and the Haute-Garonne (Toulouse). For references, see the notes to Chapter 4.

There is a voluminous literature on industrialization and the condition of the working classes. Of central importance are Coleman, *Death Is a Social Disease*, and Bernard Lécuyer, "Les maladies professionnelles dans les 'Annales d'hygiène publique et de médecine légale,' ou une première approche de l'usure du travail," *Mouvement social* 124 (1984): 45–69. The main sources for public health history are Villermé's *Tableau de l'état physique et moral des ouvriers*, and Pierre Thouvenin, "De l'influence que l'industrie exerce sur la santé des populations dans les grands centres manufacturiers," *Annales d'hygiène publique* 36 (1846): 16–46, 277–86; 37 (1847): 83–111. On occupational hygiene the best source is Michel Valentin, *Travail des hommes et savants oubliés: Histoire de la médecine du travail, de la sécurité et de l'ergonomie* (Paris: Editions Docis, 1978). For the regulation of industrial establishments the definitive work is Adolphe Trébuchet, *Code administratif des établissemens dangereux, insalubres, et incommodes* (Paris: Béchet jeune, 1832). Recent works on French industrialization and the working classes are Peter Stearns, *Paths to Authority: The Middle Class and the Industrial Labor Force in France, 1820–1848* (Chicago: University of Illinois Press, 1978); William Sewell, *Work and Revolution in France: The Language of Labor from the Old Regime to 1848* (New York: Cambridge University Press, 1980); William Reddy, *The Rise of Market Culture: The Textile Trade and French Society, 1750–1900* (New York: Cambridge University Press, 1984); and Katherine Lynch, *Family, Class and Ideology in Early Industrial France: Social Policy and the Working Class Family, 1825–1848* (Madison: University of Wisconsin Press, 1988). Lynch also deals with employment of children and child labor reform, as do Colin Heywood in *Childhood in Nineteenth-Century France: Work, Health and Education Among the "Classes Populaires"* (Cambridge: Cambridge University Press, 1988) and Lee Shai Weissbach in *Child Labor Reform in Nineteenth-Century France: Assuring the Future Harvest* (Baton Rouge: LSU Press, 1989).

On urban public health, especially in Paris, the main works are the reports of the Paris health council, cited in detail in the notes, and the articles of Parent-Duchâtelet, most published originally in the *Annales d'hygiène publique* and then published in the collection *Hygiène publique*. On Parent-Duchâtelet, see Ann F. La Berge "A. J. B. Parent-Duchâtelet: Hygienist of Paris, 1821–1836," *Clio Medica* 12 (1977): 279–301; Jill Harsin, *Policing Prostitution in Nineteenth-Century Paris* (Princeton, NJ: Princeton University Press, 1985), pp. 96–130; and Alain Corbin, "Présentation" to Alexandre Parent-Duchâtelet, *La Prostitution à Paris au XIXe siècle*, texte présenté et annoté par Alain Corbin (Paris: Seuil, 1981), pp. 9–42. Other important contemporary works include the memoirs of Rambuteau, prefect of the Seine, and Gisquet, prefect of police: Claude Rambuteau, *Mémoires du Comte de Rambuteau publiées par son petit-fils* (Paris: Calmann-Lévy, 1905), and Henri Gisquet, *Mémoires de M. Gisquet, ancien préfet de police écrits par lui-même*, 4 vols. (Paris: Marchant, 1840). General works on the history of Paris with information on public health include David Pinkney, *Napoleon III and the Rebuilding of Paris* (Princeton NJ: Princeton University Press, 1958); Bertier de Sauvigny, *Nouvelle histoire de Paris: La Restauration* (Paris: Hachette, 1979); and the very rich nineteenth-century work by Maxime du Camp, *Paris. Ses organes. Ses fonctions et sa vie dans le seconde moitié du XIXe siècle*, 6 vols. (Paris: Hachette, 1868–75). For public health and medical care in the communes surrounding Paris, see Evelyn Ackerman, *Health Care in the Parisian Countryside, 1800–1914* (New Brunswick, NJ: Rutgers University Press, 1990). On cholera in Paris, essential are Benoiston de Châteauneuf, *Rapport sur la marche et les effets du choléra-morbus*, and Sussman, "From Yellow Fever to Cholera." Delaporte, *Disease and Civilization*, and Bourdelais and Raulot, *Une peur bleue*, all cited previously, can also be profitably consulted. On cultural perceptions of smell and implications for public health, the definitive work is Alain Corbin, *Le miasme et la jonquille: L'odorat et l'imaginaire social, 18–*

19e siècle (Paris: Aubier Montaigne, 1982). On water and water supply, the principal work is Jean-Pierre Goubert, *The Conquest of Water: The Advent of Health in the Industrial Age* (Princeton, NJ: Princeton University Press, 1989). A comprehensive article on the late-nineteenth-century Parisian sanitary revolution is Gérard Jacquemet, "Urbanisme Parisien: La bataille du tout à l'ègout à la fin du XIXe siècle," *Revue d'histoire moderne et contemporaine* 46 (1979): 505–48. For Parisian public health regulation, see in addition to the reports of the Paris health council, Elouin, Adolphe Trébuchet, and Labat, *Nouveau dictionnaire de police*, 2 vols. (Paris: Béchet jeune, 1835). The classic work on the laboring and dangerous classes, and the resultant problems of public health and public order is Honoré Frégier, *Des classes dangereuses de la population dans les grandes villes et les moyens de les rendre meilleures*, 2 vols. (Paris: Baillière, 1840), which no doubt inspired the twentieth-century work by Louis Chevalier, *Classes laborieuses et classes dangereuses à Paris*. On unhealthy dwellings and establishments, consult Adolphe Trébuchet, *Code administratif des établissements dangereux, insalubres ou incommodes* and Ann-Louise Shapiro, *Housing the Poor of Paris, 1852–1902* (Madison: University of Wisconsin Press, 1985). A number of good works are available on social welfare and public health problems associated with prostitution, wet nursing, and foundlings. On prostitution, the principal works are Parent-Duchâtelet, *De la prostitution dans la ville de Paris*; the recent monograph by Jill Harsin, *Policing Prostitution in Nineteenth-Century Paris*, already cited; and Parent-Duchâtelet, *La Prostitution à Paris au XIXe siècle*, ed. Alain Corbin, also previously cited. For a comparative point of view and to show continuity of thought with regard to prostitution Allan Brandt's *No Magic Bullet: A Social History of Venereal Disease in the United States since 1880* (New York: Oxford University Press, 1987) should be consulted. The two basic works on wet nursing are George Sussman, *Selling Mothers' Milk: The Wet-Nursing Business in France, 1715–1914* (Chicago: University of Illinois Press, 1982), and Fanny Faÿ-Sallois, *Les nourrices à Paris au XIXe siècle* (Paris: Payot, 1980). On foundlings the definitive nineteenth-century work is Jean-François Terme and Jean-Baptiste Monfalcon, *Histoire des enfants trouvés* (Paris: Paulin, 1840). A good recent monograph is Rachel Fuchs, *Abandoned Children: Foundlings and Child Welfare in Nineteenth-Century France* (Albany: State University of New York Press, 1984).

This is not the place to cite the wide and varied literature available on the American and British public health movements. But some of the most important works include, on American public health: John Duffy, *The Healers: The Rise of the Medical Establishment* (New York: McGraw-Hill, 1976) and his recent work, *The Sanitarians* (Chicago: University of Illinois Press, 1990). The now-classic work on public health in nineteenth-century America is Charles Rosenberg, *The Cholera Years* (Chicago: University of

Chicago Press, 1962). Contemporary works central for an understanding of American public health in the nineteenth century include *Origins of Public Health in America: Selected Essays, 1820–1835* (New York: Arno Press, 1972), *The First American Medical Association Reports on Public Hygiene in American Cities* (New York: Arno Press, 1977, reprint; originally published 1849); John Griscom, *The Sanitary Condition of the Laboring Class of New York* (New York: Arno Press, 1970, reprint of the 1845 edition) and Lemuel Shattuck et al., *Report on the Sanitary Condition of Massachusetts, 1850* (Cambridge MA: Harvard University Press, 1948).

The single most important secondary source on the British public health movement is Michael W. Flinn's "Introduction" to Edwin Chadwick, *Report on the Sanitary Condition of the Labouring Population of Great Britain. 1842*, ed. M. W. Flinn (Edinburgh: Edinburgh University Press, 1965). Other essential works include Margaret Pelling, *Cholera, Fever, and English Medicine*, already cited; John M. Eyler, *Victorian Social Medicine: The Ideas and Methods of William Farr* (Baltimore: Johns Hopkins University Press, 1979); and Anthony Wohl, *Endangered Lives: Public Health in Victorian Britain* (Cambridge, MA: Harvard University Press, 1983). On Chadwick, the standard biographies are Samuel E. Finer, *The Life and Times of Sir Edwin Chadwick* (London: Methuen, 1952), and Richard A. Lewis, *Edwin Chadwick and the Public Health Movement, 1832–1854* (London: Longmans, Green, 1952).

On public health in France after 1850, key works include Ambroise Tardieu, *Dictionnaire d'hygiène publique et de salubrité*, 3 vols. (Paris: Baillière, 1862); Maxime Vernois, *Traité pratique d'hygiène industrielle et administrative*, 2 vols. (Paris: Baillière, 1860); and Adolphe Trébuchet, *Rapport général sur les travaux du Conseil de l'hygiène publique et de salubrité du département de la Seine depuis 1849 jusqu'à 1858 inclusivement* (Paris: Imprimerie municipale, 1861). Secondary works include Martha Hildreth, *Doctors, Bureaucrats and Public Health in France, 1888–1902* (New York: Garland, 1987); Ann-Louis Shapiro, *Housing the Poor of Paris*; Robert Nye, *Crime, Madness and Politics in Modern France: The Medical Concept of National Decline* (Princeton, NJ: Princeton University Press, 1984); and Jane Ellen Crisler, "Saving the Seed: The Scientific Preservation of Children in the Third Republic" (Ph.D. dissertation, University of Wisconsin, 1984). Also important are Claire Salomon-Bayet, ed., *Pasteur et la révolution pastorienne*, and Bruno Latour, *The Pasteurization of France* (Cambridge, MA: Harvard University Press, 1987) in which the work of the early-nineteenth-century hygienists is discussed as a necessary pre-science to Pasteurism.

Additional sources on all these topics are located in the notes for each chapter.

INDEX